Keto
RESTAURANT
favorites

(more than 175 tasty
classic recipes made fast,
fresh, and healthy)

First Published in 2017 by Victory Belt Publishing Inc.

ISBN-13: 978-1-628602-58-6

Front and back cover photography by Hayley Mason and Bill Staley

Interior design by Charisse Reyes

Printed in Canada

TC 0117

TABLE OF CONTENTS

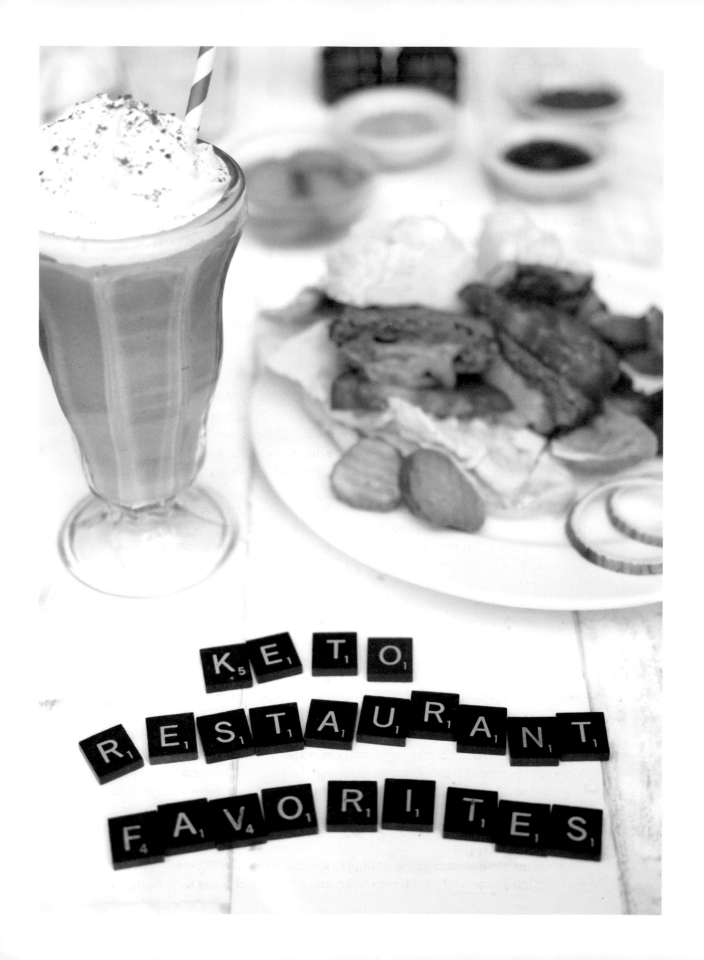

Introduction

When did it become so common to eat out? Eating out used to be a rare treat. Now, if you walk into a restaurant during the lunch hour, it is usually packed! People are attracted to fast food because of the low cost and the convenience, and even children are drawn to the brilliant marketing that large restaurant chains put out there. Sometimes it just seems so much easier to eat out rather than go grocery shopping and cook at home.

But eating out comes with a price—literally as well as figuratively.

Restaurants Are Expensive

I hear many complaints about the cost of healthy eating, but the cost of eating out is much higher. My family of four went to brunch the other day, and we all got eggs and salmon with extra hollandaise, a side of chorizo, and a side of bacon. Craig ordered organic coffee while the boys and I drank water. The bill? Sixty-three dollars! For eggs! Seriously, people. It's almost comical that I had gasped at the idea of paying four dollars for a dozen eggs at the grocery store the day before.

I understand that some people are on a tight food budget and worry about spending more on groceries to cook at home. I get that; I count my pennies, too! However, there are six very busy coffee shops in my small town that are always packed with customers ordering four-dollar mochas. There are lines outside of Chipotle to buy eight-dollar burritos when you can make them at home for a lot less. Restaurants are thriving, and eating out costs way more than eating in.

And let's talk about what we're actually getting for all that extra money we're spending to eat out rather than cook at home. In 2011, a lawsuit against Taco Bell alleged that its taco meat was only 35 percent beef. Taco Bell fired back proudly that its meat was 88 percent beef and 12 percent seasonings—but those seasonings include things like chemicals to change its texture and taste, sugars, artificial colors and flavors, and preservatives. These are not the nutrients that our body needs to thrive. Worse, according to a 2008 study, fast food meat in general contains, in addition to skeletal muscle, peripheral nerve tissue, cartilage, bone, and plant material. If that doesn't deter you from eating that junk, I don't know what will.

Even though real, whole foods from quality sources may seem expensive at first, most people tell me that they end up saving money on their grocery bills because they aren't buying pricey processed junk—which only leaves them hungrier and craving more junk.

If you're thinking that you're willing to spend extra on eating out because you don't have time to cook, I have a suggestion: instead of going to the gym and walking on a boring treadmill for thirty minutes, then being pressed for time and stressed out because nothing is ready for dinner, walk around the grocery store while you shop for food and then dance while you cook your family a healthy dinner. It's cheaper than driving to Applebee's, and it's so much healthier!

Fast Food Is Addictive

Have you seen the 2004 movie *Supersize Me*? I'm not usually one for documentaries, but Morgan Spurlock sure made his movie worth watching! He decided to eat nothing but food from McDonald's for one month and filmed the entire experiment. The first time he was asked if he wanted to "supersize" his meal at McDonald's, Spurlock enthusiastically agreed; he had a rule that if he was offered a supersized meal, he had to say yes. He received his meal, happily walked back to his car, and gobbled down a giant burger, fries, and soda. Before he even left the parking lot, he felt queasy, and his "not-so-happy meal" eventually came back up.

But something interesting happened as the days went by: he began to crave the same high-sugar meals that had once made him sick. At the beginning of the experiment, the food was clearly toxic to his system, but toward the end, he felt irritable, anxious, and depressed unless he was getting that same food in regular doses. In other words, he was going through physical withdrawal.

Large fast-food chains spend a lot of money on developing food additives and smells that are literally addictive, and sadly, it's working. Spurlock's experience was so dramatic that nutrition experts use his movie to prove an important fact: not only is fast food unhealthy, but it also can make us addicts.

The first things that come to mind when we hear "physical addictions" are probably alcohol, cigarettes, and drugs. But research shows that some of the ingredients in fast food can have a similar addictive effect. Fast-food burgers, overstuffed burritos, french fries, soft drinks, milkshakes, and even fast-food chicken breasts are loaded with sugar and highly processed carbohydrates. Eating foods with a lot of sugar triggers the release of a brain chemical called dopamine, a "feel-good" neurotransmitter that's also triggered by drugs like heroin and cocaine. When our brains get that hit of dopamine, it's pleasurable, and we're inclined to repeat the experience. But over time, our brains adjust to the trigger and release less and less dopamine in response to it. That means we need more of the feel-good foods to get the same pleasurable experience, and we seek them out more and more—even though they're bad for us.

Even if you plan on choosing a healthy option, once you enter a fast-food restaurant, the overwhelming smells attract you to the less-healthy options instead. (Do you really want a salad, or do you want those delicious-smelling french fries?) Immediately after you eat your meal, the spike in dopamine creates a feeling of euphoria, but soon after, your blood sugar crashes and your mood plummets. You crave more sugar-filled foods to restore those good feelings. Fast-food fans tend to overeat in order to feed their addictions.

Studies also show that when you eat a lot of fast food, overeating itself becomes habitual because you're not getting the nutrients you need, even though a single fast-food meal packs as many calories as the average person should consume in a whole day. Unfortunately, fast food is extremely calorie-dense but devoid of nutrients. Most of the products on the menu come from "food products," far removed from the farms, fields, and orchards where food naturally comes from. This means that they are less nutritious and leave our brains and bodies unsatisfied.

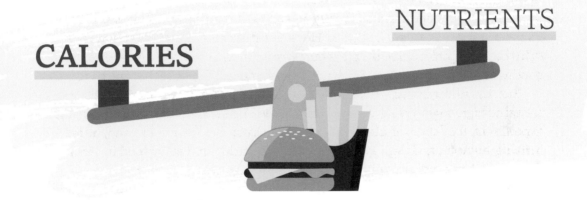

THE DANGERS OF TRANS FAT

Trans fat is a kind of fatty acid that's primarily produced during a manufacturing process called hydrogenation. This process adds hydrogen to oils in order to make them solid at room temperature. The resulting oils—partially hydrogenated oils—are often used in processed and packaged foods, especially deep-fried foods and baked goods like cookies and crackers.

Trans fat has been known to cause health problems for a long time. It's associated with heart disease, high cholesterol, and type 2 diabetes. It also promotes weight gain, causes inflammation, and ages cells.

In fact, the damaging effects of trans fat are so well known that the FDA has banned trans fat from all foods starting in 2018. But there are two loopholes: companies can ask the FDA for a waiver to continue using oils that contain trans fat, and any company can include less than 0.5 gram of trans fat per serving in its foods—and still claim that it has zero trans fat.

So it's a good idea to keep checking ingredient labels for partially hydrogenated oils and avoid fast food, especially fried fast food, because those small amounts of allowed trans fat can add up.

Is it worth it? We all know that fast food isn't ideal for our waistlines, but here are some other health issues to consider:

Acne
The boost of insulin after a meal high in refined carbohydrates and sugar leads to a boost of sebum on the skin, which results in acne.

Flatulence and Leakage
Gluten, dairy, and corn are added to most fast-food items. They're also common food allergens, and they can lead to GI problems.

Toxic Liver
Toxic chemicals in cheap meats and overly processed grains can impede weight loss by disturbing the endocrine system, slowing metabolism, and increasing inflammation and stress on the liver.

Cholesterol and High Blood Pressure
The overwhelmingly high amounts of carbohydrates and poor-quality ingredients in fast food inflame and harden arteries, which is the cause of these detrimental health issues.

FAST FOOD

Fatigue
The high amounts of carbs in fast food give an initial boost of energy as blood sugar spikes, but after the spike, blood sugar crashes, which means a drop in energy.

Kidney Stones
The amount of sodium in fast food trumps any food item in the grocery store. Hospitals are seeing triple the number of teenagers with kidney stones than they saw in the 1980s. This is directly linked to the overconsumption of sodium!

Bad Breath and Body Odor
Consuming the man-made chemicals in fast food has been shown to produce undesired smells in breath and sweat glands.

What We're Really Eating

At the most basic level, eating is about giving our bodies the nutrients they need. Unfortunately, eating out often means getting less valuable nutrients and more inflammatory agents, toxins, and chemicals.

Most fast food is filled with corn, wheat, soy, and dairy because they are cheap, government-subsidized fillers—even the grilled chicken breasts are filled with carbohydrates. Unfortunately, these fillers also happen to be the main food allergens. Many people are sensitive to them without even knowing it—if you happen to be one of those who has a "delayed food intolerance," your body reacts to these ingredients with an inflammatory response that can ultimately cause high blood pressure, high cholesterol, fatigue, and digestive problems, long after you've eaten the ingredient.

Even at fine restaurants, you can't be sure if you're getting real food, with real, wholesome ingredients. I recently ate at a local crab restaurant, and when the crab arrived, I asked for real butter. The young waiter scurried to the back, and when he returned to our table he said, "We don't have any butter, but we do have this vegetable oil blend."

What? A restaurant with no butter? We packed up our crab to go and picked up butter at a market so we could enjoy a picnic outside. Crab just isn't right without butter!

It's not just about flavor. (Though, does anything taste better than real butter?) It's also about health. Vegetable oil is full of unsaturated fats, and when these are heated, they can become oxidized. Oxidized fats can cause inflammation, which is at the root of many chronic illnesses. Vegetable oils are also highly processed with chemicals, and those chemicals can be harmful for health. Real butter, on the other hand, is full of healthy saturated fats that don't oxidize when exposed to heat. It's also full of vitamins, and it's free of chemicals and inflammatory agents. (That's especially true if you use grass-fed butter, which I recommend.)

This is just one example, of course. There are lots of ways that restaurants can use ingredients that you might not want to consume, without your even being aware that they're in a dish.

For all these reasons—the expense of eating out, the effects of fast food on our health, the presence of harmful fillers and artificial ingredients in restaurant food—we need to take a step back from eating out and return to cooking healthy meals at home. We need to know what we're putting into our bodies, and we need to make choices that will improve, not damage, our health.

I'm a big believer in home cooking, but I'm just as big a believer in a specific kind of eating: the ketogenic diet. Home cooking and the ketogenic diet go together beautifully.

The Ketogenic Diet for Better Health

When our dog, Teva, started losing her hair in patches, the first thing the veterinarian asked me was, "What are you feeding her?" Yes! What a good question! But I have never been asked that question at the doctor. Not once—not even when I was a teenager suffering from IBS and acid reflux. I was just given a prescription. Nothing frustrates me more than getting a bandage for the symptoms and not steps to address the underlying cause of my issues, which is why helping people find the right foods to nourish them is so important to me. I want people to start feeling amazing—to eliminate migraines, get off cholesterol-lowering drugs, increase serotonin naturally, balance hormones to alleviate PMS, and do it with food and natural supplements. That is how I became a happy and healthy person after years of irritable bowel syndrome, estrogen dominance, and low moods.

Good health starts with food, and understanding the role the ketogenic diet plays in good health starts with understanding exactly what makes a ketogenic diet different from any other kind of diet.

Food is what gives us energy, but there are two ways we can use that energy: we can burn sugar (glucose) or we can burn fat.

Most of us primarily burn sugar. But the body can't store much glucose—it stores way more fat. If you use glucose as your main fuel source, you are going to crave foods high in carbohydrates. (Glucose is a form of carbohydrate, and the body breaks down all other forms of carbs into glucose.)

If we are addicted to glucose, we eat it constantly during the day (that's why so many of us eat every two hours to "fuel our metabolism"). But eating high amounts of carbohydrates causes insulin—which moves glucose from the bloodstream into cells—to be chronically elevated. That eventually makes our cells stop listening to insulin's messages, and we become insulin resistant. (Eventually, if that gets bad enough, we even develop type 2 diabetes.) Plus, in order to store the excess carbs, the body turns them into fat.

What is even more disturbing is what occurs during sleep. If you are a sugar burner, you still need to burn glucose while you sleep; you may not be using much energy, but your body still needs to keep your organs working, maintain your body temperature, and so on, and all that requires fuel. Since you are not eating while you're asleep, your body gets that glucose by tearing down your lean muscle mass and bones. The biggest cause of osteoporosis has nothing to do with calcium; it is that we are breaking down our bones during sleep to feed our glucose addiction.

If we burn fat instead of glucose, so many of these problems are resolved. Because our bodies can store a lot of fat, we don't need to be constantly eating to get more energy. Our bodies can use both the fat we eat and the fat stored on them for fuel. That has a secondary effect: not only are we less hungry, we also lose weight! When we're primarily fat burners, we're burning stored fat and eating less, which means the pounds drop off.

Before I found peace with keto, I ran at least eleven miles a day and was still fifty pounds overweight. I often ran in the morning and then went for another run in the afternoon. I ate Special K with skim milk for breakfast and dinner and carrots dipped in mustard and dried fruit for lunch—and still I was too heavy for my frame. No wonder: I was eating lots of carbs and sugar and very little fat. Finding true health is not about calories in, calories out. Our bodies are more complex than that. You do not have to push yourself to the limit at the gym in order to lose weight!

Becoming a fat burner also means that blood sugar and insulin levels stabilize—no more spikes and crashes—so we don't develop insulin resistance or type 2 diabetes. In fact, insulin sensitivity improves, because we're not constantly flooding the body with insulin to deal with high blood sugar.

To become a fat burner, we have to teach our bodies to prefer fat as a fuel. And the way to do this is to stop providing it with glucose. That means cutting way, way down on—almost eliminating—carbohydrates and increasing your consumption of healthy fats. This, in essence, is the ketogenic diet.

It's called "ketogenic" because it increases the production of ketones, molecules that the body produces when it breaks down fat and that it uses for energy. The ketogenic diet raises levels of ketones in the blood; being in "ketosis" means that your ketone levels are above 0.5 mmol. (You can test this with a blood ketone meter.)

In my books *Keto Adapted, Quick and Easy Ketogenic Cooking,* and *The 30-Day Ketogenic Cleanse,* I focus on how to measure your intake of macronutrients and know when you're in ketosis. That's not my goal here. Instead, here I want to give you healthy, delicious, keto-friendly alternatives to your favorite restaurant meals. You don't have to sacrifice the restaurant foods you love in the name of good health. And in fact, adapting to a ketogenic diet will make these home-cooked dishes even tastier.

How I Got Back to Basics, and Back to Flavor

Most Americans are consuming copious amounts of fake flavorings without even knowing it. Chemical-laden "food" from fast-food restaurants (and sometimes even fine-dining restaurants) is ruining our taste buds and deceiving our senses. These fake flavors do not make us feel fulfilled, either; they only cause us to crave more: the can't-eat-just-one-chip phenomenon.

Flavor determines what we eat on a daily basis—we all want to eat delicious food! However, "foods" filled with flavor enhancers aren't satisfying our search for tasty fare, nor are they doing our bodies any good.

It is possible to break that cycle and end the addiction to fake food. Before I found keto, I was caught up in this madness, too. But I changed my palate, and so can you! I don't like to hear clients say, "I can't give up certain foods," or "I never can give up coffee," or "My husband will never give up beer." I know it's a cliché, but never say never. I say that because I was the pickiest eater as a child. When I was a little girl, my birthday parties were often held at the local Hardee's. I loved their hamburgers, french fries, and ketchup, with a tasty malt to go alongside my flavor bomb of a meal. I grew up eating way too much junk, which ruined my palate at a young age.

It only got worse as I got older. When I was a teenager, I had the best job ever: I worked at a beautiful coffee shop in Medford, Wisconsin, before and after school. I loved making and serving yummy muffins and cinnamon rolls to eager customers. The best part was, because we served everything freshly made, I was allowed to take home the leftover muffins at the end of the day. My love for mochas and other coffee drinks also intensified since I could have as many as I wanted. I was filling my body with sugar, caffeine, and gluten, which caused me to become lethargic and depressed and started me down the path to polycystic ovary syndrome (PCOS).

All that changed when I finally found the ketogenic diet. Going back to the basics of whole foods instead of processed and packaged foods and cutting out carbohydrates not only made me healthier, it also reset my palate, so I could enjoy the deliciousness of natural flavors again. As you remove sugar, carbohydrates, and the flavor additives often found in fast food and processed foods, your palate will start to change and you will no longer be addicted to those foods. And with the flavorful ingredients found in the homemade restaurant remakes in this book— such as tasty real butter, fish sauce, and herbs and spices—you will create much more flavorful food that will nourish not only your body but your soul!

This book is meant to help you feel encouraged and empowered to take control of your diet and health. If you are willing to take the time to prepare your own meals using keto-friendly ingredients, you will feel like the amazing self you are meant to be. You deserve this!

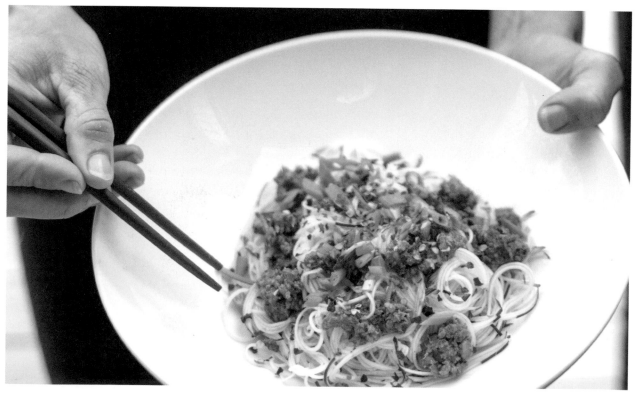

MY FIRST RESTAURANT MEMORY

It may sound like I'm not a fan of restaurants, but actually, some of my favorite memories are of fish fries at a restaurant called High View in Medford. If you have ever been to Wisconsin in the spring, you know that Friday night means fish fry. Just about every restaurant in Wisconsin hosts a fish fry on Friday nights during Lent, including bars and churches.

Every Friday at about 5:30 p.m., my parents would drive my little brother and me to High View, a quaint and lovely restaurant on a small lake. My brother and I would run out of the station wagon with our fishing poles in hand while my parents entered the restaurant to visit with friends. My brother and I were more interested in catching fish than eating it; I never liked fish growing up, unless it came out of a box labeled "fish sticks." (Remember, I was the pickiest eater! Find my keto fish sticks recipe on page 322.) We would fish until my dad came to tell us that our food was ready. We ran in quickly to eat so we could get back to fishing.

When I turned sixteen, I became a hostess and waitress at High View. Every waitress remembers those difficult guests who are hard to please, and my mom was the first customer I remember making me work hard for my tip. I never brought enough lemon for her broiled fish. I laugh at it now; my parents were my best tippers!

It's not that we need to avoid restaurants altogether—going out to eat with family and friends can be a wonderful experience. But we do need to make it a special occasion, not an everyday one. And we can still make sure that when we eat out, we pick the foods that will truly nourish us. See my tips for dining out on keto on pages 14 and 15.

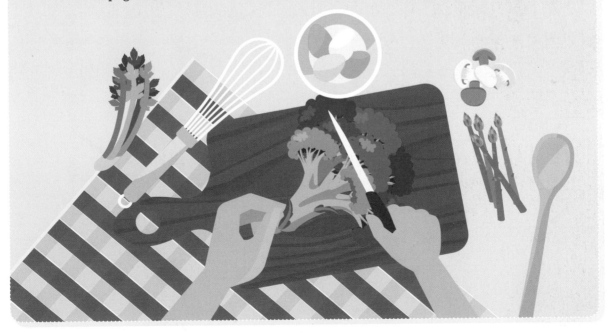

TOP TIPS FOR EATING KETO AT RESTAURANTS

If you're eating out while maintaining the keto lifestyle, here are my top picks for keto-friendly restaurant meals.

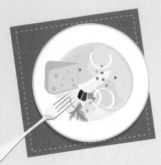

Omelet

Many places serve omelets for lunch as well as breakfast, which I adore. Just choose keto-friendly fillings, such as mushrooms, onions, cheeses, and meats. My favorite omelet is ham and Emmentaler cheese, with a side of house made hollandaise for dipping. But some large breakfast chains such as IHOP add pancake batter to their omelets. That's right—they add sugar, carbs, and wheat to the omelet base for "fluffiness." Yuck!

Tip: Ask them to cook your omelet in butter instead of vegetable oil.

Poached Eggs Benedict

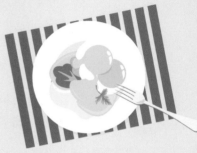

Skip the bun and ask for extra hollandaise. Because the eggs are poached, you don't have to worry about what oils might be used to fry them.

Tip: Make sure the hollandaise is made from scratch, not from a mix.

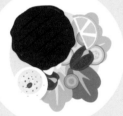

Hamburger on a Side Salad

Skip the bun. Order a hamburger with a large side salad with a sugar-free salad dressing (ranch, blue cheese, or Italian). Bonus points if you bring your own salad dressing. But beware of hidden sugars in ingredients such as barbecue sauce; even caramelized onions can be made with soda.

Sandwich on a Side Salad

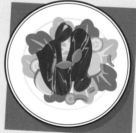

Skip the bread and fries and sub in a large salad instead. I have even ordered a Reuben over a large salad. Beware of hidden sugars in dressings such as Thousand Island.

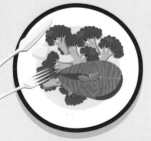

Salmon with Broccoli

Skip the rice or potatoes and ask for a non-starchy vegetable instead, such as broccoli. Smother it in extra butter.

Steak and Mushrooms

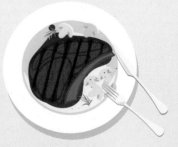

Again, skip the starchy potatoes and ask for a ketogenic vegetable such as sautéed mushrooms. Skip the steak sauce, too—it's filled with sugar. Bonus points if you choose a ketogenic cut of steak. For a helpful chart on the best cuts, see page 23.

Chicken Alfredo and Other Pasta Dishes

Ask them to skip the pasta and put the sauce over sautéed broccoli. Even at popular chain Italian restaurants I have enjoyed chicken Alfredo and shrimp scampi over broccoli instead of pasta.

Tip: Make sure the Alfredo sauce is not made with a roux, which has added flour as a thickener.

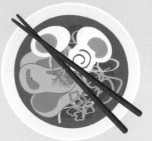

Ramen and Pho

I love getting pho at one Vietnamese restaurant in Minneapolis. I ask them to not put any noodles in the soup; instead they add extra cabbage, which is sliced extra thin and reminds me of noodles. Be aware of what type of soy sauce the restaurant is using. Are they using true fermented soy sauce or Americanized sauce, which has gluten added?

Thai Food

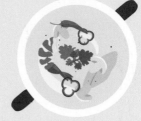

I adore going to Thai restaurants; everything is so fresh. I often replace the noodles with sautéed cabbage noodles. Tom ka gai (coconut chicken soup) is one of my favorites. Beware of added sugars, though!

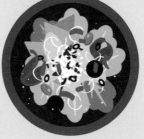

Nachos with Lettuce

I love nachos, and one local restaurant called San Pedro makes these awesome nachos from chip-sized crispy romaine lettuce—no tortilla chips needed! The toppings are loaded with flavor. I have asked for this at a variety of restaurants and they all have been very open to my request.

Sushi

Sushi can be a great choice if you skip all the rice and get sashimi. Craig once overheard a sushi chef saying that he adds more than three quarts of sugar to each batch of rice, which equals 34 grams of added sugar in each cup of rice! We never eat rice anyway, but that sure is another reason not to. Also, be aware of the type of soy sauce the restaurant is using. Are they using true fermented soy sauce or Americanized sauce, which has gluten added? Bonus points if you bring your own coconut aminos to use in place of soy sauce.

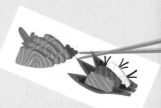

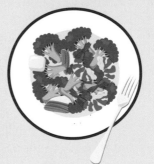

Crab, Lobster, or Shrimp with Butter

This is always a tasty choice as long as the butter is really butter and not a vegetable oil mixture. Ask for a side salad or sautéed keto vegetable, such as broccoli, on the side.

Sausages and Brats with a Side of Sauerkraut

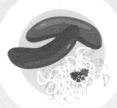

Beware of Bavarian sauerkraut, which has added sugar.

Fast Food

The only fast-food restaurant I recommend is Chipotle. Get lettuce layered with your choice of meat and topped with sautéed bell peppers, salsa, and guacamole (sour cream and cheese if you're not dairy sensitive).

These are just a few ideas—I've ordered all of these dishes at restaurants. I've never been to a restaurant where I couldn't find a keto-friendly option on the menu or modify a dish to make it keto-friendly. Try looking at the menu online beforehand and plan out what you are going to order before you go. Stick to your plan and do not get tempted or influenced by friends who order unhealthy options or waiters who make unhealthy suggestions.

"Food can be the most powerful form of medicine or the slowest form of poison." —Ann Wigmore

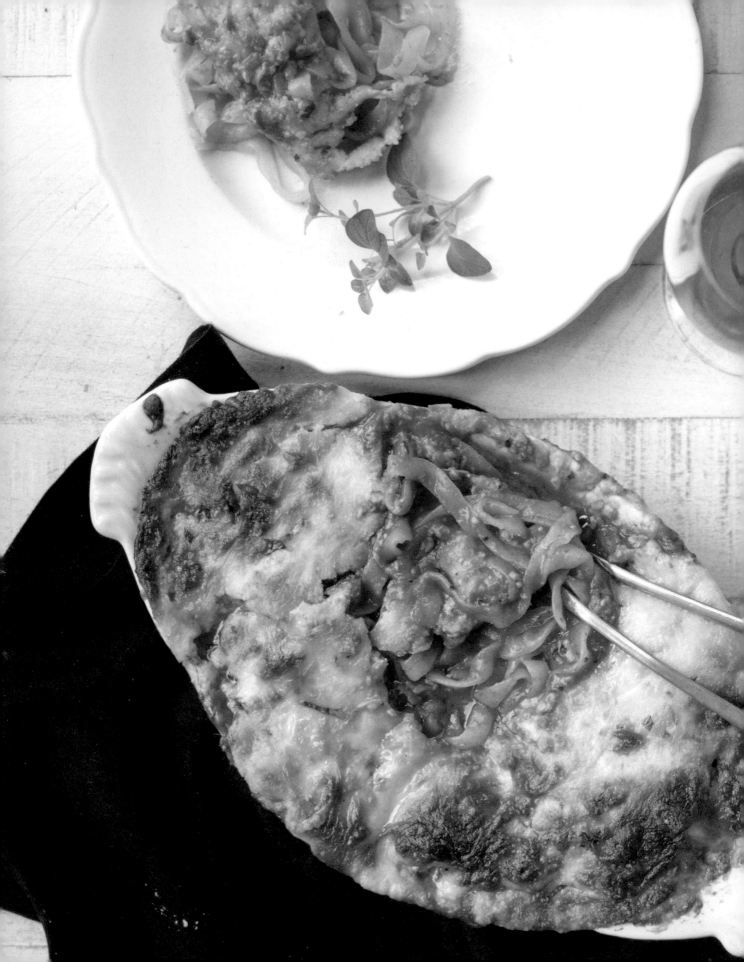

part 1

THE KETOGENIC KITCHEN

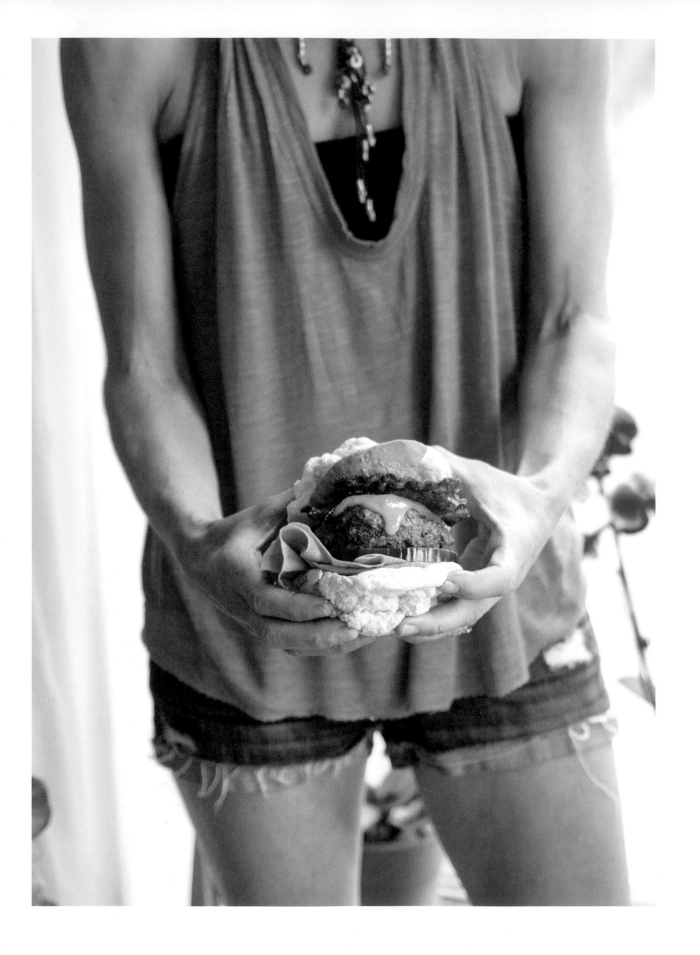

Ingredients

The key to any healthy diet is eating real, whole foods. When following a keto-genic diet, you'll want to seek out keto-friendly ingredients and avoid those that aren't keto-friendly.

Fats

On a keto diet, you need lots of healthy fat to burn as fuel. But as important as it is to seek out healthy fats, it's just as critical to avoid unhealthy fats.

Healthy Fats

Fats with high amounts of saturated fatty acids (SFAs)—such as MCT oil, coconut oil, butter, ghee, tallow, and lard—are best: they are stable and anti-inflammatory, protect against oxidation, and have many other important health benefits. Organic and grass-fed or pastured sources are always best.

On page 20 is a list of the best fats and oils to use, with their SFA and PUFA content (see page 21 for more on PUFAs). When you see "keto fat" mentioned in a recipe in this book, know that it's fine to use any of these fats—just make sure to take into account whether you need it for a hot or a cold use.

If you're not dairy-sensitive, the following are great healthy, keto-friendly dairy fats to include in your diet:

- **Butter:** 50% SFA, 3.4% PUFA
- **Ghee*:** 48% SFA, 4% PUFA
- **Heavy cream:** 62% SFA, 4% PUFA
- **Cheddar cheese:** 64% SFA, 3% PUFA
- **Cream cheese:** 56% SFA, 4% PUFA
- **Sour cream:** 58% SFA, 4% PUFA
- **Crème fraîche:** 64% SFA, 3% PUFA

*You may be able to tolerate ghee even if you're dairy-sensitive because the milk proteins have been removed.

MCT OIL

MCT stands for medium-chain triglycerides, which are chains of fatty acids. MCTs are found naturally in coconut oil, palm oil, and dairy, and they're particularly helpful on a keto diet because the body uses them quickly and any MCTs not immediately utilized are converted to ketones. MCT oil is extracted from coconut or palm oil and contains higher, concentrated levels of MCTs, so it's great for adding ketones to your diet. Whenever MCT oil appears in a recipe in this book, it's generally my first choice, but to make the recipes as accessible as possible, I've provided alternative oil choices as well.

Many of the recipes in this book also use Parmesan cheese. I call for either grated or powdered Parmesan. Fresh pregrated Parmesan cheese available at supermarket cheese counters usually has a light and fluffy texture and can be a convenient option in recipes that call for powdered Parmesan. To make powdered Parmesan at home, see page 363.

Fat	SFA	PUFA	Notes
Almond oil	8.2%	17%	• Has a mild, neutral flavor • Works great for sweet dishes and Thai dishes • Use in nonheat applications, such as salad dressings • Can also be used on the skin
Avocado oil	11%	10%	• Has a mild, neutral flavor • Works great for savory and sweet dishes • Can be heated
Beef tallow	49.8%	3.1%	• Has a mild beef flavor • Works great for savory dishes • Can be heated
Cocoa butter	60%	3%	• Has a mild coconut flavor • Works great for sweet and savory dishes • Can be heated
Coconut oil	92%	1.9%	• Has a strong coconut flavor • Works great for sweet dishes and Thai dishes • Can be heated • Can also be used on the skin
Duck fat	25%	13%	• Has a rich duck flavor • Works great for frying savory foods • Can be heated
Extra-virgin olive oil*	14%	9.9%	• Has a strong olive flavor • Works great for Italian salad dressings • Use in nonheat applications, such as salad dressings
Hazelnut oil	10%	14%	• Has a mild hazelnut flavor • Works great for sweet dishes and Thai dishes • Use in nonheat applications, such as salad dressings
High-oleic sunflower oil	8%	9%	• Has a mild sunflower seed flavor • Works great for sweet dishes and Thai dishes • Use in nonheat applications, such as salad dressings
Lard	41%	12%	• Has a mild flavor • Works great for frying sweet or savory foods • Can be heated
Macadamia nut oil	15%	10%	• Has a mild nutty flavor • Works great for salad dressings • Use in nonheat applications, such as salad dressings
MCT oil**	97%	less than 1%	• Has a neutral flavor • Works great for savory dishes and baked goods • Can be heated using low to moderate heat (no higher than 320°F)
Palm kernel oil***	82%	2%	• Has a neutral flavor • Works great for baking • Can be heated

*Extra-virgin olive oil is great for cold applications, such as salad dressings, but should not be used for cooking; heat causes the oil to oxidize, which is harmful to your health.

**MCT oil can be found at most health food stores, but if you have trouble finding it, you can use avocado oil, macadamia nut oil, or extra-virgin olive oil instead, keeping in mind that avocado oil is the most neutral-flavored of the three.

***Be sure to purchase sustainably sourced and processed palm kernel oil. There are ecological concerns associated with some palm oils.

Bad fats

Two kinds of fats should be avoided on a ketogenic diet: trans fats and polyunsaturated fatty acids (PUFAs).

Trans fats are the most inflammatory fats; in fact, they are among the worst substances for our health that we can consume. Many studies have shown that eating foods that contain trans fats increases the risk of heart disease and cancer.

Here is a list of trans fats to avoid at all costs:
- Hydrogenated or partially hydrogenated oils (check ingredient labels for these sneaky fats)
- Margarine
- Vegetable shortening

PUFAs should also be limited because they are prone to oxidation. Many cooking oils are high in PUFAs. Here is a list of the most common ones:

Oil	PUFA
Grapeseed oil	70.6%
Sunflower oil	68%
Flax oil	66%
Safflower oil	65%
Soybean oil	58%
Corn oil	54.6%
Walnut oil	53.9%
Cottonseed oil	52.4%
Vegetable oil	51.4%
Sesame oil	42%
Peanut oil	33.4%
Canola oil	19%

PURCHASING KETO-FRIENDLY INGREDIENTS

You can purchase keto-friendly pantry products on my website, MariaMindBodyHealth.com/store. They're also available in most grocery stores.

To save money, I recommend buying ingredients in bulk—including perishables like meat and fresh veggies. They can be frozen (a chest freezer is a great investment) and thawed later. Remember, choosing top-quality organic foods is always best.

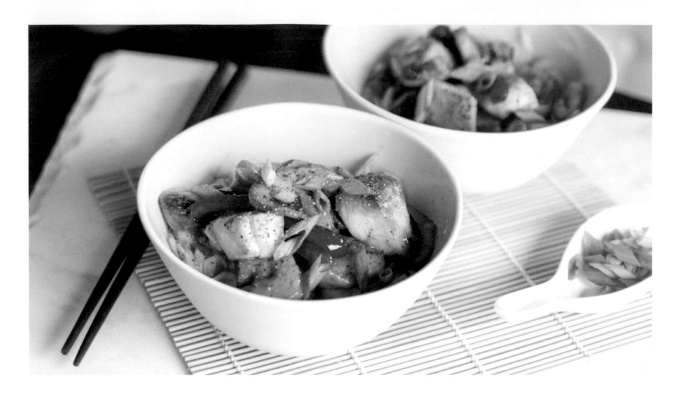

Proteins

It's always best to choose humanely raised, grass-fed or pastured meat and eggs and wild-caught seafood. Not only do they offer more nutrients, but they also haven't been exposed to added hormones, antibiotics, or other potential toxins.

For help choosing sustainably sourced seafood, check out the Monterey Bay Aquarium Seafood Watch app and website, seafoodwatch.org.

BEEF	WILD MEATS	POULTRY	FISH	SEAFOOD/ SHELLFISH
BUFFALO	· Bear	· Chicken	· Ahi/mahi mahi	· Clams
GOAT	· Boar	· Duck	· Catfish	· Crab
LAMB	· Elk	· Game hen	· Halibut	· Langostino
PORK	· Rabbit	· Goose	· Herring	· Lobster
	· Venison	· Ostrich	· Mackerel	· Mussels
		· Partridge	· Salmon	· Oysters
	EGGS	· Pheasant	· Sardines	· Prawns
	· Chicken eggs	· Quail	· Snapper	· Scallops
	· Duck eggs	· Squab	· Swordfish	· Shrimp
	· Goose eggs	· Turkey	· Trout	· Snails
	· Ostrich eggs		· Tuna	
	· Quail eggs		· Walleye	
			· Whitefish (cod, bluegill)	

NUTRITIONAL INFO (per 4 ounces)								
Beef Cuts	CALORIES	FAT (G)	PROTEIN (G)	CARBS (G)	FIBER (G)	% FAT	% PROTEIN	% CARBS
Rib-eye steak	310	25.0	20.0	0	0	73%	26%	0%
Rib roast	373	28.0	27.0	0	0	69%	30%	0%
Beef back ribs	310	26.0	19.0	0	0	75%	25%	0%
Porterhouse steak	280	22.0	21.0	0	0	70%	30%	0%
T-bone steak	170	12.2	15.8	0	0	64%	36%	0%
Top loin steak	270	20.0	21.0	0	0	67%	31%	0%
Tenderloin roast	180	8.0	25.0	0	0	40%	56%	0%
Tenderloin steak	122	3.0	22.2	0	0	60%	40%	0%
Tri-tip roast	340	29.0	18.0	0	0	77%	21%	0%
Tri-tip steak	200	11.0	23.0	0	0	50%	46%	0%
Top sirloin steak	240	16.0	22.0	0	0	60%	37%	0%
Top round steak	180	9.0	25.0	0	0	45%	56%	0%
Bottom round roast	220	14.0	23.0	0	0	57%	42%	0%
Bottom round steak	220	14.0	23.0	0	0	57%	42%	0%
Eye round roast	253	13.4	32.0	0	0	48%	51%	0%
Eye round steak	182	9.0	25.0	0	0	45%	55%	0%
Round tip roast	199	12.0	22.9	0	0	54%	46%	0%
Round tip steak	150	6.0	23.5	0	0	36%	63%	0%
Sirloin tip center roast	190	7.0	31.0	0	0	33%	65%	0%
Sirloin tip center steak	190	7.0	31.0	0	0	33%	65%	0%
Sirloin tip side steak	190	6.0	34.0	0	0	28%	72%	0%
Skirt steak	255	16.5	27.0	0	0	58%	42%	0%
Flank steak	200	8.0	32.0	0	0	36%	64%	0%
Shank cross cut	215	6.7	38.7	0	0	28%	72%	0%
Brisket flat cut	245	14.7	28.0	0	0	54%	46%	0%
Chuck 7-bone pot roast	240	14.0	28.0	0	0	53%	47%	0%
Chuck boneless pot roast	240	14.0	28.0	0	0	53%	47%	0%
Chuck steak boneless	160	8.0	22.0	0	0	45%	55%	0%
Chuck eye steak	250	18.0	21.0	0	0	65%	34%	0%
Shoulder top blade steak	204	13.0	22.0	0	0	57%	43%	0%
Shoulder top blade flat iron	204	13.0	22.0	0	0	57%	43%	0%
Shoulder pot roast	185	7.0	30.7	0	0	34%	66%	0%
Shoulder steak	204	12.0	24.0	0	0	53%	47%	0%
Shoulder center ranch steak	152	8.0	24.0	0	0	40%	60%	0%
Shoulder petite tender	150	7.0	22.0	0	0	42%	59%	0%
Shoulder petite tender medallions	150	7.0	22.0	0	0	42%	59%	0%
Boneless short ribs	440	41.0	16.0	0	0	84%	15%	0%

NUTRITIONAL INFO (per 4 ounces)								
Pork Cuts	CALORIES	FAT (G)	PROTEIN (G)	CARBS (G)	FIBER (G)	% FAT	% PROTEIN	% CARBS
Chop	241	12.0	33.0	0	0	45%	55%	0%
Loin	265	15.5	30.8	0	0	53%	46%	0%
Pork hocks	285	24.0	17.0	0	0	76%	24%	0%
Leg ham	305	20.0	30.4	0	0	59%	40%	0%
Rump	280	16.2	32.8	0	0	52%	47%	0%
Tenderloin	158	4.0	30.0	0	0	23%	76%	0%
Middle ribs (country style)	245	16.0	25.0	0	0	59%	41%	0%
Loin back ribs (baby back ribs)	315	27.0	18.0	0	0	77%	23%	0%
Belly	588	60.0	10.4	0	0	92%	7%	0%
Shoulder	285	23.0	19.0	0	0	73%	27%	0%
Butt	240	18.0	19.0	0	0	68%	32%	0%
Bacon	600	47.2	41.8	0	0	71%	28%	0%

NUTRITIONAL INFO (per 4 ounces)								
Poultry	CALORIES	FAT (G)	PROTEIN (G)	CARBS (G)	FIBER (G)	% FAT	% PROTEIN	% CARBS
Chicken breast, skinless	138	4.0	25.0	0	0	26%	72%	0%
Chicken breast, skin-on	200	8.4	31.0	0	0	38%	62%	0%
Chicken leg, skinless	210	9.5	30.7	0	0	41%	58%	0%
Chicken leg, skin-on	255	15.2	29.4	0	0	54%	46%	0%
Chicken thigh, skinless	165	10.0	19.0	0	0	55%	46%	0%
Chicken thigh, skin-on	275	17.6	28.3	0	0	58%	41%	0%
Chicken wings	320	22.0	30.4	0	0	62%	38%	0%
Chicken drums	178	9.9	22.0	0	0	50%	49%	0%
Game hen	220	16.0	19.0	0	0	65%	35%	0%
Pheasant	200	10.5	25.7	0	0	47%	51%	0%
Turkey	175	9.9	21.0	0	0	51%	48%	0%
Goose	340	24.9	28.5	0	0	66%	34%	0%
Duck	228	13.9	26.3	0	0	55%	46%	0%

NUTRITIONAL INFO (per 4 ounces)								
Fish	CALORIES	FAT (G)	PROTEIN (G)	CARBS (G)	FIBER (G)	% FAT	% PROTEIN	% CARBS
Tuna (yellowfin)	150	1.5	34.0	0	0	9%	91%	0%
Tuna (canned)	123	0.8	27.5	1.5	0	6%	89%	5%
Salmon	206	9.0	31.0	0	0	39%	60%	0%
Anchovies	256	15.9	28.0	0	0	56%	44%	0%
Sardines	139	7.5	18.0	0	0	49%	52%	0%
Barramundi	110	2.0	23.0	0	0	16%	84%	0%
Trout	190	8.6	28.0	0	0	41%	59%	0%
Walleye	156	7.5	22.0	0	0	43%	56%	0%
Cod	113	1.0	26.0	0	0	8%	92%	0%
Sea bass	135	3.0	27.0	0	0	20%	80%	0%
Halibut	155	3.5	30.7	0	0	20%	79%	0%
Mackerel	290	20.3	27.0	0	0	63%	37%	0%
Arctic char	208	10.0	29.0	0	0	43%	56%	0%

NUTRITIONAL INFO (per 4 ounces)								
Seafood/Shellfish	CALORIES	FAT (G)	PROTEIN (G)	CARBS (G)	FIBER (G)	% FAT	% PROTEIN	% CARBS
Scallops	97	1.0	19.0	3.0	0	9%	78%	12%
Mussels	97	2.8	13.5	4.5	0	26%	56%	19%
Clams	82	1.1	15.0	3.0	0	12%	73%	15%
Shrimp	135	2.0	25.8	1.7	0	18%	78%	4%
Oysters	58	1.9	6.5	3.1	0	29%	33%	38%
Crab	107	2.0	22.0	0.0	0	17%	82%	0%
Lobster	116	1.8	25.0	0.0	0	14%	86%	0%
Caviar	260	12.0	31.0	8.0	0	42%	48%	12%

FINDING THE BEST-QUALITY EGGS

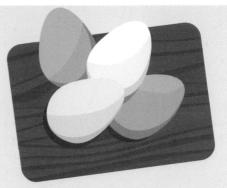

Eggs are an amazingly nutritious food, especially the yolks, which are full of choline, healthy fats, and a ton of flavor. And high-quality eggs—those from healthy, happy, humanely raised hens—are even more nourishing and tastier. So which eggs are the best quality?

Brown or White Eggs: There's absolutely no difference in quality between brown and white eggs; the only thing that determines the color of an egg is the breed of the hen. Do not choose eggs based on color.

Egg Grades: Eggs can be grade AA, A, or B. There is little to no difference in the taste, though, and no difference in nutritional value. Grade AA eggs have the thickest, firmest whites and high, round yolks. This grade of egg is virtually free of defects and is best for frying, poaching, or methods where presentation is important. Grade A eggs are the same quality as grade AA, but the whites are categorized as "reasonably" firm. Most grade B eggs are sold to restaurants, bakeries, and other food institutions and are used to make liquid, frozen, and dried egg products.

Vegetarian-Fed: The only thing this label means is that the hens are fed a diet based on corn (which is usually genetically modified). To ensure that the hens consume a strictly vegetarian diet, they are kept in cages. But chickens are natural omnivores: they evolved to eat insects, worms, and grubs as well as grass and grains. They weren't meant to be vegetarians!

Certified Organic: This label means that the hens are not kept in cages but in barns. They are required to have access to the sun, but that doesn't necessarily mean they can go outside; there may be a small window in the barn for sunlight. The hens are fed an organic, vegetarian diet that is free from antibiotics and pesticides. This label is regulated with inspections.

Free-Range or Cage-Free: This sounds like a good choice, right? Well, all this label really means is that the hens are not caged. However, there is no requirement to let the hens outside, there are no mandatory inspections to regulate this claim, and there are no guidelines for what the birds are fed.

Omega-3 Enriched: This label indicates that the hens' feed has extra omega-3 fatty acids added to it in the form of flaxseed. But eggs already are a good source of omega-3s, so there's no need to seek out eggs bearing this label.

Since most of the terms used on egg labels don't really help us figure out which eggs are healthiest, here are some guidelines to follow when egg shopping:

1. Be conscious of antibiotic and hormone use. While the USDA prohibits the use of hormones for egg production and the use of therapeutic antibiotics is illegal unless the hens are ill, these rules aren't always enforced. The only way to ensure that the hens were not given antibiotics is to purchase organic eggs.

2. To guarantee that you get truly free-range eggs, purchase eggs from pastured hens. Pastured hens are able to eat their natural diet of greens, seeds, worms, and bugs, and studies show that their eggs may contain more omega-3 fatty acids, vitamins, and minerals.

3. Smaller eggs tend to have thicker shells than larger eggs and therefore are less likely to become contaminated by bacteria.

4. Be cautious of unregulated labels. Terms like "natural" and "cage-free" are frequently used, but these claims may not necessarily be valid. Claims on egg packaging with the USDA shield have been verified by the United States Department of Agriculture, so look for the shield when purchasing eggs from a store.

Nuts and Seeds

Most nuts and seeds are fine on a keto diet, but they can take some people with metabolic syndrome out of ketosis. If you are extremely metabolically damaged and your goal is to lose weight, I highly recommend that you consume ketogenic dishes that use nuts, seeds, or nut flour in moderation, not every day. There are so many recipes to choose from in this book that you should never feel deprived! Nuts are also constipating, so if you suffer from lack of stool elimination, I suggest that you limit or cut out nuts, as well as dairy.

- Almonds
- Brazil nuts
- Hazelnuts
- Macadamia nuts
- Pecans
- Pumpkin seeds
- Sesame seeds
- Sunflower seeds
- Walnuts

Cashews, chestnuts, and pistachios have too many carbohydrates and therefore are not allowed on a ketogenic diet.

Veggies

Fresh vegetables are packed with nutrients and are an important part of a ketogenic diet, but to make sure you stay in ketosis, it's important to choose nonstarchy vegetables, which are lower in carbs than starchy vegetables. The following are some of the nonstarchy vegetables that I use most:

- Arugula
- Asparagus
- Bok choy
- Broccoli
- Cabbage
- Cauliflower
- Celery
- Collard greens
- Endive
- Garlic
- Kale
- Kelp
- Lettuces: red leaf, Boston, romaine, radicchio
- Mushrooms
- Onions: green, yellow, white, red
- Peppers: bell peppers, jalapeños, chiles
- Seaweed
- Swiss chard
- Watercress

Herbs and Spices

Spices and fresh herbs are the most nutritious plants you can consume. For example, everyone thinks spinach is an amazingly nutritious food, but fresh oregano has eight times the amount of antioxidants! Sure, we don't eat a cup of oregano, but it goes to show that a little bit of an herb provides a huge benefit. Here are some of my favorite herbs and spices:

- Anise
- Annatto
- Basil
- Bay leaf
- Black pepper
- Caraway
- Cardamom
- Cayenne pepper
- Celery seed
- Chervil
- Chili pepper
- Chives
- Cilantro
- Cinnamon

- Cloves
- Coriander
- Cumin
- Curry
- Dill
- Fenugreek
- Galangal
- Garlic
- Ginger
- Lemongrass
- Licorice
- Mace
- Marjoram
- Mint

- Mustard seeds
- Oregano
- Paprika
- Parsley
- Peppermint
- Rosemary
- Saffron
- Sage
- Spearmint
- Star anise
- Tarragon
- Thyme
- Turmeric
- Vanilla beans

Fruit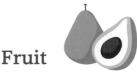

We tend to think of fruit as a health food, but in reality, most fruits are full of carbs and sugar. In fact, studies prove that the produce we consume today is lower in nutrients and much higher in sugar than it was in Paleolithic times. In general, high-sugar fruits like bananas, grapes, and mangoes should be avoided on a ketogenic diet.

But that doesn't mean you have to avoid all fruits! I once made a keto fruit salad filled with cucumbers, olives, eggplant, and capers, all covered in a Greek vinaigrette. So yes, fruits are certainly allowed; just seek out those that are low in sugar.

- Avocados
- Cucumbers
- Eggplants
- Lemons
- Limes

- Olives
- Seasonal wild berries (in moderation)
- Tomatoes

Beverages

It probably goes without saying that sodas and fruit juices should be avoided—they're full of sugar that will raise your blood glucose and kick you out of ketosis. But that doesn't mean you're limited to drinking just water! The following are all liquids that you can consume on a ketogenic diet.

- Unsweetened almond milk
- Unsweetened cashew milk
- Unsweetened coconut milk
- Unsweetened hemp milk
- Decaf coffee (make sure it is not chlorinated)
- Decaf caffè Americano (espresso with water)
- Decaf green tea
- Mineral water
- Water (reverse osmosis is best)

The Pantry

In addition to the whole foods discussed above, some pantry items are essential for making the recipes in this book.

Baking Products

See page 30 for recommended sweeteners.

- Baking powder
- Baking soda
- Blanched almond flour
- Coconut flour
- Egg white protein powder (check carbs and added ingredients—I recommend Jay Robb brand)
- Extracts and essential oils, including pure vanilla extract, for flavoring
- Guar gum
- Maca powder
- Pecan meal
- Unsweetened baking chocolate
- Unsweetened cocoa powder

Sauces and Flavor Enhancers

- Coconut aminos or wheat-free tamari
- Coconut vinegar
- Fish sauce

EGG REPLACER

The only keto egg replacer that I recommend is unflavored gelatin. Chia and flax seeds are not recommended because of their estrogenic properties as well as their high total carb count.

Other Foods

It is always better to buy fresh, but here are some keto-friendly foods that are also great jarred, canned, or prepackaged:

- Banana peppers
- Boxed beef and chicken broth
- Canned full-fat coconut milk
- Canned salmon
- Canned tuna
- Capers
- EPIC bars (made from grass-fed meat—but check for added sugars)
- Fermented pickles*
- Fermented sauerkraut*
- Marinara sauce (check for unhealthy oils and added sugar)**
- Mikey's English Muffins
- Nori wraps
- Olives (choose jars over cans)
- Organic dried spices
- Paleo mayo
- Pickled eggs
- Pickled herring
- Pizza sauce (check for unhealthy oils and added sugar)**
- Pure Wraps
- Roasted bell peppers
- Sardines
- Tomato paste**
- Tomato sauce**

Not only is fermenting a great way to preserve food, but it also creates beneficial gut bacteria and helpful digestive enzymes. Fermented sauerkraut is particularly rich in B vitamins.
**When it comes to tomato products, opt for jarred (the best choice) or BPA-free canned products. The linings of cans often contain BPA, a chemical that's associated with several health problems and may affect children's development, and tomatoes' high acidity can cause more BPA to leach into the food.*

Natural Sweeteners

In my recipes, I always use natural sweeteners. Just as sugarcane and honey are found in nature, so are erythritol and the stevia herb.

However, I prefer not to use sweeteners such as honey, maple syrup, and agave in my recipes because, even though they're natural, they raise blood sugar, which not only causes inflammation but will also take you out of ketosis.

Fructose is particularly problematic. More than glucose, it promotes a chemical reaction called glycation, which results in advanced glycation end products (AGEs). AGEs form a sort of crust around cells that has been linked to a wide range of diseases, from diabetes and heart disease to asthma, polycystic ovary syndrome, and Alzheimer's. Fructose also contributes to nonalcoholic fatty liver disease. For these reasons, I avoid sweeteners that are high in fructose: table sugar, high-fructose corn syrup, honey, agave, and fruit.

The following is a list of the natural sweeteners that I recommend, all of which have little effect on blood sugar.

- **Erythritol:** Erythritol is a sugar alcohol that is found naturally in some fruits and fermented foods. Erythritol is generally available in granulated form, though sometimes you can find it powdered. If you purchase a granulated product, such as Sukrin or Wholesome! All-Natural Zero, I recommend grinding it to a powder before use.

- **Swerve and other blended sweeteners:** These products combine two zero-calorie natural sweeteners, usually erythritol (see above) and oligosaccharides, which are found in many plants. They do not affect blood sugar and measure cup for cup just like table sugar. I use the powdered form of Swerve (the one labeled "confectioners") because it dissolves particularly well. Other blends I recommend are Pyure (erythritol and stevia), Norbu (erythritol and monk fruit), Natvia (erythritol and stevia), Lakanto (erythritol and monk fruit), and Zsweet (erythritol and stevia).

- **Stevia:** Stevia is available as a powder or a liquid. Because stevia is so concentrated, many companies add bulking agents like maltodextrin to the powdered form so that it's easier to bake with. Stay away from those products. Look for products that contain just stevia or stevia combined with another natural, keto-friendly sweetener.

- **Stevia glycerite:** Stevia glycerite is a thick liquid form of stevia that is similar in consistency to honey. Do not confuse it with liquid stevia, which is much more concentrated. Stevia glycerite is about twice as sweet as sugar, making it a bit less sweet than liquid or powdered stevia. I prefer stevia glycerite because, unlike powdered and liquid stevia, it has no bitter aftertaste. Stevia glycerite is great for cooking because it maintains its flavor when heated. However, it doesn't caramelize or create bulk, so most baking recipes call for combining it with another sweetener.

- **Monk fruit:** Also known as lo han kuo, monk fruit comes in pure liquid and powdered forms. Since it is 300 times sweeter than sugar, the powdered form is typically bulked up with another sweetener so that it measures cup for cup like sugar. Check the ingredients for things like maltodextrin, and buy brands that add only keto-friendly sweeteners, such as erythritol.

- **Xylitol:** Xylitol is a naturally occurring low-calorie sweetener found in fruits and vegetables. It has a minimal effect on blood sugar and insulin. Xylitol has been known to kick some people out of ketosis, so if you're using it in baking or cooking, monitor your ketones closely and stop using it if you find that you're no longer in ketosis.

- **Yacón syrup:** Yacón syrup is a thick syrup that is pressed from the yacón root and tastes a bit like molasses. I use yacón syrup sparingly—a tablespoon here and there to improve the texture and flavor of my sauces— both because it is very expensive and because it has some fructose in it.

Using Sweeteners in the Recipes in This Book

If you're trying keto for the first time, the recipes in this book should have just the right amount of sweetness. But as you continue with a ketogenic lifestyle, you may find that food naturally begins to taste sweeter, and you may want to reduce the amount of sweetener used in the recipes.

Whenever a recipe requires a powdered sweetener, my go-to choice is the powdered (confectioners) form of Swerve because it gives a smoother finished product and better overall results. That said, you can always pulverize a granular form of erythritol, such as Wholesome! All-Natural Zero, in a blender or coffee grinder to get a powdered texture.

If a recipe calls for a specific sweetener or type of sweetener (such as powdered or liquid), do not substitute any other sweeteners; these recipes rely on these particular sweeteners. For example, in recipes where the sweetener has to melt, some products won't work—so it's important to use exactly what's called for.

If a sweetener in an ingredient list is followed by "or equivalent," such as "¼ cup Swerve confectioners'-style sweetener or equivalent amount of liquid or powdered sweetener," you are free to use any keto-friendly sweetener, liquid or powdered. For example, you could use liquid stevia, stevia glycerite, monk fruit, Zsweet, or xylitol.

If you prefer to use a keto-friendly sweetener other than Swerve, here are the conversions:

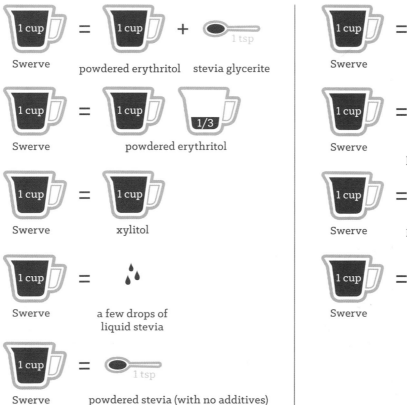

MARIA EMMERICH   31

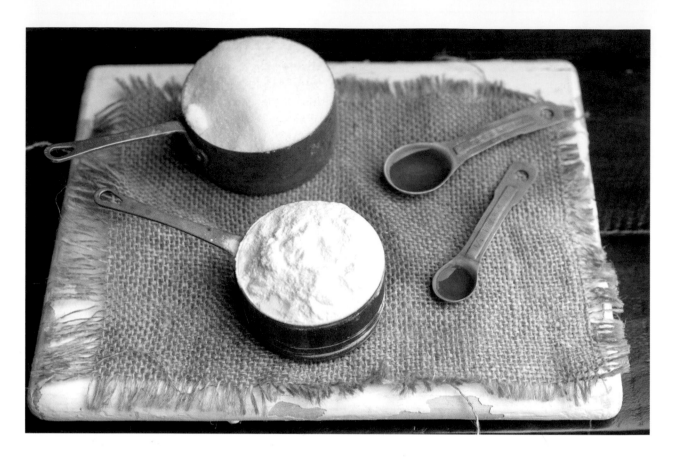

Advanced Tip: Blending Sweeteners for the Tastiest Keto Treats

For newcomers to the keto lifestyle, I try to keep my recipes as simple as possible and to limit the number of ingredients I use. For example, in recipes that are sweetened, I usually just call for Swerve or an equivalent. But the truth is, you'll get better results if you use a blend of different natural sweeteners.

For example, if a recipe calls for 1 cup of confectioners'-style Swerve, I use:

½ cup confectioners'-style Swerve

1 teaspoon stevia glycerite

10 to 15 drops liquid monk fruit

Adding a pinch of salt will also increase the sweetness because salt is a flavor enhancer.

So if you think that desserts made with Swerve have too much of an aftertaste or a cooling effect on your mouth, I highly recommend that you try making baked goods and keto ice cream with this combination of sweeteners.

The less Swerve/erythritol you use in keto ice cream, the less hard your ice cream will freeze. Sometimes the divine taste of natural organic heavy cream is enough, and all you need to add is a teaspoon of stevia glycerite. Then your ice cream won't harden like a rock. Slowly add the natural sweetener to the ice cream and adjust the sweetness before churning or making ice pops or push pops.

Substitutions for High-Carb Foods

Many everyday foods are high in sugar and carbs, which is why I've found healthier substitutions to use in my recipes. I was that girl who could never stop at ½ cup of pasta or one chip, so I loved putting together this information—all the foods in each photo have the same amount of carbs, so they make it shockingly clear just how much healthier these replacements are. As Craig and I prepped the ingredients to photograph, Craig had to keep making more and more and more zucchini noodles just to equal the carbs in a measly ½ cup of whole-wheat pasta!

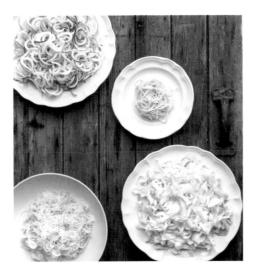

½ cup whole-wheat pasta = noodles from 3 stalks broccoli OR 5 cups zoodles (page 360) OR 5 cups cabbage pasta (page 361)

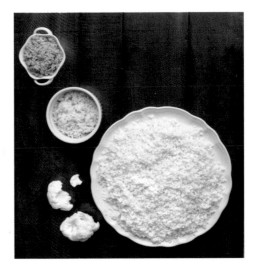

½ cup white rice = ½ cup quinoa = 4 cups riced cauliflower (page 363)

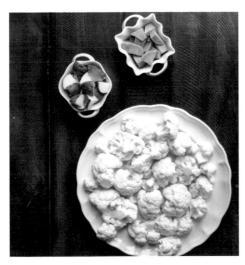

¾ cup diced sweet potato = 1 cup diced white potato = 4 cups mashed cauliflower

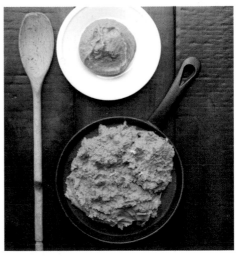

½ cup refried beans = 1½ cups of my healthified refried "beans" made with eggplant or zucchini (page 234)

Avoiding Foods That Contain Gluten

As you're probably well aware, a ketogenic diet typically omits gluten. But you may not realize that gluten lurks in many unexpected places!

Once when we were visiting family, someone asked if I wanted a Bloody Mary, explaining that the mix she had bought was gluten-free. I don't drink alcohol, so I passed, but the offer prompted my brother to ask if Bloody Marys typically contain gluten. Yep, many mixes include Worcestershire sauce (or the bartender will add a few drops to the mix), and Worcestershire sauce contains gluten.

During that same visit, my aunt made stuffed mushrooms and claimed that they were gluten-free because she hadn't added any crackers or breadcrumbs, but when I asked her for her recipe, she said that she adds a few dashes of Worcestershire sauce. This hidden gluten can be quite problematic for people with serious allergies! So I put a list together for you, whether you want to get rid of all gluten from your diet or you have a guest coming for dinner who suffers from a gluten allergy.

Foods You Wouldn't Expect to Contain Gluten, but Sometimes Do

- Beverage mixes
- Bologna
- Candy (even sugar-free candy)
- Chewing gum
- Cold cuts
- Commercially prepared broth
- Commercially prepared soup
- Custard
- Enchilada sauce
- Gravy
- Hot dogs
- Ice cream (even low-carb ice cream)
- Nondairy creamer
- Pudding (even sugar-free pudding)
- Root beer (even sugar-free root beer)
- Salad dressings
- Soy sauce
- Taco seasoning
- Vegetables in commercially prepared sauces, such as Alfredo

Ingredients That Often Contain Hidden Gluten

- Barley
- Barley grass
- Binders
- Some blue cheese
- Bouillon
- Bran
- Brewer's yeast
- Bulgur
- Chilton
- Couscous
- Durum
- Emulsifiers
- "Fillers"
- Hydrolyzed plant protein
- Hydrolyzed vegetable protein
- Kamut
- Kasha
- Malt
- Malt flavoring
- Malt vinegar
- Matzo
- Modified food starch
- Monosodium glutamate (MSG)
- "Natural" flavor
- Rye
- Seitan
- Semolina
- Soy sauce
- Spelt
- Some spice mixes
- Stabilizer
- Suet
- Teriyaki sauce
- Textured vegetable protein (TVP)
- Wheat grass
- Wheat protein

Tools

For the most part, the recipes in this book require tools that are part of a basic kitchen setup: standard pots, pans, baking sheets, and so on. However, some of the recipes, particularly the desserts, rely on specialized tools, and there are some tools that will simply make your life in the kitchen easier.

Spiral slicer

For: vegetable noodles, especially zucchini noodles

A spiral slicer makes it easy to cut vegetables into noodles—see, for instance, the recipe for Zoodles on page 360.

I'm often asked what my favorite spiral slicer is. It depends on the thickness of the noodle. For a thicker noodle, I love the Veggetti Pro Table-Top Spiralizer. If you prefer a thin, angel hair–like noodle, I recommend the Joyce Chen Saladacco Spiral Slicer.

8-inch crepe pan or nonstick skillet

For: crepes, omelets, and wraps

Does such a thing as a healthy nonstick pan exist? Nonstick cookware can be very handy when cooking crepes, omelets, or wraps, but most nonstick pans are coated with Teflon and other chemicals that we want to avoid. Instead, you can use a well-seasoned cast-iron pan or a stainless-steel pan coated with lots of keto-friendly oil.

I've also found that the glazed ceramic pans from Ceramcor have a great nonstick surface without any chemicals. They can be cleaned as you would any other pan—the surface is very hard to scratch. They are super-durable and heavy-duty. However, there is a little learning curve with these pans. Because they are ceramic, they take longer to heat up. For omelets, I turn my burner on low for 2 or 3 minutes to warm the pan, then I add my cooking fat; I turn off the heat when I flip the omelet (ceramic pans, like cast-iron pans, hold heat longer). The omelet slides right out!

High-speed blender

For: pureeing and making shakes, salad dressings, dips, and ice cream

A high-speed blender is perfect for processing liquids. High-powered blenders, such as those from Blendtec and Vitamix, have better performance, durability, and speed—but they're also more expensive than regular blenders.

Ice cream maker

For: making ice cream and sorbet

Ice cream treats are my favorite! You will always find keto ice cream and other frozen treats in my freezer. I adore my Cuisinart ICE-21 1.5 Quart Frozen Yogurt/ Ice Cream Maker. About ten years ago, I got my first ice cream maker from Cuisinart, and when it broke due to overuse, they sent me a new motor for free!

Immersion (stick) blender

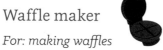

For: pureeing and blending

I can't believe I went so long without an immersion blender! I'm not a gadget person like my husband is—I like simplicity and I'm not a fan of clutter—so when Craig first asked if I wanted an immersion blender (also known as a stick blender), I politely said, "No thank you." But I have to tell you, when I started to use one, I was immediately hooked! It is so easy to use, and I can't believe the power behind this little tool. I love to use it for making pureed soups, shakes, and homemade mayo, sauces, and salad dressings.

Waffle maker

For: making waffles

I love to keep grain-free waffles in the freezer for easy breakfasts. My advice is to spend the money on a quality waffle maker. I adore my Waring Pro WMK600 Double Belgian Waffle Maker.

Slow cooker (6-quart)

For: slow cooking over low heat over several hours

If you don't have a lot of time for hands-on cooking, a slow cooker is a great tool that can save you time and effort. You can prep the ingredients the night before, turn it on before you leave for work in the morning, and come home to a wonderful home-cooked meal. A 4-quart slow cooker is handy for smaller quantities.

Double boiler

For: making and reheating sauces

A double boiler is a great tool for making sure you don't overheat sauces and cause them to separate or burn. But if you don't have a double boiler, you can use a heatproof bowl set over a pot of simmering water. I even reheat my hollandaise this way when we go camping.

Whipped cream canister

For: making sweetened whipped cream

This is definitely a frivolous gadget, but also one of the most fun to use! I keep mine filled with heavy cream presweetened with a keto sweetener (see page 336 for the suggested ratio) so I always have whipped cream at the ready. The brand I use is iSi.

How to Use the Recipes in This Book

In addition to 175 delicious keto comfort food recipes, this book has some handy features to help you along your keto journey.

Icons

I've marked the recipes with a number of icons, as applicable.

First, there are icons highlighting those recipes that are free of dairy, nuts, and/or eggs, which are problematic for some people:

If a recipe isn't free of a particular allergen but a substitution or an omission will make it free of that allergen, you will see the word OPTION below the icon, like this:

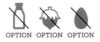

OPTION OPTION OPTION

Keto Meters and Nutritional Information

Keto meters indicate where each recipe ranks on the keto "scale": low, medium, or high. Note that in a few cases, a dish's ranking may vary based on whether you include an optional ingredient or component, such as a keto sauce.

M   M   M

L ⌒ H   L ⌒ H   L ⌒ H

KETO   KETO   KETO

I've also included nutritional information for each recipe, listing the total calories along with the fat, protein, carbohydrate, and fiber counts in grams. You'll find this information helpful as you fine-tune your personal keto targets for these macronutrients.

NUTRITIONAL INFO (per serving)				
calories	fat	protein	carbs	fiber
26	1g	0.3g	2g	2g

If you're wondering whether the recipes in this book are recipes that you can enjoy every day on your ketogenic diet, the answer is yes, most of them are. There are a few dishes, such as Garlic Bread (page 134), that I would eat only on special occasions. The keto meters can help you decide when and how often to make certain recipes; dishes marked as high are everyday comfort foods to enjoy anytime, while dishes marked as low should be reserved for special occasions. Those recipes marked as medium are generally best for weekends or overfeeding days.

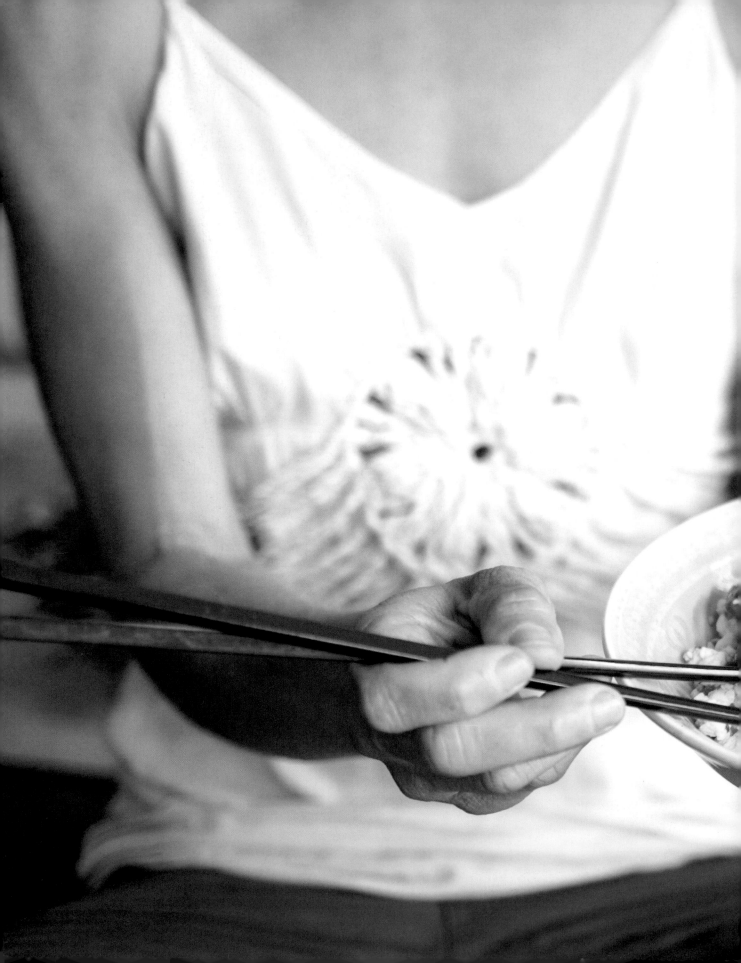

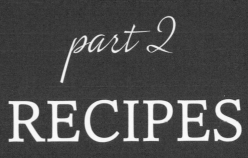

part 2

RECIPES

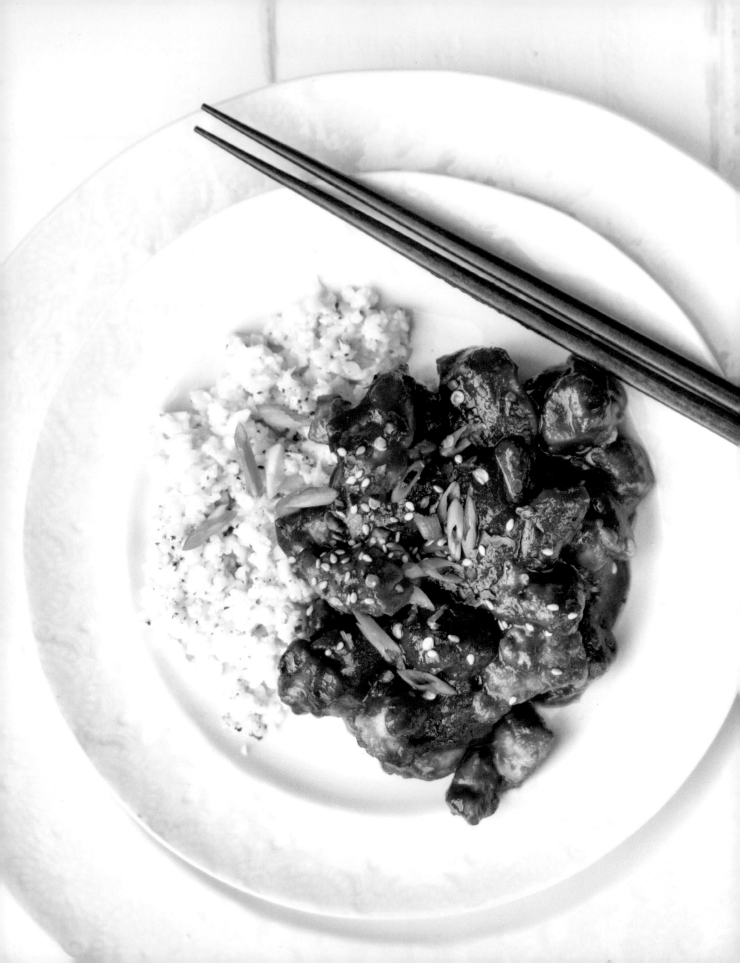

Chinese, Japanese, and Korean *Delights*

Stir-Fry Sauce

(L—M—H KETO ⊘ ⊘ ⊘) prep time: 3 minutes   yield: 2¼ cups (3 tablespoons per serving)

¼ cup wheat-free tamari, or 1 cup coconut aminos

2 teaspoons unseasoned rice vinegar

2 teaspoons toasted (dark) sesame oil

2 teaspoons Swerve confectioners'-style sweetener or equivalent amount of liquid or powdered sweetener (see page 31)

2 teaspoons grated fresh ginger

1 teaspoon crushed red pepper

1 clove garlic, smashed to a paste or minced

1 cup chicken bone broth, homemade (page 356) or store-bought, hot

½ teaspoon guar gum (optional, for thickening; see note)

1. Place the tamari, vinegar, oil, sweetener, ginger, crushed red pepper, and garlic in a small bowl and mix well.

2. If using store-bought broth, place the hot broth in a small bowl. Sift in the guar gum and whisk until well combined; let sit for 1 minute or until thickened.

3. While whisking, add the broth to the tamari mixture. Use immediately or store in an airtight container in the refrigerator for up to 1 week.

note: *If you use a true bone broth with plenty of collagen in it, you won't need to add guar gum to thicken the sauce. Naturally thick homemade bone broth is your best bet, but there are a few good store-bought bone broths available. My favorite is Kettle and Fire brand.*

NUTRITIONAL INFO (per serving)				
calories	fat	protein	carbs	fiber
126	14g	0.1g	1g	1g

Ginger Sauce

(L—M—H KETO ⊘ ⊘ ⊘) prep time: 3 minutes   yield: 1 cup (2 tablespoons per serving)

½ cup MCT oil, avocado oil, or olive oil

¼ cup thinly sliced scallions, plus extra for garnish

2 tablespoons fresh lime juice

1½ teaspoons wheat-free tamari, or 2 tablespoons coconut aminos

1 tablespoon grated fresh ginger

½ teaspoon fine sea salt

½ teaspoon ground black pepper

Place the ingredients in a small bowl and stir until well combined. Taste and adjust the seasoning to your liking. Use immediately or store in an airtight container in the refrigerator for up to 1 week or in the freezer for up to 1 month.

tip: *I store large pieces of ginger root in my freezer for making sauces like this one, which pairs nicely with Gyoza (page 58).*

NUTRITIONAL INFO (per serving)				
calories	fat	protein	carbs	fiber
26	1g	0.3g	2g	2g

Asian Dipping Sauce

(LMH KETO 🚫 🚫 🚫) prep time: 5 minutes   yield: 10 tablespoons (2 tablespoons per serving)

¼ cup coconut vinegar or unseasoned rice vinegar

1 tablespoon wheat-free tamari, or ¼ cup coconut aminos

1 tablespoon Swerve confectioners'-style sweetener or equivalent amount of liquid or powdered sweetener (see page 31)

1 teaspoon toasted (dark) sesame oil

1 clove garlic, minced

½ teaspoon grated fresh ginger

¼ teaspoon crushed red pepper

2 scallions, green parts only, thinly sliced on the diagonal

Place the vinegar, tamari, sweetener, oil, garlic, ginger, and crushed red pepper in a small bowl. Stir well to combine. Add the scallions just before serving. Store in an airtight container in the refrigerator for up to 5 days.

NUTRITIONAL INFO (per serving)				
calories	fat	protein	carbs	fiber
25	1g	0.2g	4g	2g

Sweet-and-Sour Sauce

(LMH KETO 🚫 🚫 🚫) prep time: 4 minutes   cook time: 3 minutes   yield: 2½ cups (¼ cup per serving)

1 (7-ounce) can tomato paste

1½ cups chicken bone broth, homemade (page 356) or store-bought

⅓ cup Swerve confectioners'-style sweetener or equivalent amount of liquid or powdered sweetener (see page 31)

¼ cup coconut vinegar

1 tablespoon fresh lime juice or lemon juice

¾ teaspoon fish sauce (see note)

½ teaspoon fine sea salt

½ teaspoon garlic powder

⅛ teaspoon grated fresh ginger

¼ teaspoon guar gum (optional, for thickening)

Place the tomato paste, broth, sweetener, vinegar, lime juice, fish sauce, salt, garlic powder, and ginger in a medium-sized saucepan over medium heat. Stir well to combine. Bring the mixture to a boil, stirring often. Boil for 3 minutes, stirring occasionally, until thickened to your liking. Remove from the heat and let cool. Sift in the guar gum, if using, and whisk until well combined. Pour the sauce into a jar and refrigerate until ready to use. Store in an airtight container in the refrigerator for up to 5 days or in the freezer for up to 1 month.

note: *Fish sauce isn't typically used in Chinese cooking, but I love the umami taste that it adds, so I've included it here. If you prefer, replace the fish sauce with an equal amount of coconut aminos.*

NUTRITIONAL INFO (per serving)				
calories	fat	protein	carbs	fiber
28	1g	1g	3g	1g

Zero-Carb Fried "Rice"

(L M H KETO 🥛 🥜)   **prep time:** 3 minutes   **cook time:** 11 minutes   **yield:** 4 servings

8 large eggs

½ cup coconut milk

2 tablespoons beef bone broth, homemade (page 356) or store-bought

½ teaspoon wheat-free tamari, or 2 teaspoons coconut aminos

1 teaspoon fine sea salt

½ teaspoon ground black pepper

3 strips bacon, diced

1 clove garlic, minced

¼ cup diced onions

Thinly sliced scallions, for garnish

1. Crack the eggs into a medium-sized bowl. Add the coconut milk, broth, tamari, salt, and pepper and whisk until well combined.

2. In a large skillet over medium heat, cook the bacon until crisp, about 2 minutes. Using a slotted spoon, remove the bacon but leave the fat in the pan. Add the garlic and onions and sauté until the onions are translucent, about 2 minutes.

3. Add the egg mixture to the skillet and cook until the mixture thickens and small curds form, all the while scraping the bottom of the pan and whisking to keep large curds from forming. This will take about 7 minutes. Stir in the reserved bacon.

4. Place the "rice" on a platter. Garnish with scallions and serve.

note: *If the "rice" releases excess liquid, soak it up with a paper towel before serving.*

NUTRITIONAL INFO (per serving)				
calories	fat	protein	carbs	fiber
255	19g	16g	3g	1g

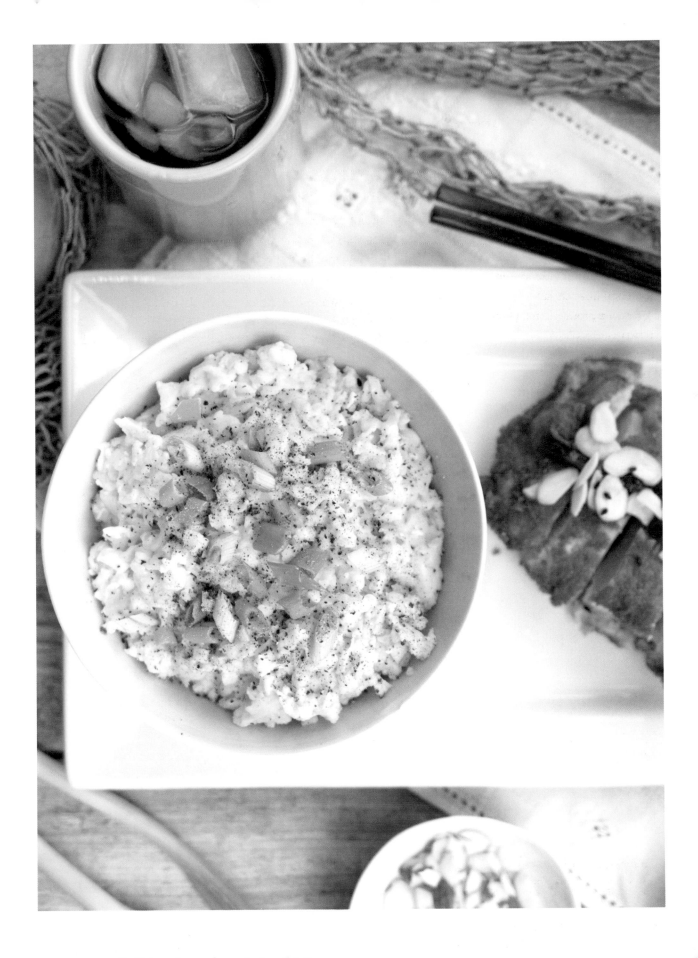

Cauliflower Fried Rice

(L M H KETO | OPTION) prep time: 5 minutes   cook time: 12 minutes   yield: 4 servings

One staple that every cook should have in the refrigerator is fish sauce, a special in-gredient that takes good food to amazing. Fish sauce (along with mushrooms and aged cheeses) has "umami," a satisfying, appetizing taste produced by glutamate and ribonu-cleotides, chemicals that occur naturally in various foods. Red Boat brand is traditionally fermented and does not contain wheat like other brands do. A bottle will last a long time since you use only a small amount per dish.

2 cups cauliflower florets (about 1½ pounds)

2 tablespoons coconut oil (or ghee or unsalted butter if not dairy-sensitive)

⅓ cup chopped onions (about 1 small)

1 clove garlic, smashed to a paste or minced

2¼ teaspoons wheat-free tamari, or 3 tablespoons coconut aminos

1 teaspoon fish sauce

⅛ teaspoon fine sea salt

⅛ teaspoon ground black pepper

1 large egg, lightly beaten

2 tablespoons chopped scallions, for garnish

1. Place the cauliflower in a food processor and pulse until the cauli-flower resembles grains of rice. Heat the oil in a large cast-iron skil-let over medium-high heat. Add the onions and sauté for 1 minute, or until softened. Add the garlic and sauté for another minute, or until fragrant.

2. Stir in the riced cauliflower, tamari, fish sauce, salt, and pepper. Reduce the heat to medium and cook for 5 minutes, stirring occa-sionally. Add the egg; stir until the egg is completely set, about 3 minutes. Serve garnished with the scallions.

3. Store in an airtight container in the refrigerator for up to 3 days. To reheat, place in a lightly greased sauté pan over medium heat for about 2 minutes, stirring often.

NUTRITIONAL INFO (per serving)				
calories	fat	protein	carbs	fiber
255	19g	16g	3g	1g

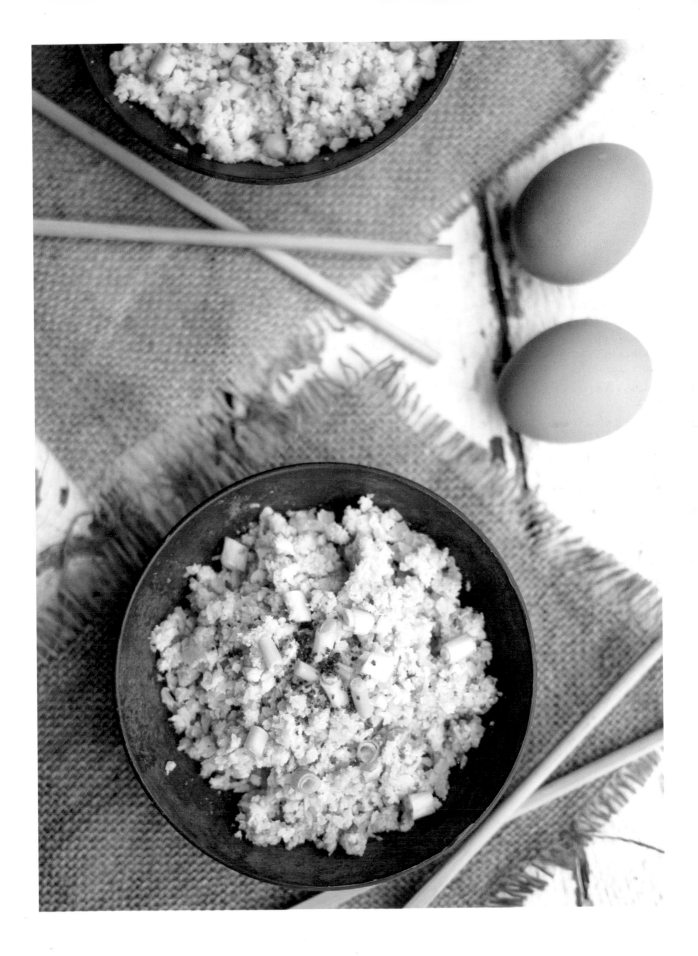

Scallion Pancakes

prep time: 5 minutes   cook time: 8 minutes
yield: 8 pancakes (2 pancakes per serving)

Serve these pancakes with Soo Guy (page 84) or other dishes from this chapter.

—pancakes

2 raw large eggs

2 hard-boiled eggs

4 ounces cream cheese (Kite Hill cream cheese style spread for dairy-free)

¼ cup sliced scallions

2 tablespoons toasted (dark) sesame oil

1 tablespoon Swerve confectioners'-style sweetener or equivalent amount of liquid or powdered sweetener (see page 31)

Pinch of fine sea salt

1 tablespoon coconut oil, for the pan

—dipping sauce

2 tablespoons unseasoned rice vinegar

2 tablespoons Swerve confectioners'-style sweetener or equivalent amount of liquid or powdered sweetener

1½ teaspoons wheat-free tamari, or 2 tablespoons coconut aminos

½ teaspoon grated fresh ginger

1 tablespoon finely sliced scallions, green parts only, for garnish

1. Make the pancakes: Place the raw eggs, hard-boiled eggs, cream cheese, scallions, sesame oil, sweetener, and salt in a blender and blend until smooth. Heat the coconut oil in a large skillet over medium heat. When the oil is hot, pour ¼ cup of the batter into the skillet. Fry until golden brown and set, about 2 minutes. Flip and continue to cook until the pancake is done all the way through, about 2 minutes. Remove from the skillet and sprinkle with salt, if desired. Repeat with the remaining batter to make a total of 8 pancakes, adding more oil to the skillet as needed.

2. Make the dipping sauce: Place the vinegar, sweetener, tamari, and ginger in a small bowl and stir well to combine. Taste and adjust the seasoning to your liking.

3. To serve, cut the pancakes into triangles, drizzle with the sauce, and garnish with scallions. Store the pancakes and sauce in separate airtight containers in the refrigerator for up to 4 days. To reheat the pancakes, place in a lightly greased skillet over medium heat for about 5 minutes.

NUTRITIONAL INFO (per serving)				
calories	fat	protein	carbs	fiber
236	20g	9g	3g	0.2g

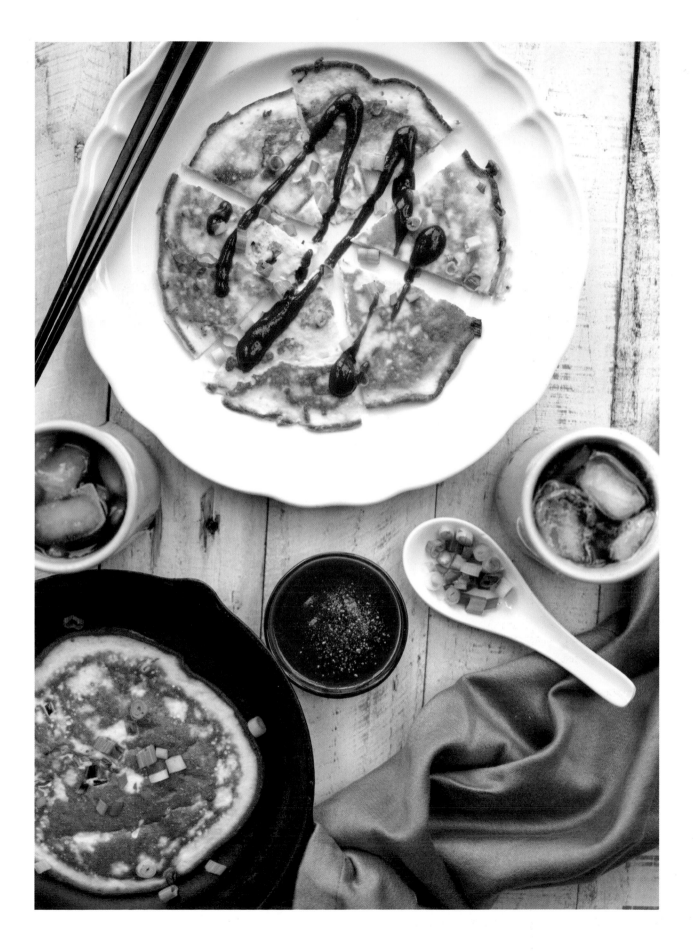

Break-Your-Fast Ramen

(L M H KETO ⌷ ◈ ◗ OPTION)   prep time: 5 minutes   cook time: 20 minutes   yield: 4 servings

In many cultures, soup, such as ramen, is a common way to break-your-fast. This tasty soup will keep you nice and warm all day long!

1 tablespoon toasted (dark) sesame oil

1 tablespoon coconut oil

½ cup minced onions (about 1 medium)

12 ounces ground pork

1 teaspoon fine sea salt

½ teaspoon ground black pepper

1 cup thinly shredded cabbage

2 cloves garlic

1 tablespoon crushed red pepper, or 1½ teaspoons chili powder

4 cups chicken bone broth, homemade (page 356) or store-bought (homemade will make a thicker soup)

1 tablespoon grated fresh ginger

1 tablespoon tomato paste

1 tablespoon coconut vinegar or unseasoned rice vinegar

1½ teaspoons wheat-free tamari, or 2 tablespoons coconut aminos

1 teaspoon fresh lime juice

4 large eggs (omit for egg-free)

1 tablespoon distilled white vinegar

Sliced scallions, for garnish

Crushed red pepper, for garnish (optional)

1. Heat the sesame and coconut oils in a large pot over medium-high heat. Add the onions and sauté for 1 minute, or until they are starting to soften. Add the ground pork, salt, and pepper and cook, stirring occasionally to break up the pork, until it is cooked through, about 3 minutes. Add the cabbage, garlic, and crushed red pepper. Reduce the heat to low and simmer for 4 minutes, or until the cabbage is starting to soften.

2. Stir in the broth, ginger, tomato paste, coconut vinegar, and tamari. Increase the heat to medium-high and cook for 8 minutes. Add the lime juice; taste and season with additional salt, if desired.

3. Make the poached eggs: Fill a medium-sized pot halfway full with water and add the white vinegar (vinegar helps the egg whites hold together). Bring the water to a boil, then rapidly swirl the water in a circle with a spoon. Crack an egg into a ramekin or small bowl. Gently tip the ramekin, let the egg slide into the boiling water, and poach for about 3 minutes, until the egg is done to your liking. Remove the egg from the water with a slotted spoon and set on a paper towel to drain. Repeat with the remaining eggs.

4. Divide the soup among 4 bowls. Place a poached egg in each bowl and garnish with scallions and crushed red pepper, if using. Store in an airtight container in the refrigerator for up to 5 days. To reheat, place the soup in a saucepan over medium heat for about 2 minutes, stirring often, then add a poached egg to each serving.

NUTRITIONAL INFO (per serving)				
calories	fat	protein	carbs	fiber
459	36g	25g	9g	3g

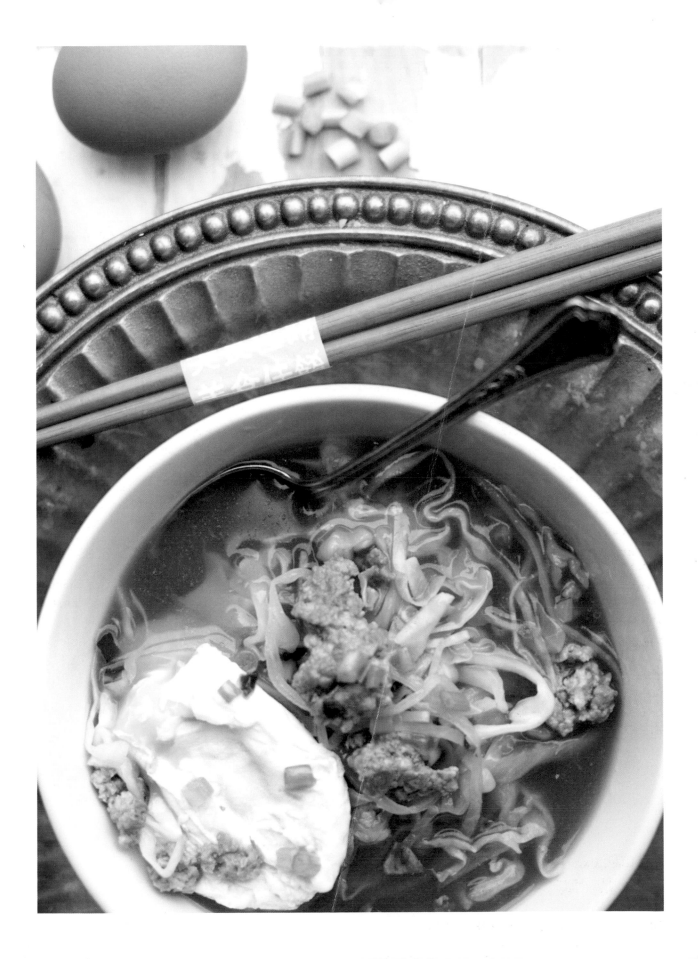

Cucumber Kimchi

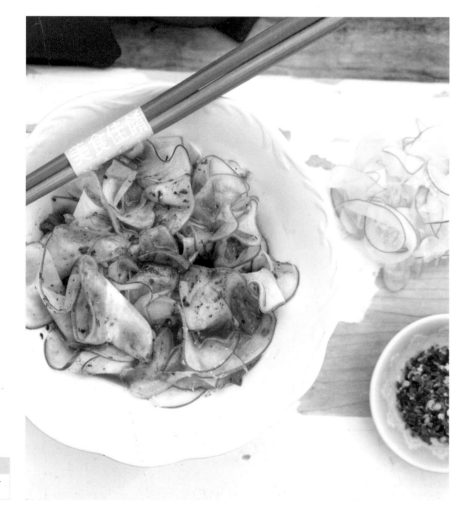

(L M H KETO) prep time: 3 minutes, plus 2 days to ferment if a stronger flavor is desired

yield: 8 servings

1 pound cucumbers (about 2 medium), very thinly sliced

¼ cup sliced scallions

1½ tablespoons fine sea salt

1 tablespoon Swerve confectioners'-style sweetener or equivalent amount of liquid or powdered sweetener (see page 31)

1 tablespoon fish sauce

2 teaspoons crushed red pepper

2 teaspoons grated fresh ginger

2 cloves garlic, smashed to a paste or minced

1. Place the ingredients in a large bowl and stir well to combine.

2. Divide the mixture evenly among 4 quart-size jars, leaving 1 inch of space at the top of each jar. Allow to rest for 1 hour for the juices to release. Eat immediately if you prefer a milder-flavored kimchi, or loosely cover the jars and allow the kimchi to ferment on the countertop for 2 days before chilling it in the refrigerator. The flavors will develop over time. Cover and refrigerate until ready to consume. Open the jars every 2 to 3 days to release accumulated gas.

NUTRITIONAL INFO (per serving)				
calories	fat	protein	carbs	fiber
12	0.2g	1g	2g	1g

Gyoza Meatballs

prep time: 8 minutes   **cook time:** 20 minutes
yield: 8 servings as an appetizer, 4 as a meal

These freezer-friendly meatballs taste great with Stir-Fry Sauce (page 42), as shown in the photo below, or in Gyoza Meatball Soup (page 74).

1 pound ground pork or ground chicken

1 large egg, lightly beaten

¼ cup finely chopped button mushrooms

2 tablespoons finely chopped scallions

1 teaspoon grated fresh ginger

1 clove garlic, smashed to a paste

¾ teaspoon wheat-free tamari, or 1 tablespoon coconut aminos

1. Preheat the oven to 400°F.

2. Place the ingredients in a large bowl and use your hands to mix together until well combined. Form the mixture into 1½-inch balls and place on a rimmed baking sheet.

3. Bake the meatballs for 20 minutes, or until browned and cooked through. Store in an airtight container in the refrigerator for up to 4 days or in the freezer for up to 1 month.

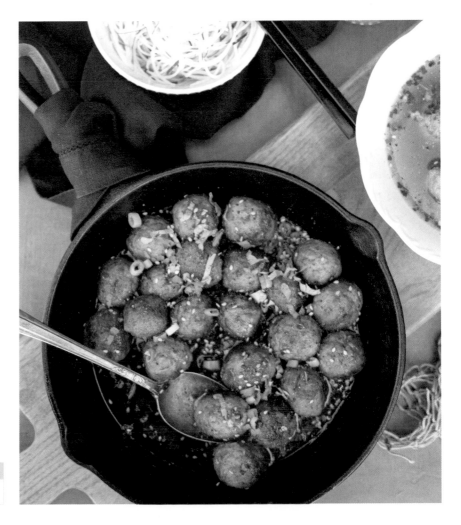

NUTRITIONAL INFO (per serving)				
calories	fat	protein	carbs	fiber
318	25g	21g	1g	1g

Pot Stickers

(L M H KETO) ( ) (OPTION) **prep time:** 8 minutes (not including time to make dipping sauce)
cook time: 12 minutes **yield:** 16 pot stickers (2 pot stickers per serving)

—filling

1 pound ground pork

1 cup thinly shredded green cabbage

¼ cup thinly sliced scallions

¾ teaspoon wheat-free tamari, or 1 tablespoon coconut aminos

1 teaspoon fine sea salt

1 teaspoon grated fresh ginger

¼ teaspoon ground black pepper

½ teaspoon toasted (dark) sesame oil

3 cloves garlic, minced

—wrappers

1¼ cups blanched almond flour, or ¾ cup coconut flour

3½ tablespoons psyllium husk powder (no substitutes)

1 teaspoon fine sea salt

2 large eggs (4 eggs if using coconut flour)

1½ cups boiling water or chicken bone broth, homemade (page 356) or store-bought

1 tablespoon coconut oil, for frying

1 batch Asian Dipping Sauce (page 43), for serving

1. Make the filling: Heat a large cast-iron skillet over medium heat. Place the ingredients for the filling in the skillet and sauté, breaking up the pork with a spatula, for about 5 minutes, until the pork is browned and cooked through. Remove from the heat and set aside.

2. Make the wrappers: In a medium-sized bowl, combine the flour, psyllium husk powder, and salt. Stir in the eggs until a thick dough forms. Add 1 cup of the boiling water to the bowl and mix until well combined. Let sit for 1 to 2 minutes, until the dough firms up and is easy to work with.

3. Lightly grease two 6-inch square pieces of parchment paper. Form the dough into 16 balls (about 1¼ inches in diameter). Place a ball in the center of one of the greased pieces of parchment. Top with the other piece of parchment. Using a rolling pin, roll out the dough into a circle about ⅛ inch thick. This dough is very forgiving, so if you don't roll it out into a neat circle, use your hands to perfect the wrapper. If you have a tortilla press, place the dough, sandwiched between the pieces of parchment paper, in the press and press down until the dough flattens to the edge of the press.

4. Fill the wrappers: Place 1 heaping tablespoon of filling in the center of a dough circle. Fold the wrapper sides to form a crescent shape. Pinch the dough together at the middle and begin gathering and folding the dough to create pleats, pinching to seal as you go. Repeat with the remaining wrappers and filling.

5. Heat the coconut oil in a large cast-iron skillet over medium-high heat. Working in two or three batches so you don't crowd the skillet, place the pot stickers in the skillet. Cook for 2 minutes per side, or until browned on both sides. Repeat with the rest of the pot stickers, adding more oil if needed. Return half of the fried pot stickers to the skillet and add the remaining ½ cup of boiling water. Cover and cook for 4 minutes, or until the wrappers are cooked through. Repeat with the remaining pot stickers.

6. Serve the pot stickers with the dipping sauce. Store in an airtight container in the refrigerator for up to 4 days or in the freezer for up to 1 month. To reheat, place in a preheated 400°F oven for 5 minutes, or until the skin gets crispy and the filling is heated through.

NUTRITIONAL INFO (per serving)				
calories	fat	protein	carbs	fiber
322	25g	15g	12g	7g

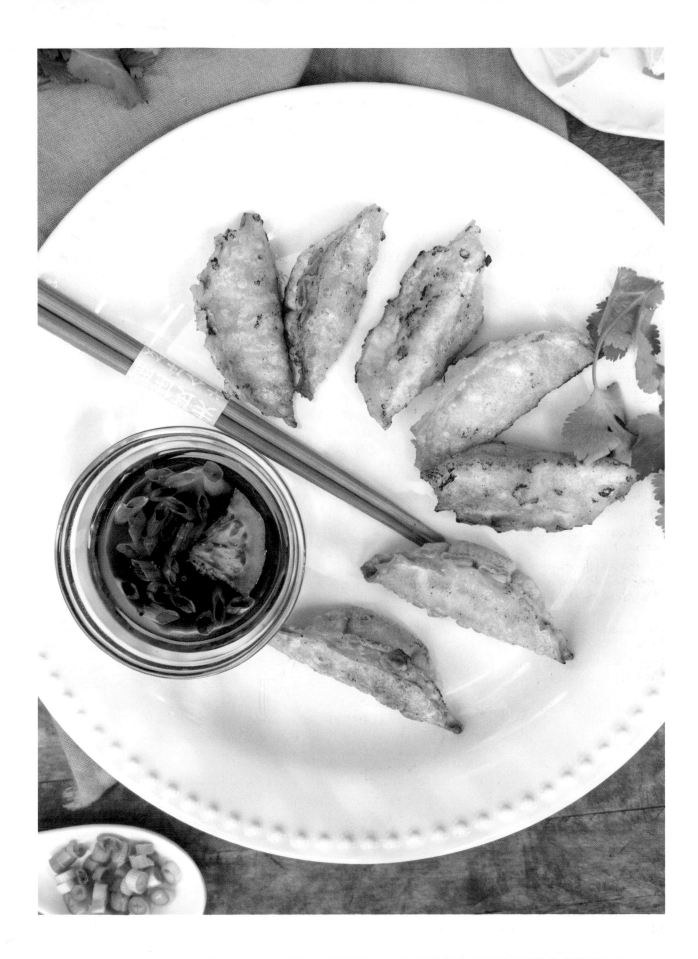

Crab Rangoon Puffs

(L M H KETO | OPTION | ⊘)   **prep time:** 10 minutes (not including time to make sauce)   **cook time:** 15 minutes
yield: 24 puffs (2 puffs per serving)

—puffs

3 large eggs

½ teaspoon cream of tartar

½ cup unflavored egg white protein powder (or whey protein powder if not dairy-sensitive)

3 ounces cream cheese (or reserved egg yolks if dairy-free), at room temperature

—filling

1 (8-ounce) package cream cheese (Kite Hill brand cream cheese style spread if dairy-free), at room temperature

1 (6-ounce) can crabmeat, drained

2 scallions, thinly sliced

1 clove garlic, minced

1 teaspoon grated fresh ginger

½ teaspoon wheat-free tamari, or 2 teaspoons coconut aminos

Sweet-and-Sour Sauce (page 43), for serving

Thinly sliced scallions, green part only, for garnish

1. Preheat the oven to 375°F. Line a rimmed baking sheet with parchment paper and lightly grease the parchment, or grease the wells of a 24-well mini muffin pan.

2. Make the puffs: Separate the eggs, putting the whites in a large bowl; reserve the egg yolks for use in Step 3, if dairy-free, or for another recipe. Add the cream of tartar to the egg whites and whip with a hand mixer until very stiff peaks form. Then add the protein powder while the mixer is running on low, or fold it in with a spatula.

3. Using a spatula, gradually fold the 3 ounces of cream cheese into the egg white mixture, being careful not to deflate the whites. (*Note:* If dairy-free, lightly beat the reserved egg yolks, then gently fold them in.)

4. Form the dough into 24 balls about 2 inches in diameter. Place the balls on the baking sheet or mini muffin pan. Bake for 10 minutes, or until golden. Turn off the oven and leave the puffs inside with the oven door shut for another 5 minutes, or until cool.

5. Meanwhile, make the filling: Place the cream cheese, crabmeat, scallions, garlic, ginger, and tamari in a medium-sized bowl. Using a hand mixer, mix the filling ingredients together until well combined. Transfer the filling to a pastry bag fitted with a tip or in a large zip-top plastic bag with ¼ inch snipped off one corner.

6. Slice the puffs in half. Fill each half with about 1½ tablespoons of the filling. To prevent the puffs from getting soggy, fill them the day you plan to eat them, just before serving. Serve with the sauce and garnish with scallions. Store extra puffs and filling in separate airtight containers in the refrigerator for up to 4 days.

NUTRITIONAL INFO (per serving)				
calories	fat	protein	carbs	fiber
138	10g	9g	2g	0.3g

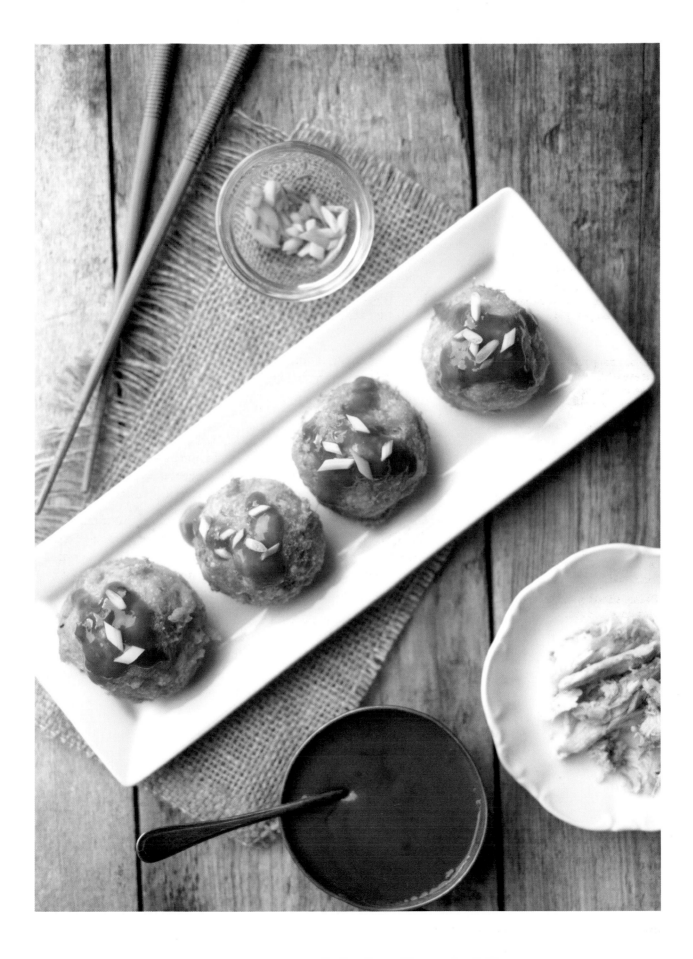

Gyoza (Japanese Dumplings)

(L M→H KETO ⃠ ⃠ ⃠) prep time: 7 minutes (not including time to make sauce) cook time: 5 minutes
yield: 12 dumplings (2 dumplings per serving)

This unique recipe uses chicken skins for the wrappers, which tastes amazing! Ask your butcher to special-order a bag of chicken skins. Otherwise, pick up a package of bone-in, skin-on chicken thighs, remove the skins for the wrappers, and use the chicken for the filling. If you go that route, you'll need to debone the meat and grind it yourself. I love having a grinder attachment on my stand mixer for tasks like this; however, if you do not have a grinder attachment, you can chop the chicken into tiny pieces by hand.

—filling

4 ounces ground chicken or ground pork

½ cup thinly shredded cabbage

2 tablespoons thinly sliced scallions

1 clove garlic, minced

¾ teaspoon wheat-free tamari, or 1 tablespoon coconut aminos

¼ teaspoon grated fresh ginger

¼ teaspoon fine sea salt

—wrappers

Chicken skins from 12 chicken thighs (see note, above)

½ cup avocado oil or coconut oil, for frying

¼ cup Ginger Sauce (page 42) or Sweet-and-Sour Sauce (page 43), for serving

Chopped fresh chives, for garnish (optional)

1. Make the filling: Heat a large cast-iron skillet over medium heat. Place the ground chicken, cabbage, scallions, garlic, tamari, ginger, and salt in the skillet; sauté, breaking up the chicken with a spatula, for about 5 minutes, until the chicken is cooked through. Remove from the heat and set aside.

2. Make the wrappers: Place the chicken skins on a cutting board with the inside facing up and flatten and stretch them out as large as you can. Lay a chicken skin wrapper flat in front of you. Place 1 tablespoon of the filling in the center of the skin. Fold the skin over the filling to make a dumpling and seal the dumpling with a toothpick. Repeat with the remaining wrappers and filling.

3. Heat the oil in a 4-inch-deep (or deeper) cast-iron skillet over medium heat to 375°F. The oil should be 3 inches deep; add more oil if needed. Working in two or three batches so you don't crowd the skillet, place the dumplings in the skillet. Fry for 3 to 5 minutes, or until the dumplings are browned on all sides and the chicken skin is crisp. Remove to a plate and repeat with the remaining dumplings.

4. Serve with the sauce and garnish with chives, if desired. Store in an airtight container in the refrigerator for up to 4 days or in the freezer (before frying) for up to 1 month. To reheat, place in a preheated 400°F oven for 5 minutes, or until the skin gets crispy and the filling is heated through.

NUTRITIONAL INFO (per serving)				
calories	fat	protein	carbs	fiber
397	39g	10g	2g	1g

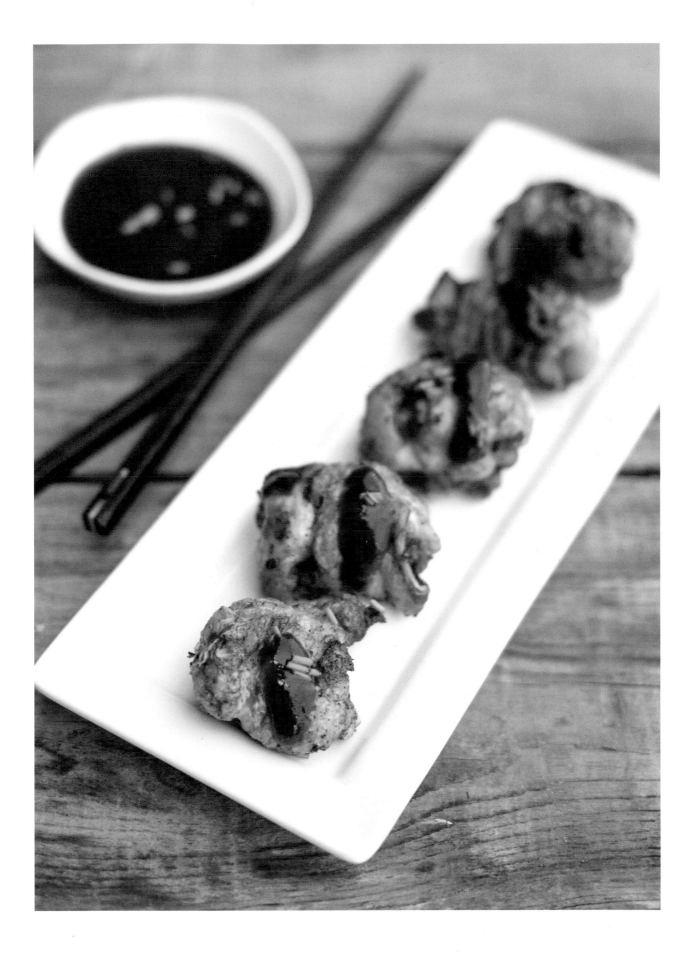

Cream Cheese Wontons

(L M H KETO / OPTION) prep time: 10 minutes   cook time: 4 minutes   yield: 16 wontons (2 per serving)

—sweet and tangy dipping sauce

½ cup Swerve confectioners'-style sweetener or equivalent amount of liquid or powdered sweetener (see page 31)

½ cup coconut vinegar

1½ teaspoons wheat-free tamari, or 2 tablespoons coconut aminos

1 tablespoon tomato paste

1 clove roasted garlic (page 359), or 1 clove raw garlic, smashed to a paste

1 teaspoon grated fresh ginger

¼ teaspoon guar gum (optional, for thickening)

1½ cups coconut oil, for frying

—filling

1 (8-ounce) package cream cheese (Kite Hill brand cream cheese style spread if dairy-free), at room temperature

2 ounces canned crabmeat, drained

1 teaspoon finely chopped scallions

¼ teaspoon grated fresh ginger

½ teaspoon fine sea salt

—wrappers

16 large slices prosciutto, very thinly sliced (see note)

1. Make the sauce: Heat the sweetener, vinegar, tamari, tomato paste, garlic, and ginger in a small saucepan over low heat until simmering. Sift in the guar gum, if using, and whisk until well combined.

2. Heat the oil in a 4-inch-deep (or deeper) cast-iron skillet over medium heat to 350°F. The oil should be 3 inches deep; add more oil if needed.

3. Make the filling: In a small bowl, combine the cream cheese, crabmeat, scallions, ginger, and salt and mix well.

4. Assemble the wontons: Lay a slice of prosciutto on a sheet of parchment paper with the short end of the prosciutto facing you. Spoon 1 heaping tablespoon of the filling onto the bottom left corner of the prosciutto. Fold the prosciutto in a triangle over the filling (like you are making a paper football to fling across a classroom). Continue folding in a triangle, making sure that the filling is well covered. Continue all the way to the top of the prosciutto. Repeat until all of the wrappers are filled. (See the photo sequence, opposite, for guidance.)

5. Carefully place half of the wontons in the hot oil and fry for about 2 minutes, until golden brown. Remove the wontons from the oil and repeat with the remaining wontons. Serve the wontons with the sauce.

6. Store the wontons and sauce in separate airtight containers in the refrigerator for up to 4 days. The wontons can be frozen for up to 1 month. To reheat the wontons, place in a preheated 400°F oven for 5 minutes, or until the skin is crispy and the filling is heated through.

note: *This recipe works best with ultra-thin slices of prosciutto. Prepackaged prosciutto is usually not as thinly sliced as what's needed here. Your best bet is to ask your butcher to slice some for you.*

tip: *Once cool, you can strain the oil and store it in a jar in the refrigerator for future frying.*

NUTRITIONAL INFO (per serving)				
calories	fat	protein	carbs	fiber
182	14g	10g	2g	1g

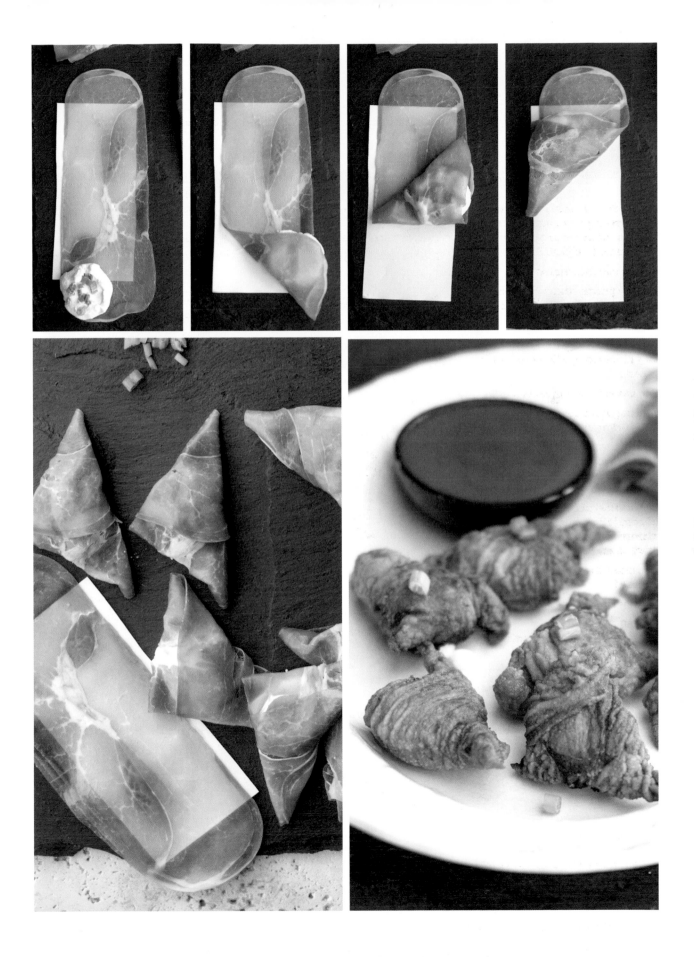

Crab Rangoon Fritters

(L M H / KETO / OPTION / OPTION) prep time: 8 minutes   cook time: 8 minutes   yield: 16 fritters (2 per serving)

—cream cheese filling

1 (8-ounce) package cream cheese (Kite Hill brand cream cheese style spread if dairy-free), at room temperature

¼ cup dried chives

—crab fritters

1 pound canned lump crabmeat, drained and squeezed of excess moisture

½ cup powdered Parmesan cheese (see page 363) (or 2 tablespoons coconut flour if dairy-free)

1 tablespoon mayonnaise, homemade (page 357) or store-bought

1 large egg

1 teaspoon grated fresh ginger

1 clove garlic, smashed to a paste or minced

¼ cup lard or coconut oil, for frying

—dipping sauce

¼ cup chicken bone broth, homemade (page 356) or store-bought

¼ cup plus 2 tablespoons Swerve confectioners'-style sweetener or equivalent amount of liquid or powdered sweetener (see page 31), or more to your desired sweetness

2 tablespoons wheat-free tamari, or ½ cup coconut aminos

2 cloves garlic, minced

1½ teaspoons grated fresh ginger

1 teaspoon fresh lime juice

⅓ teaspoon guar gum (optional, for thickening)

Thinly sliced scallions, for garnish

1. Make the filling: In a small bowl, combine the cream cheese and chives. For easy handling, refrigerate the filling mixture.

2. Make the fritter coating: In a large bowl, combine the crabmeat, powdered Parmesan, mayonnaise, egg, ginger, and garlic until blended.

3. In a small pot, heat the lard over medium-high heat. The lard should be 3 inches deep; add more lard if needed. Line a plate with paper towels.

4. Form the filling mixture into 1-tablespoon balls. Take 2 tablespoons of the fritter mixture and form it tightly around a cheese ball. Repeat with the rest of the fritter mixture until all the cream cheese balls are coated.

5. When the lard is between 360°F and 375°F (or it sizzles when you start to drop a fritter into it), use a spoon to place a few balls at a time into the pot. Cook until golden brown, about 4 minutes. Remove the fritters from the pot and place onto the paper towel–lined plate. Repeat with the remaining balls.

6. Make the dipping sauce: Combine the broth, sweetener, tamari, garlic, ginger, and lime juice in a small saucepan over medium-high heat. Cook until the sweetener is dissolved. Sift in the guar gum, if using (make sure to sift it or it will clump up), and whisk until well combined. Remove from the heat. Taste and adjust the seasoning to your liking.

7. Transfer the fritters to a platter and serve with the dipping sauce. Garnish with scallions. Store the fritters and sauce in separate air-tight containers in the refrigerator for up to 4 days. To reheat, place in a preheated 350°F oven for about 5 minutes.

NUTRITIONAL INFO (per serving)				
calories	fat	protein	carbs	fiber
149	10g	11g	2g	1g

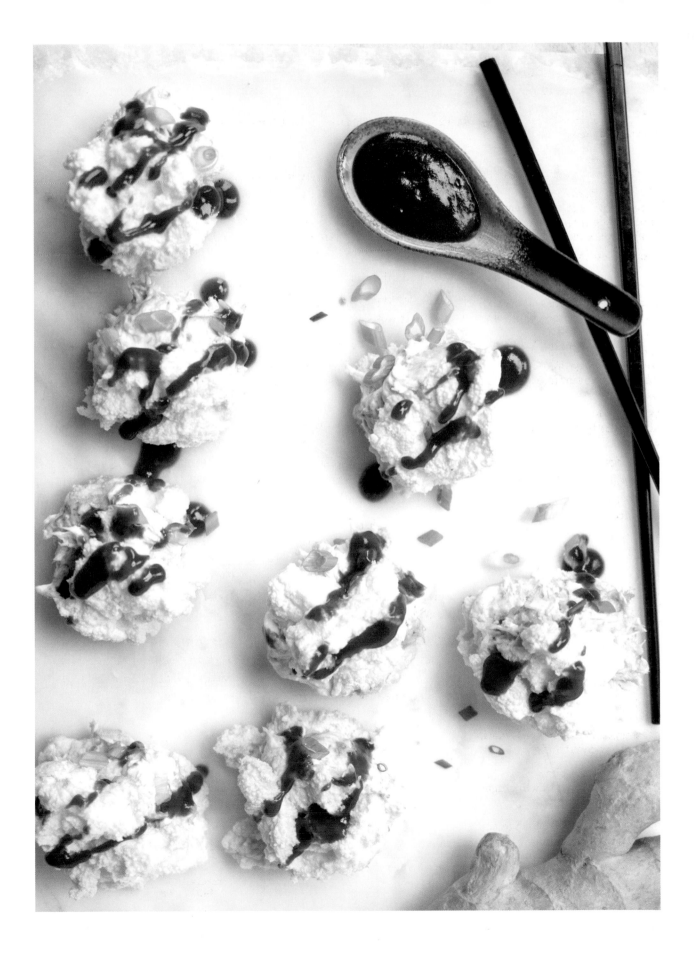

General Tso's Chicken Drummies

(L →M H KETO) prep time: 5 minutes   cook time: 30 minutes
yield: 8 servings (about 3 drummies per serving)

This recipe uses a lot of coconut oil, but you can use it more than once. I keep a large mason jar of oil in the refrigerator that is reserved for frying. Once you are done with the frying, let the oil cool, strain it, and save it for future use.

2 cups coconut oil, for frying

2 pounds (about 24) chicken drumettes and/or wings

Fine sea salt and ground black pepper

—sauce

½ teaspoon toasted (dark) sesame oil

¼ cup chicken bone broth, homemade (page 356) or store-bought

3 tablespoons coconut vinegar or unseasoned rice vinegar

2¼ teaspoons wheat-free tamari, or 3 tablespoons coconut aminos

3 tablespoons Swerve confectioners'-style sweetener or equivalent amount of liquid or powdered sweetener (see page 31)

¼ cup chopped scallions

3 small dried chiles, chopped

¼ teaspoon guar gum (optional, for thickening)

Sliced scallions, green part only, for garnish (optional)

Crushed red pepper, for garnish (optional)

1. Heat the oil in a 4-inch-deep (or deeper) cast-iron skillet over medium heat to 350°F. The oil should be 3 inches deep; add more if needed. Fry about 6 drumettes or wings at a time until golden brown on all sides and cooked through, about 8 minutes. Transfer the fried chicken to a platter and sprinkle with salt and pepper. Repeat with the remaining chicken.

2. Make the sauce: Place the sesame oil, broth, vinegar, tamari, sweetener, scallions, and chiles in a small saucepan over medium-high heat. Sift in the guar gum, if using, and whisk until well combined. Cook for 3 to 5 minutes, until thickened. Remove from the heat.

3. Serve the chicken with the sauce. Garnish with scallions and crushed red pepper, if desired. Store the chicken and sauce in separate airtight containers in the refrigerator for up to 4 days. To reheat the chicken, place in a preheated 375°F oven for about 5 minutes.

NUTRITIONAL INFO (per serving)				
calories	fat	protein	carbs	fiber
350	24g	31g	2g	1g

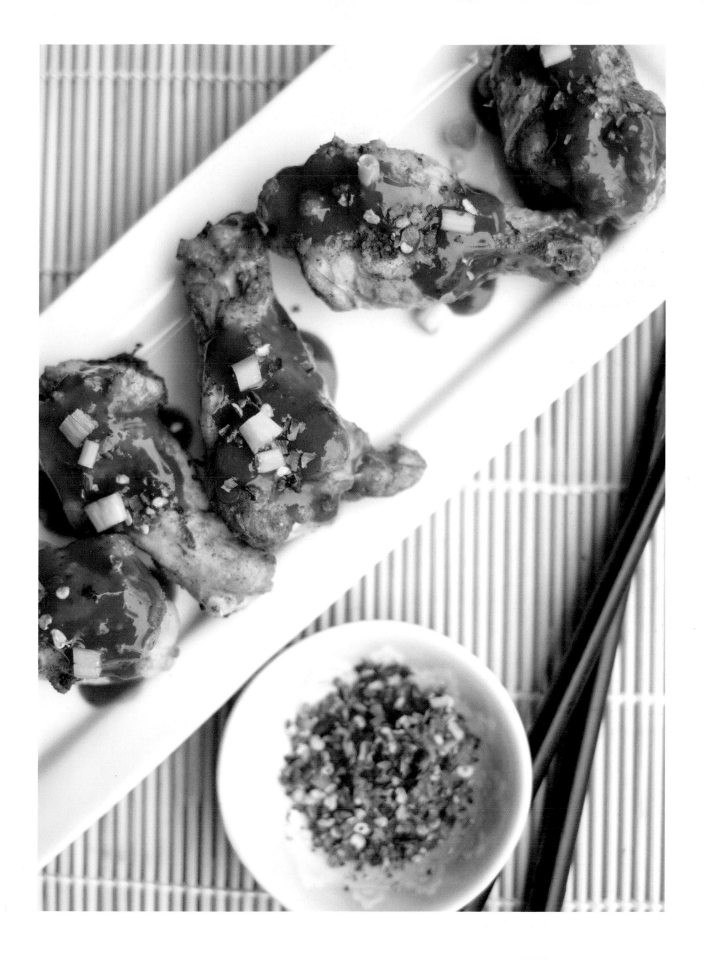

Chinese Sticky Rib Bites

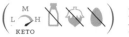 prep time: 5 minutes, plus time to marinate   cook time: 1 hour 20 minutes
yield: 8 servings

Sticky spareribs are a standard at almost every Chinese takeout restaurant. And believe me, these ribs do not disappoint! Just make sure to grab a lot of napkins!

2 pounds pork spareribs

½ cup chicken bone broth, homemade (page 356) or store-bought

⅓ cup Swerve confectioners'-style sweetener or equivalent amount of liquid or powdered sweetener (see page 31)

¼ cup tomato sauce

1½ tablespoons wheat-free tamari, or ⅓ cup coconut aminos

1 tablespoon coconut vinegar or apple cider vinegar

½ teaspoon Chinese five-spice powder

¼ teaspoon toasted (dark) sesame oil

⅛ teaspoon liquid smoke (optional)

1 clove garlic, smashed to a paste

Sliced scallions, for garnish

1 tablespoon toasted sesame seeds, for garnish

1. Slice the spareribs into individual ribs. In a large bowl, whisk together the broth, sweetener, tomato sauce, tamari, vinegar, five-spice powder, sesame oil, liquid smoke (if using), and garlic. Place the ribs in the bowl and stir well to coat. Cover the bowl and place in the refrigerator to marinate for 2 hours or overnight.

2. Preheat the oven to 350°F. Remove the ribs from the marinade and place them on a wire rack set inside a rimmed baking sheet; reserve the marinade. Lay a sheet of parchment paper over the ribs, then place a sheet of foil on top and crimp the edges of the foil around all sides of the pan to seal tightly. Bake for 1 hour.

3. Remove the ribs from the oven and increase the oven temperature to 450°F. Remove the cover, brush the ribs with the marinade, and bake, uncovered, for 10 minutes more. Repeat and bake for another 10 minutes. Remove the ribs from the oven, garnish with scallions and sesame seeds, and serve. Store in an airtight container in the refrigerator for up to 4 days. To reheat, place in a preheated 350°F oven for about 5 minutes.

NUTRITIONAL INFO (per serving)				
calories	fat	protein	carbs	fiber
316	26g	18g	3g	1g

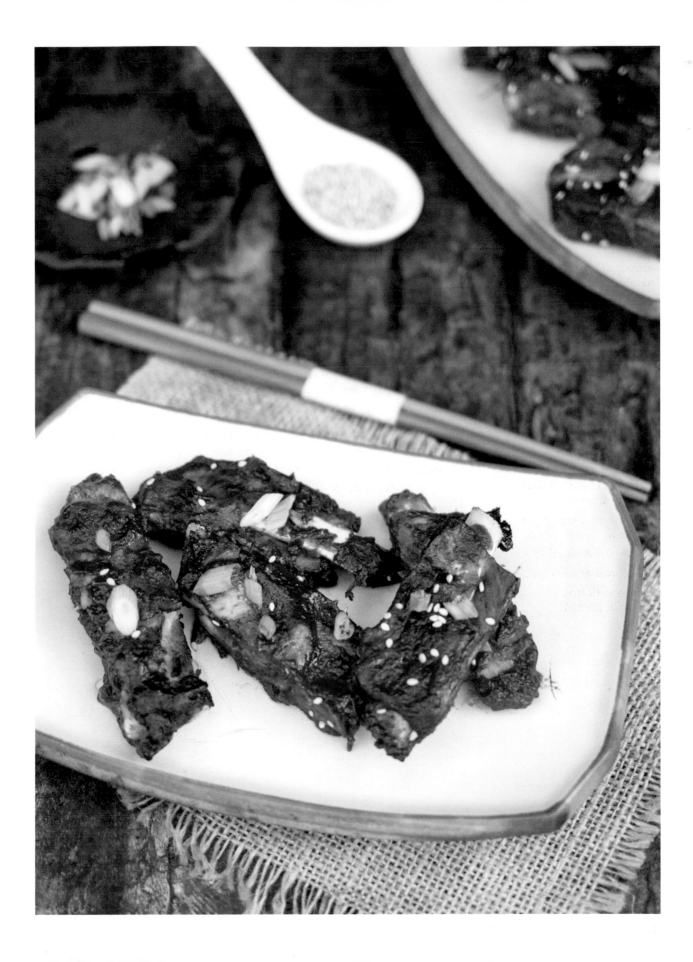

Po Ho Thng

prep time: 3 minutes   cook time: 5 minutes   yield: 8 servings

This aromatic mint soup is traditionally sipped throughout the meal because the minty flavor freshens the palate between courses. It also soothes the stomach. If you've made egg drop soup, the technique used to make this soup will be familiar to you. Just as in egg drop soup, whisked eggs are drizzled into hot broth to form "ribbons" of egg.

8 cups chicken bone broth, homemade (page 356) or store-bought

2 cups loosely packed fresh mint leaves, plus extra for garnish

3 large eggs, lightly beaten

½ teaspoon fine sea salt

¼ teaspoon ground black pepper

1. Bring the broth to a boil in a large pot. Add the mint and remove from the heat. Allow to steep for 3 minutes, or longer for a more intense minty flavor. Remove the mint leaves.

2. Add the eggs in a steady stream, stirring slowly in one direction. The eggs will cook in the hot broth. Stir in the salt and pepper and serve garnished with fresh mint leaves, if desired. Store in an airtight container in the refrigerator for up to 5 days. To reheat, place in a saucepan over medium heat for about 2 minutes, stirring often.

NUTRITIONAL INFO (per serving)				
calories	fat	protein	carbs	fiber
100	8g	6g	1g	0.3g

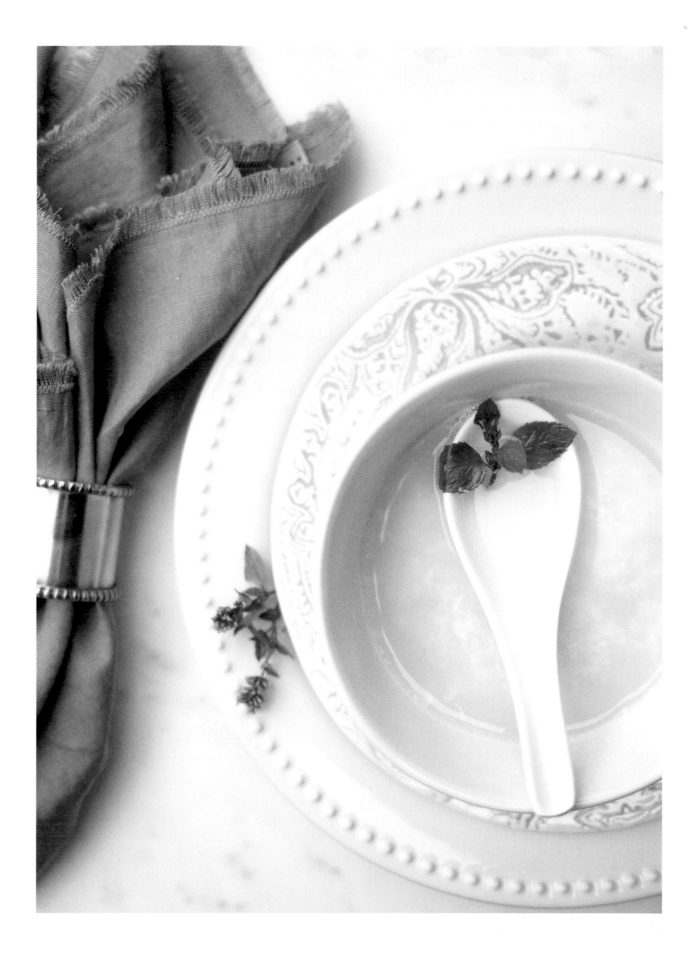

Hot-and-Sour Soup

(L M H KETO) prep time: 7 minutes   cook time: 10 minutes   yield: 6 servings

1 tablespoon coconut oil

½ pound boneless, skinless chicken thighs, cut into ½-inch cubes

Fine sea salt and ground black pepper

2 cloves garlic, smashed to a paste or minced

1 leek, thinly sliced

1 cup thinly sliced button mushrooms (about 8 ounces)

6 cups chicken bone broth, homemade (page 356) or store-bought

¼ cup unseasoned rice vinegar or coconut vinegar

1 tablespoon wheat-free tamari, or ¼ cup coconut aminos

1 tablespoon chili sesame oil

2 teaspoons grated fresh ginger

2 large eggs, lightly beaten

Sliced scallions, for garnish

Chopped cilantro leaves, for garnish

2 limes, quartered, for serving

1. In a large pot, heat the coconut oil over medium-high heat. Season the chicken on all sides with salt and pepper. Place the chicken in the pot and sear on all sides, about 3 minutes total. Reduce the heat to medium. Add the garlic, leek, and mushrooms and sauté for 4 minutes, or until the mushrooms are turning golden brown.

2. Pour in the broth. Add the vinegar, tamari, chili sesame oil, and ginger and boil for 5 minutes. Taste and adjust the seasoning to your liking.

3. Just before serving, remove the pot from the heat and drizzle the eggs into the soup while stirring in one direction. Divide the soup among 6 bowls, garnish with scallions and cilantro, and serve with a squirt of lime juice. Store in an airtight container in the refrigerator for up to 5 days. To reheat, place in a saucepan over medium heat for about 2 minutes, stirring often.

NUTRITIONAL INFO (per serving)				
calories	fat	protein	carbs	fiber
210	15g	13g	7g	3g

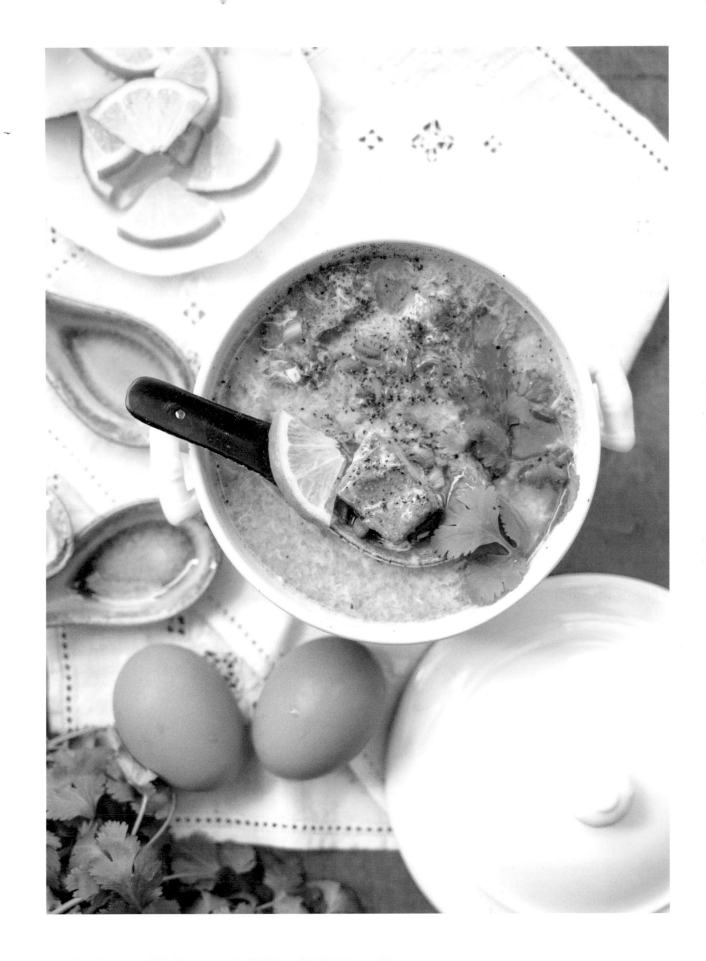

Simple Egg Drop Soup

(L M H KETO 🧂 🚫)   prep time: 5 minutes   cook time: 5 minutes   yield: 2 servings

4 cups chicken bone broth, homemade (page 356) or store-bought (see note)

¾ cup sliced button or shiitake mushrooms (about 6 ounces)

2¼ teaspoons wheat-free tamari, or 3 tablespoons coconut aminos

1 teaspoon grated fresh ginger

1 teaspoon fish sauce, or ½ scant teaspoon fine sea salt

¼ teaspoon ground black pepper

3 scallions, chopped, plus extra for garnish (optional)

4 large eggs, lightly beaten

1. Place the broth, mushrooms, tamari, ginger, fish sauce, pepper, and scallions in a large pot and bring to a boil. Cook until the mushrooms soften, about 3 minutes. Taste and adjust the seasoning to your liking.

2. Reduce the heat to low. Slowly pour in the eggs while stirring in one direction. The eggs will cook in a minute or two and form ribbons.

3. Remove the soup from the heat and divide it between 2 bowls. Garnish with additional scallions, if desired. This soup is best served fresh, but any extra can be stored in an airtight container in the refrigerator for up to 3 days. To reheat, place in a saucepan over medium-low heat until just warmed.

note: *Store-bought broth will work in this recipe, but the soup will have a thinner consistency. If you're using store-bought broth and you want a thicker soup, place ½ cup of the hot broth in a small bowl and whisk in 1 egg yolk until very smooth (reserve the egg white for adding more ribbons to the soup). After the mushrooms are cooked and you have reduced the heat to low, whisk this mixture into the soup.*

NUTRITIONAL INFO (per serving)				
calories	fat	protein	carbs	fiber
317	22g	24g	6g	1g

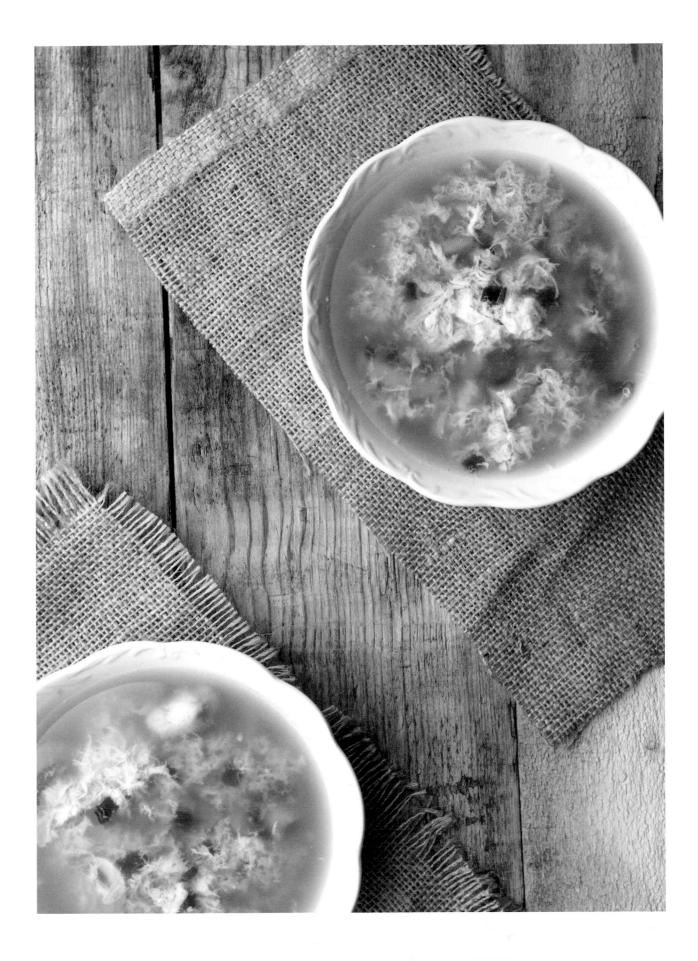

Gyoza Meatball Soup

(L M H KETO) 🍶 🚫   **prep time:** 8 minutes (not including time to make meatballs)   **cook time:** 15 minutes
           yield: 6 servings

1 teaspoon toasted (dark) sesame oil

2 tablespoons grated fresh ginger

1 clove garlic, minced

6 cups chicken bone broth, homemade (page 356) or store-bought

1 tablespoon wheat-free tamari, or ¼ cup coconut aminos

1 tablespoon fish sauce

½ teaspoon crushed red pepper

2 cups thinly shredded bok choy or Chinese (napa) cabbage (about 4 ounces)

Fine sea salt (optional)

1 batch Gyoza Meatballs (page 53)

Sliced scallions, for garnish

Chopped cilantro leaves, for garnish

2 limes, quartered, for serving

1. Preheat the oven to 400°F.

2. Make the broth: Heat the oil in a medium-sized saucepan over medium heat. Add the ginger and garlic and sauté for 1 minute, or until fragrant. Add the broth, tamari, fish sauce, crushed red pepper, and bok choy. Increase the heat to medium-high and simmer for 5 to 10 minutes, until fragrant. Taste and season with salt, if desired.

3. Just before serving the soup, add the meatballs and allow to heat through over medium-low heat. Garnish with scallions and cilantro and serve with a squirt of lime juice. Store in an airtight container in the refrigerator for up to 5 days. To reheat, place in a saucepan over medium heat for about 2 minutes, stirring often.

NUTRITIONAL INFO (per serving)				
calories	fat	protein	carbs	fiber
158	11g	8g	7g	3g

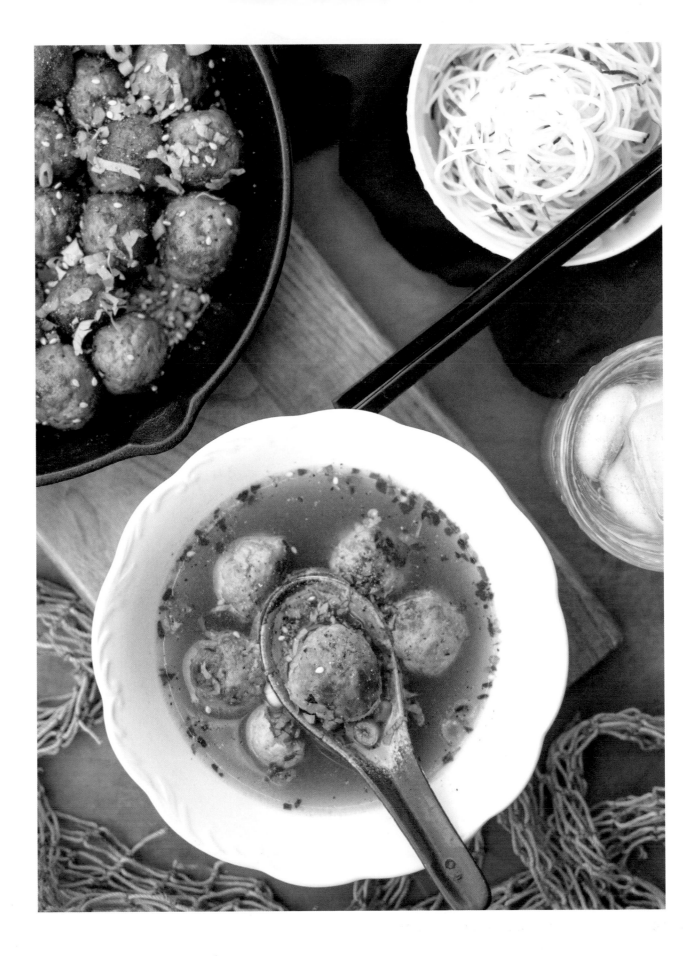

Pot Sticker Soup

(L~H M KETO [icons] OPTION) prep time: 8 minutes (not including time to make pot stickers)
cook time: 20 minutes   yield: 8 servings

I can't think of anything better than pot stickers, except perhaps pot sticker soup! This recipe is inspired by the flavors of Chinese cooking, but I added a touch of fish sauce to heighten the flavor of the soup. If you don't have fish sauce (or you don't care for it), replace it with 1 teaspoon of salt.

1 teaspoon toasted (dark) sesame oil

2 tablespoons grated fresh ginger

1 clove garlic, minced

6 cups chicken bone broth, homemade (page 356) or store-bought

1 tablespoon wheat-free tamari, or ¼ cup coconut aminos

1 tablespoon fish sauce

½ teaspoon crushed red pepper

2 cups thinly shredded bok choy or Chinese (napa) cabbage (about 4 ounces)

Fine sea salt (optional)

1 batch Pot Stickers (page 54)

Sliced scallions, for garnish

Chopped cilantro leaves, for garnish

2 limes, quartered, for serving

1. Make the broth: Heat the oil in a medium-sized saucepan over medium heat. Add the ginger and garlic and sauté for 1 minute, or until fragrant. Add the broth, tamari, fish sauce, crushed red pepper, and bok choy. Increase the heat to medium-high and simmer for 5 to 10 minutes, until the bok choy is softened. Taste and season with salt, if desired.

2. Just before serving the soup, add the pot stickers and allow to heat through over medium-low heat. Divide among serving bowls and garnish with scallions and cilantro, and serve with a squirt of lime juice. Store in an airtight container in the refrigerator for up to 5 days. To reheat, place in a saucepan over medium heat for about 2 minutes, stirring often.

NUTRITIONAL INFO (per serving)				
calories	fat	protein	carbs	fiber
386	29g	19g	14g	8g

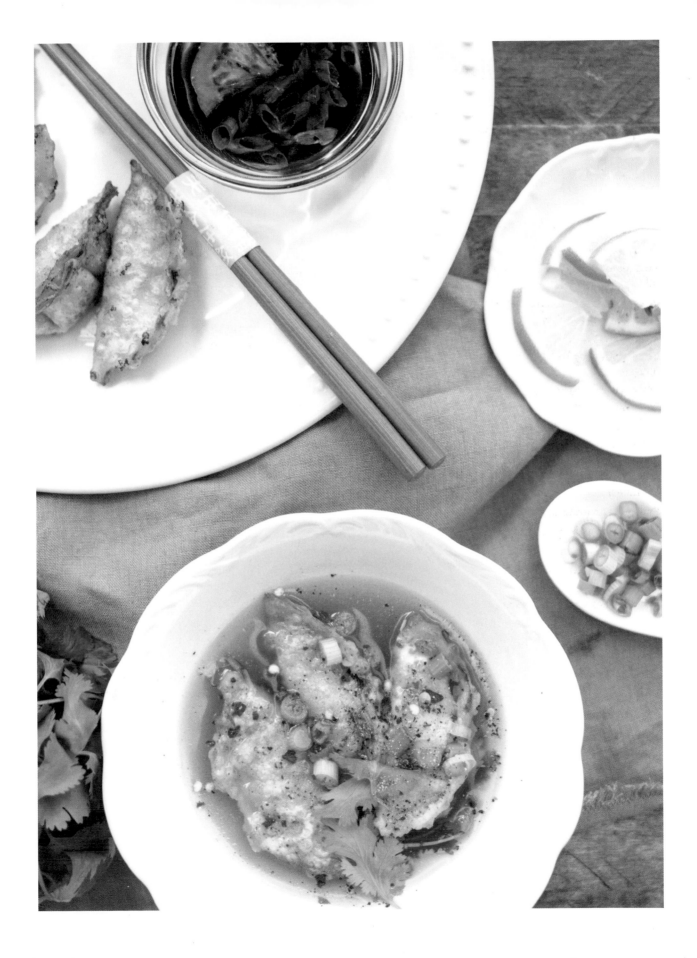

Udon Soup with Bok Choy and Poached Eggs

(L → M → H / KETO)   **prep time:** 6 minutes   **cook time:** 13 minutes   **yield:** 4 servings

4 cups chicken bone broth, homemade (page 356) or store-bought

4 bok choy leaves, roughly torn

1 cup thinly sliced Chinese (napa) cabbage

2 scallions, thinly sliced, plus extra for garnish

1 tablespoon wheat-free tamari, or ¼ cup coconut aminos

2 star anise

1 cinnamon stick

Fine sea salt (optional)

4 large eggs

1 tablespoon distilled white vinegar

1. Place the broth, bok choy, cabbage, scallions, tamari, star anise, and cinnamon stick in a medium-sized saucepan and bring to a boil. Boil for 10 minutes. Remove from the heat and discard the star anise and cinnamon stick. Taste and add salt, if desired.

2. When the soup is nearly done boiling, poach the eggs: Fill a medium-sized pot halfway full with water and add the white vinegar (vinegar helps the egg whites hold together). Bring to a gentle simmer, then rapidly swirl the water with a spoon. Crack an egg into a ramekin or small bowl. Gently tip the ramekin, let the egg slide into the boiling water, and poach for about 3 minutes, until the egg is done to your liking. Remove the egg from the water with a slotted spoon and set on a paper towel to drain. Repeat with the remaining eggs.

3. Divide the soup among 4 bowls. Add a poached egg to each bowl and garnish with scallions. Store in an airtight container in the refrigerator for up to 5 days. To reheat, place the soup in a saucepan over medium heat for about 2 minutes, stirring often, then add a poached egg to each serving.

NUTRITIONAL INFO (per serving)				
calories	fat	protein	carbs	fiber
172	11g	11g	6g	4g

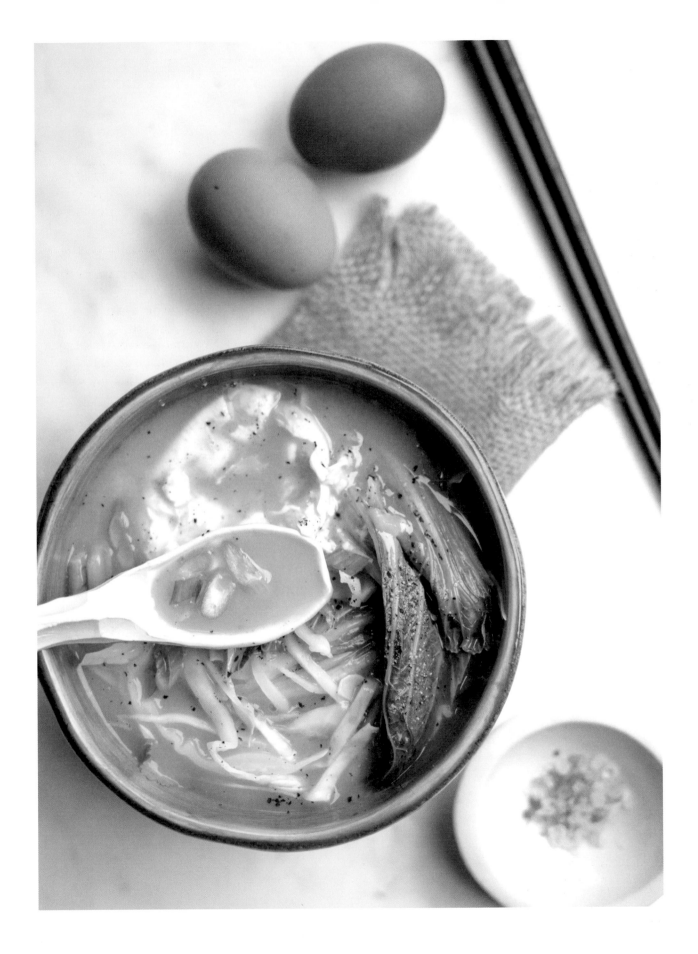

Asian Slow Cooker Short Ribs

(L → M H, KETO) prep time: 5 minutes   cook time: 5 or 8 hours   yield: 12 servings

4 pounds pork ribs

½ cup Swerve confectioners'-style sweetener or equivalent amount of liquid or powdered sweetener (see page 31)

3 tablespoons wheat-free tamari, or ¾ cup coconut aminos

2 tablespoons unseasoned rice vinegar

1 teaspoon fish sauce (optional, for umami taste)

1 teaspoon hot sauce (such as Frank's RedHot)

4 drops food-grade orange oil

6 cloves garlic, finely grated or minced

2 teaspoons finely grated fresh ginger

½ teaspoon crushed red pepper

¼ teaspoon guar gum (optional, for thickening)

Sliced scallions, for garnish

Toasted sesame seeds, for garnish

1. Place the ribs in a 4-quart slow cooker. In a medium-sized bowl, whisk together the sweetener, tamari, vinegar, fish sauce, hot sauce, orange oil, garlic, ginger, and crushed red pepper. Pour the sauce over the ribs.

2. Cook on high for 4 to 5 hours or on low for 7 to 8 hours, until the meat is tender.

3. Before serving, preheat the oven broiler to high. Place the ribs on a rimmed baking sheet.

4. Transfer the sauce in the slow cooker to a small saucepan and sift in the guar gum, if using. Boil the sauce over high heat for about 4 minutes, until thickened a little. Baste the ribs with a few table-spoons of the sauce.

5. Broil the ribs for about 3 minutes, until the sauce is bubbling and slightly caramelized. Serve the ribs with extra sauce and garnish with scallions and sesame seeds. Store in an airtight container in the refrigerator for up to 4 days or in the freezer for up to 1 month. To reheat, place on a rimmed baking sheet in a preheated 350°F oven for about 5 minutes.

NUTRITIONAL INFO (per serving)				
calories	fat	protein	carbs	fiber
605	46g	44g	1g	0.1g

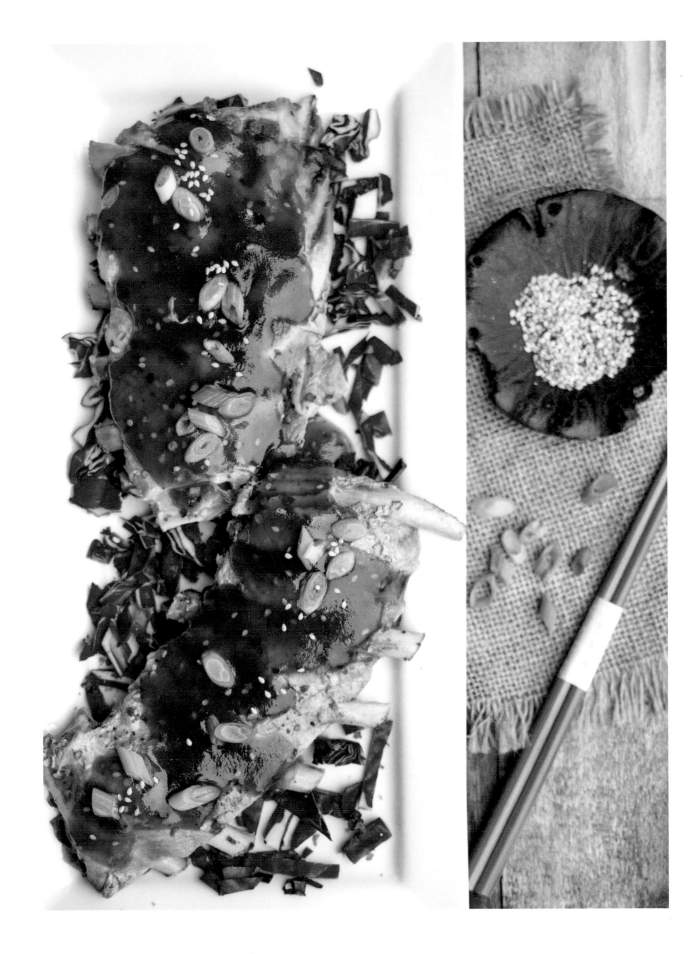

Moo Shu Pork and Pancakes

(L M H KETO OPTION) prep time: 10 minutes, plus time to marinate   cook time: about 30 minutes
yield: 4 servings

¼ cup MCT oil, avocado oil, or toasted (dark) sesame oil

¼ cup coconut vinegar or unseasoned rice vinegar

2 tablespoons Swerve confectioners'-style sweetener or equivalent amount of liquid or powdered sweetener (see page 31)

1 tablespoon wheat-free tamari, or ¼ cup coconut aminos

2 teaspoons fish sauce

¼ teaspoon ground black pepper

12 ounces pork butt, sliced across the grain into thin strips

—pancakes

2 raw large eggs

2 hard-boiled eggs

4 ounces cream cheese (Kite Hill brand for dairy-free)

1 tablespoon Swerve confectioners'-style sweetener or equivalent amount of liquid or powdered sweetener

Pinch of fine sea salt

1 tablespoon coconut oil, for the pan

—sesame scrambled eggs

1 teaspoon toasted (dark) sesame oil

4 large eggs, lightly beaten

½ teaspoon fine sea salt

—stir-fry

¼ cup coconut oil

4 cups thinly shredded Chinese (napa) cabbage (about 1 pound)

2 cups sliced mushrooms (about 2 ounces)

4 scallions, thinly sliced, plus extra for garnish

2 cloves garlic, minced

1 teaspoon grated fresh ginger

1. Marinate the pork: Combine the MCT oil, vinegar, sweetener, tamari, fish sauce, and pepper in a large bowl. Place the pork butt in the marinade and mix until the strips are well coated. Cover the bowl, place in the refrigerator, and marinate for 20 minutes or overnight.

2. Make the pancakes: Place the raw eggs, hard-boiled eggs, cream cheese, sweetener, and salt in a blender and puree until very smooth. Heat the coconut oil in a large skillet over medium-high heat until a drop of water sizzles in the skillet. Pour three 3-inch circles of batter into the skillet. Cook for 3 to 5 minutes per side, until golden brown. Remove from the heat. Repeat with the remaining batter to make a total of 8 pancakes, adding more oil to the skillet if needed.

3. Make the scrambled eggs: Heat the sesame oil in a small sauté pan over medium heat. Add the eggs and salt and scramble gently for 1 minute, or until cooked through. Remove from the heat and set aside.

4. Make the stir-fry: Heat the coconut oil in a large cast-iron skillet or wok over medium-high heat. Add the cabbage, mushrooms, scallions, garlic, ginger, and marinated pork (reserving the marinade). Stir-fry for 5 minutes, or until the pork is cooked through. Add the scrambled eggs and the reserved marinade and heat until the marinade simmers and is warmed through, another 2 minutes.

5. To serve, transfer the pork mixture to a serving bowl and garnish with scallions. Divide the pork mixture among the pancakes and roll up the pancakes to enclose the filling.

6. Store the pork mixture in the refrigerator for up to 3 days. To reheat the pork, place in a preheated 350°F oven for 5 about minutes. Store the pancakes in an airtight container in the refrigerator for up to 3 days or in the freezer for up to 1 month. To reheat the pancakes, place in a lightly greased skillet over medium heat for about 1 minute per side, or place in a preheated 350°F oven for about 2 minutes.

busy family tip: *To cut the total cooking time for the pancakes in half, use two large skillets or one large griddle pan to cook 6 pancakes at a time.*

NUTRITIONAL INFO (per serving)				
calories	fat	protein	carbs	fiber
655	56g	31g	7g	2g

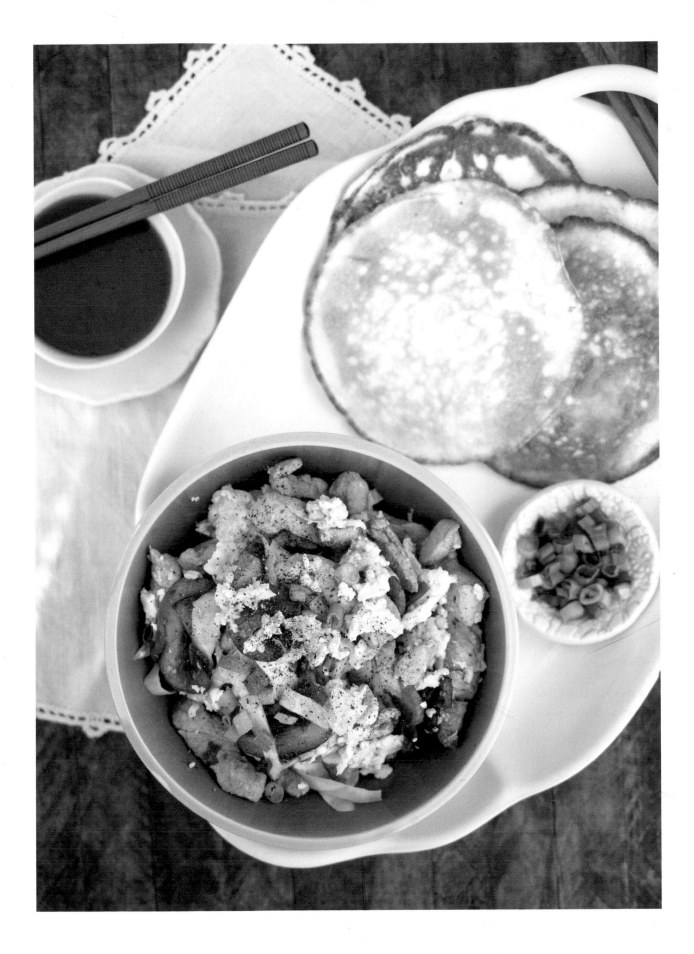

Crispy Almond Chicken (Soo Guy)

(L M H / KETO) prep time: 10 minutes (not including time to make sauce)   cook time: 8 minutes
yield: 2 servings

This chicken dish tastes fantastic with Zero-Carb Fried "Rice" (page 44), as pictured.

1 boneless, skinless chicken breast (about 10 ounces)

—wet coating

2 large eggs, separated, at room temperature

Fine sea salt and ground black pepper

—dry coating

½ cup powdered Parmesan cheese (see page 363)

Ground black pepper

2 tablespoons avocado oil or coconut oil, for frying

½ batch Sweet-and-Sour Sauce (page 43), for serving

Sliced almonds, for garnish

Black or white sesame seeds, for garnish

1. Slice the chicken into 1-inch-wide strips.

2. Crack the eggs into a shallow baking dish. Beat in 1 tablespoon of water and season with a pinch each of salt and pepper. Place the powdered Parmesan in another shallow baking dish, add a pinch of pepper, and mix until well combined.

3. Dip each chicken strip in the eggs and let any excess drip off, then dredge both sides of the chicken in the Parmesan mixture. Set the coated chicken strips aside.

4. Heat the oil in a large cast-iron skillet over medium-high heat. When the oil is hot, dip each coated chicken strip into the egg mixture once more to coat the whole strip. Fry the chicken on all sides until light golden brown, 3 to 4 minutes per side.

5. Serve the chicken immediately with the sweet-and-sour sauce. Garnish with sliced almonds and sesame seeds. Store the chicken in an airtight container in the refrigerator for up to 4 days. To reheat, place in a lightly greased skillet for about 5 minutes.

NUTRITIONAL INFO (per serving)				
calories	fat	protein	carbs	fiber
494	33g	52g	2g	1g

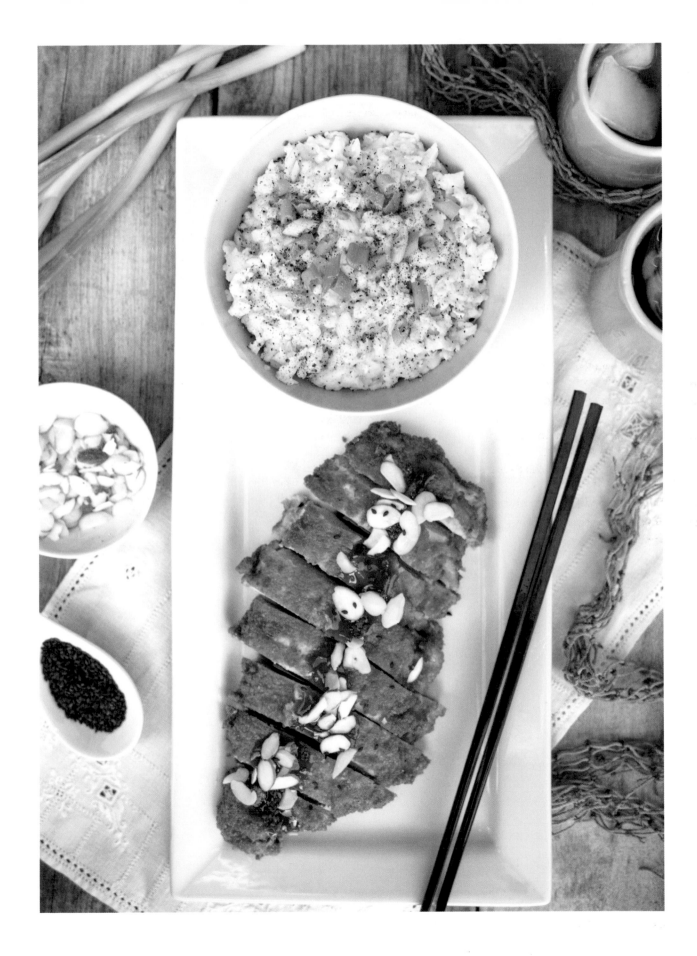

Chicken Chow Mein

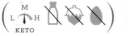 prep time: 8 minutes, plus time to marinate   cook time: 7 minutes
yield: 2 servings

The thing about these tasty "noodles" is that I marinate them, which gives them an amazing Chinese flair! Fish sauce isn't typical to Chinese cooking, but I love the way it tastes. Replace it with salt if you prefer.

½ pound boneless, skinless chicken thighs, cut into very thin slices

1 small Chinese (napa) cabbage, very thinly sliced

1 baby bok choy (½ pound), very thinly sliced

1 tablespoon wheat-free tamari, or ¼ cup coconut aminos

1 tablespoon unseasoned rice vinegar

1 tablespoon fish sauce, or 1 teaspoon fine sea salt

1 tablespoon toasted (dark) sesame oil

1 teaspoon grated fresh ginger

2 cloves garlic, minced

2 tablespoons Swerve confectioners'-style sweetener or equivalent amount of liquid or powdered sweetener (see page 31)

1 tablespoon coconut oil, for the pan

2 scallions, chopped

1. Place the chicken, cabbage, and bok choy in a large bowl. Combine the tamari, vinegar, fish sauce, sesame oil, ginger, garlic, and sweetener in a small bowl, then pour over the chicken mixture and toss until well coated. Cover and place in the refrigerator to marinate for 30 minutes or overnight.

2. Heat the coconut oil in a large cast-iron skillet or wok over medium-high heat. When the oil is hot, stir-fry the chicken mixture until the chicken is cooked through, about 4 minutes.

3. Transfer the chow mein to a platter, top with the scallions, and serve immediately. Store in an airtight container in the refrigerator for up to 4 days. To reheat, place in a lightly greased skillet over medium heat for about 5 minutes.

NUTRITIONAL INFO (per serving)				
calories	fat	protein	carbs	fiber
346	23g	28g	9g	3g

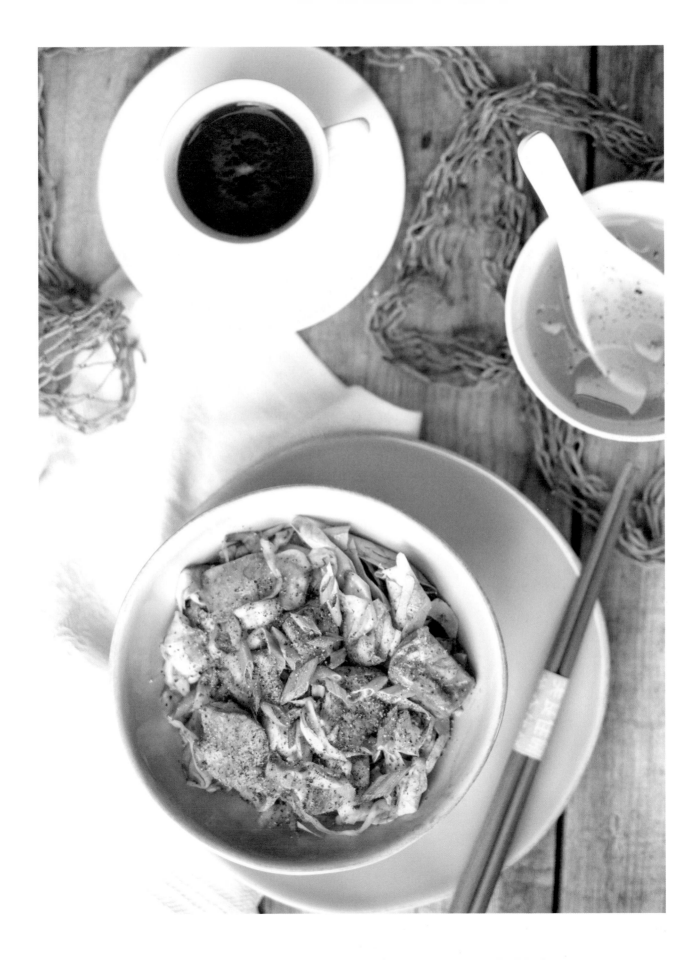

Chicken and Mushrooms

(L **M** H KETO) [icons] prep time: 8 minutes, plus time to marinate cook time: 15 minutes
yield: 4 servings

½ small head green cabbage (for "noodles"), or 2 (7-ounce) packages Miracle Noodles (see note)

4 teaspoons Swerve confectioners'-style sweetener or equivalent amount of liquid or powdered sweetener (see page 31), divided

3 tablespoons unseasoned rice vinegar, divided

2 tablespoons wheat-free tamari, or ½ cup coconut aminos, divided

1 pound boneless, skinless chicken thighs, cut into ½-inch pieces

2¼ cups chicken bone broth, homemade (page 356) or store-bought

1 tablespoon toasted (dark) sesame oil

½ teaspoon ground black pepper

½ teaspoon guar gum (optional, for thickening)

2 tablespoons coconut oil, divided

2 tablespoons grated fresh ginger

1 clove garlic, minced

8 ounces button mushrooms, stemmed and sliced

6 scallions, sliced diagonally into ½-inch pieces

½ red bell pepper, sliced

1. If using cabbage, thinly shred it and set aside.

2. In a medium-sized bowl, mix together 2 teaspoons of the sweetener, 1½ tablespoons of the vinegar, and 1 tablespoon of the tamari (or ¼ cup of the coconut aminos) until well combined. Add the chicken to the bowl and toss to coat thoroughly. Cover the bowl, place in the refrigerator, and marinate for 1 hour or overnight.

3. Make the sauce: In another medium-sized bowl, combine the broth, sesame oil, and pepper with the remaining 2 teaspoons of sweetener, remaining 1½ tablespoons of vinegar, and remaining tablespoon of tamari (or ¼ cup of coconut aminos). Sift in the guar gum, if using, and whisk until well combined. Set the sauce aside.

4. When you're ready to cook the chicken, heat 1 tablespoon of the coconut oil in a wok or large cast-iron skillet over high heat. Remove the chicken from the marinade; discard the marinade. Add the chicken to the wok and stir-fry for 4 minutes, or until the chicken is golden brown. Transfer the chicken and any juices to a plate.

5. Heat the remaining 1 tablespoon of coconut oil in the wok or skillet. If using cabbage, add it now, along with the ginger, garlic, mushrooms, scallions, and bell pepper and stir-fry for 5 to 10 minutes, depending on how soft you want the cabbage. Add the reserved sauce and then the chicken. Reduce the heat and simmer until the sauce begins to thicken a bit, about 2 minutes. If using Miracle Noodles, rinse and drain them, then add them to the wok; toss to coat well and heat through, about 1 minute.

6. Store in an airtight container in the refrigerator for up to 4 days. To reheat, place in a lightly greased skillet over medium heat for about 5 minutes, stirring occasionally.

note: *Miracle Noodles are composed of a dietary fiber called glucomannan and contain very few calories and close to zero carbohydrates. They do not have much flavor on their own, but they are great at absorbing flavors. You can shop for them in my Amazon store, under "pantry," on my site, MariaMindBodyHealth.com. Zoodles (page 360) are a good substitute.*

NUTRITIONAL INFO (per serving using cabbage pasta)				
calories	fat	protein	carbs	fiber
326	22g	26g	9g	3g

NUTRITIONAL INFO (per serving using Miracle Noodles)				
calories	fat	protein	carbs	fiber
315	22g	25g	7g	2g

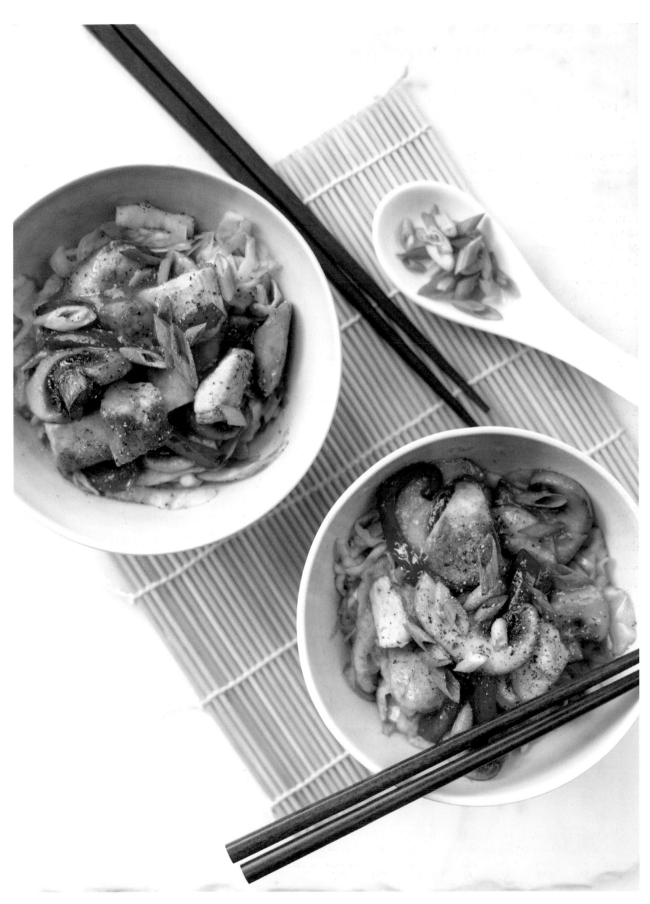

Beef and Broccoli Stir-Fry

(L M H KETO) prep time: 5 minutes   cook time: 10 minutes   yield: 3 servings

2 cups broccoli florets (about 1 pound)

¼ cup avocado oil or coconut oil

6 ounces sirloin steak, cut into thin strips

3 tablespoons beef bone broth, homemade (page 356) or store-bought (see note)

2¼ teaspoons wheat-free tamari, or 3 tablespoons coconut aminos

1 teaspoon fish sauce (optional, for umami taste)

½ teaspoon grated fresh ginger

1 clove garlic, minced

¼ teaspoon Swerve confectioners'-style sweetener or equivalent amount of liquid or powdered sweetener (see page 31)

⅛ teaspoon fine sea salt

1. Bring a medium-sized saucepan of water to a boil. Add the broccoli and boil for 3 minutes. Remove from the heat and rinse under cold running water to retain the bright green color. Set aside.

2. Heat the oil in a large cast-iron skillet over medium-high heat. Add the steak and sauté until cooked to your desired doneness, about 3 minutes for medium-rare.

3. Heat the broth, tamari, fish sauce (if using), ginger, garlic, sweetener, and salt in a small saucepan over medium heat for a few minutes, just until warm. Stir well to combine. Pour the sauce over the broccoli and beef and serve. Store in an airtight container in the refrigerator for up to 4 days. To reheat, place in a lightly greased skillet over medium heat for about 5 minutes, stirring occasionally.

note: *If using store-bought broth, add 1 egg yolk for a natural thickener. Whisk the yolk into the broth, then slowly whisk it into the hot sauce mixture; this is somewhat like how hollandaise is thickened.*

NUTRITIONAL INFO (per serving)				
calories	fat	protein	carbs	fiber
278	25g	11g	5g	2g

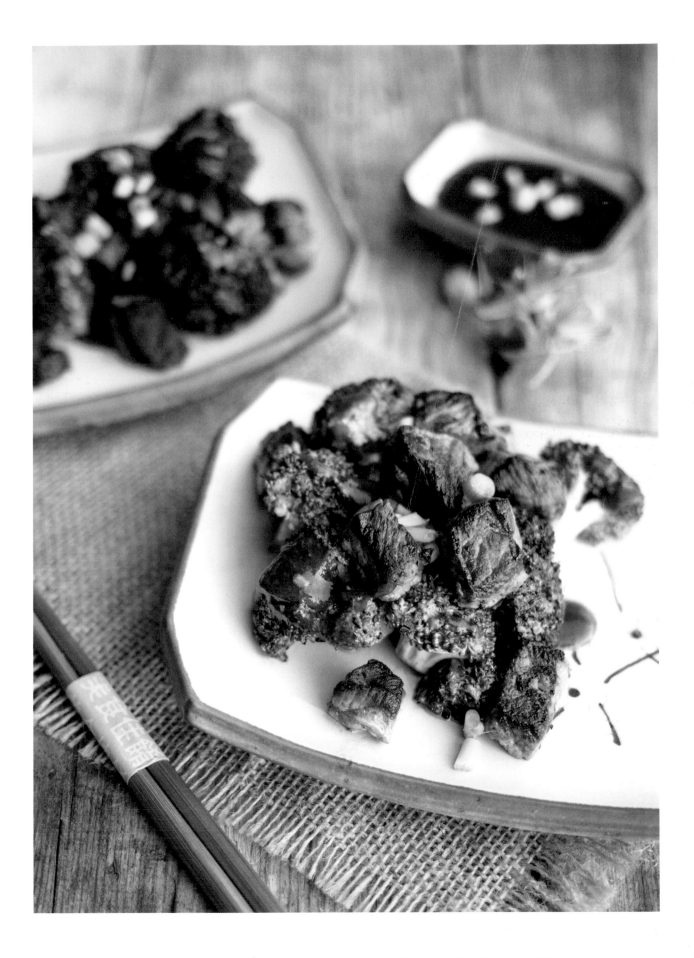

Teriyaki Salmon

(L M T H KETO) 🧴 🚫 🚫   prep time: 7 minutes, plus time to marinate   cook time: 15 minutes
yield: 2 servings

⅓ cup Swerve confectioners'-style sweetener or equivalent amount of liquid or powdered sweetener (see page 31)

¼ cup fresh lime juice (about 2 limes)

1½ tablespoons wheat-free tamari, or ¼ cup plus 2 tablespoons coconut aminos

1 tablespoon coconut vinegar or apple cider vinegar

1 tablespoon toasted (dark) sesame oil

1 teaspoon fish sauce (optional, for umami taste)

1 teaspoon stone-ground mustard

3 cloves garlic, smashed to a paste or minced

2 teaspoons grated fresh ginger

8 ounces salmon fillets, cut into 1¼-inch by 2-inch-wide strips

½ teaspoon guar gum (optional, for thickening)

Black or toasted sesame seeds, for garnish

Sliced scallions, for garnish

1. Place the sweetener, lime juice, tamari, vinegar, sesame oil, fish sauce (if using), mustard, garlic, and ginger in a medium-sized bowl and stir well to combine. Add the salmon strips and turn to coat in the marinade. Cover the bowl, place in the refrigerator, and marinate for 30 minutes or up to 2 hours.

2. Preheat the oven to 400°F. Line a rimmed baking sheet with parchment paper. Remove the salmon from the marinade and place it on the lined baking sheet; reserve the marinade. Bake for 13 to 15 minutes, until the salmon is flaky and no longer translucent in the center.

3. Meanwhile, make the sauce: Pour the marinade into a small saucepan over medium-high heat. Sift in the guar gum, if using, and whisk until well combined. Boil until thickened, about 5 minutes. Taste and adjust the seasoning to your liking; adding more sweetener or lime juice if desired. Remove the sauce from the heat and pour over the salmon.

4. Garnish with sesame seeds and scallions. Store in an airtight container in the refrigerator for up to 4 days. To reheat, place in a lightly greased skillet over medium heat for about 5 minutes, stirring occasionally.

NUTRITIONAL INFO (per serving)				
calories	fat	protein	carbs	fiber
219	11g	25g	6g	1g

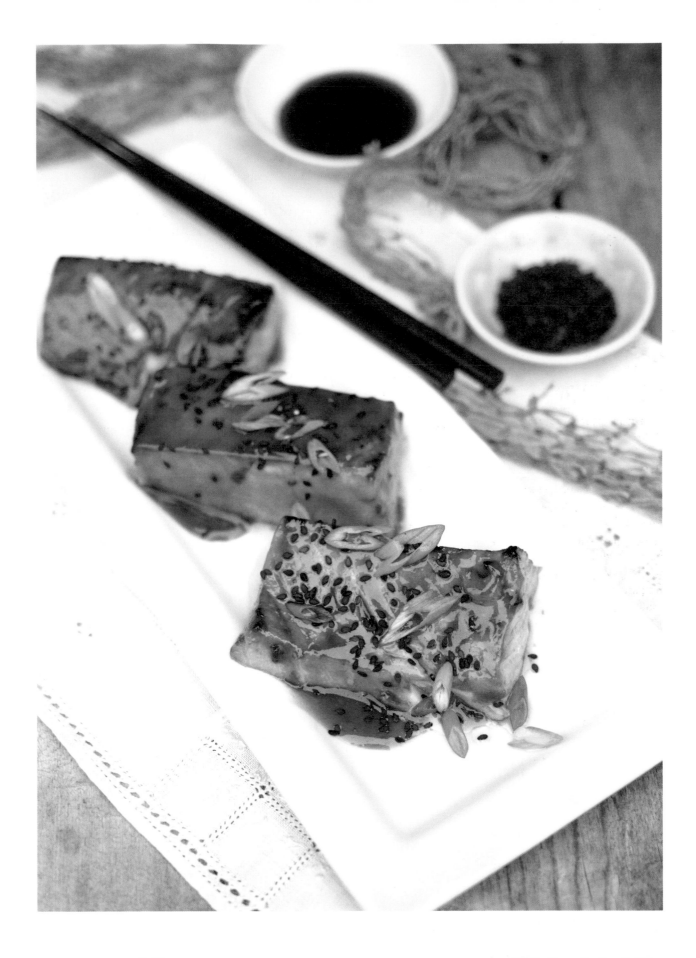

Bulgogi Wraps

L M H KETO · prep time: 7 minutes · cook time: 9 minutes · yield: 4 servings

16 large romaine or butter lettuce leaves

2 tablespoons coconut oil

8 ounces button mushrooms, quartered

1 cucumber, diced

3 scallions, thinly sliced

2 teaspoons grated fresh ginger

4 cloves garlic, minced

1 pound ground pork

2 tablespoons toasted (dark) sesame oil

2 tablespoons coconut vinegar

1½ teaspoons wheat-free tamari, or 2 tablespoons coconut aminos

½ teaspoon fine sea salt

1 cup thinly sliced purple or Chinese (napa) cabbage

2 tablespoons sliced scallions, for garnish

Crushed red pepper, for garnish

1. Clean the lettuce leaves and place on a platter.

2. Heat the coconut oil in a large cast-iron skillet over medium heat. When the oil is hot, add the mushrooms, cucumber, scallions, ginger, and garlic. Sauté until the mushrooms are soft, about 4 minutes. Add the ground pork, sesame oil, vinegar, tamari, and salt. Sauté, breaking up the pork with a spatula, until the pork is cooked through, about 5 minutes.

3. Remove from the heat and serve in romaine leaves. Top with the cabbage, scallions, and crushed red pepper. Store the filling and lettuce in separate airtight containers in the refrigerator for up to 4 days. To reheat the filling, place in a lightly greased skillet over medium heat for about 5 minutes, stirring occasionally.

tip: *I store ginger root in my freezer for easy flavor additions to meals such as this one.*

NUTRITIONAL INFO (per serving)				
calories	fat	protein	carbs	fiber
462	39g	23g	8g	2g

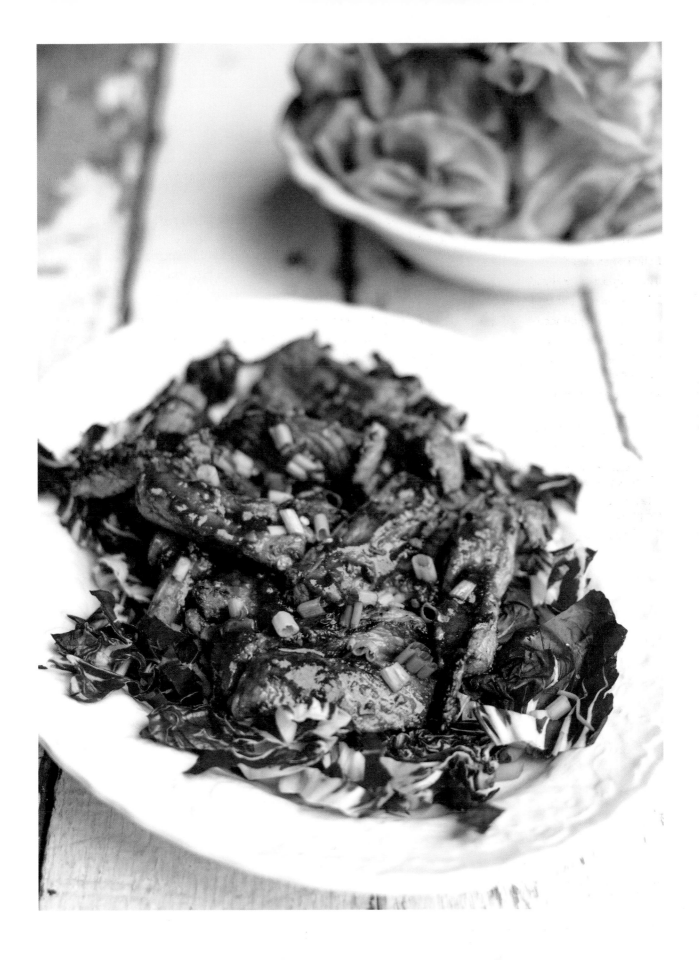

Sweet-and-Sour Chicken

(L $\overset{M}{\underset{KETO}{\curvearrowright}}$ H 🚫)   **prep time:** 10 minutes (not including time to make sauce or rice)   **cook time:** 15 minutes
yield: 4 servings

1 cup coconut oil or bacon fat, for frying

2 large eggs

1½ cups powdered Parmesan cheese (see page 363)

¼ teaspoon ground black pepper

1 pound boneless, skinless chicken thighs, cut into bite-sized nuggets

½ cup Sweet-and-Sour Sauce (page 43), warmed

1 batch Cauliflower Fried Rice (page 46) or Zero-Carb Fried "Rice" (page 44), or 2 (8-ounce) packages Miracle Rice (see note), for serving

Sliced scallions, for garnish (optional)

1. Heat the oil in a 4-inch-deep (or deeper) cast-iron skillet over medium heat to 350°F. The oil should be 1 inch deep; add more oil if needed.

2. Bread the chicken: Crack the eggs into a shallow baking dish and beat lightly with a fork. In another shallow baking dish, combine the powdered Parmesan and pepper. Dip a chicken nugget into the eggs, then into the cheese mixture. Coat each nugget well.

3. When the oil is hot, fry the nuggets in batches for about 5 minutes, until golden brown and cooked through.

4. Baste the fried chicken nuggets with the sauce. Serve over rice and garnish with scallions, if desired. Store in an airtight container in the refrigerator for up to 4 days. To reheat, place in a lightly greased skillet for about 5 minutes, stirring occasionally.

variation: oven-baked sweet-and-sour chicken. *Preheat the oven to 350°F and grease a rimmed baking sheet. Complete Step 2, then place the chicken on the baking sheet and bake for 20 to 30 minutes, until golden brown. Complete Step 4 and serve.*

note: *Miracle Rice is made from the root of an Asian plant called konjac. It is a tasty keto substitute for traditional rice that is very low in carbohydrates. You can shop for it in my Amazon store, under "pantry," on my site, MariaMindBodyHealth.com.*

NUTRITIONAL INFO (per serving)				
calories	fat	protein	carbs	fiber
521	36g	45g	8g	4g

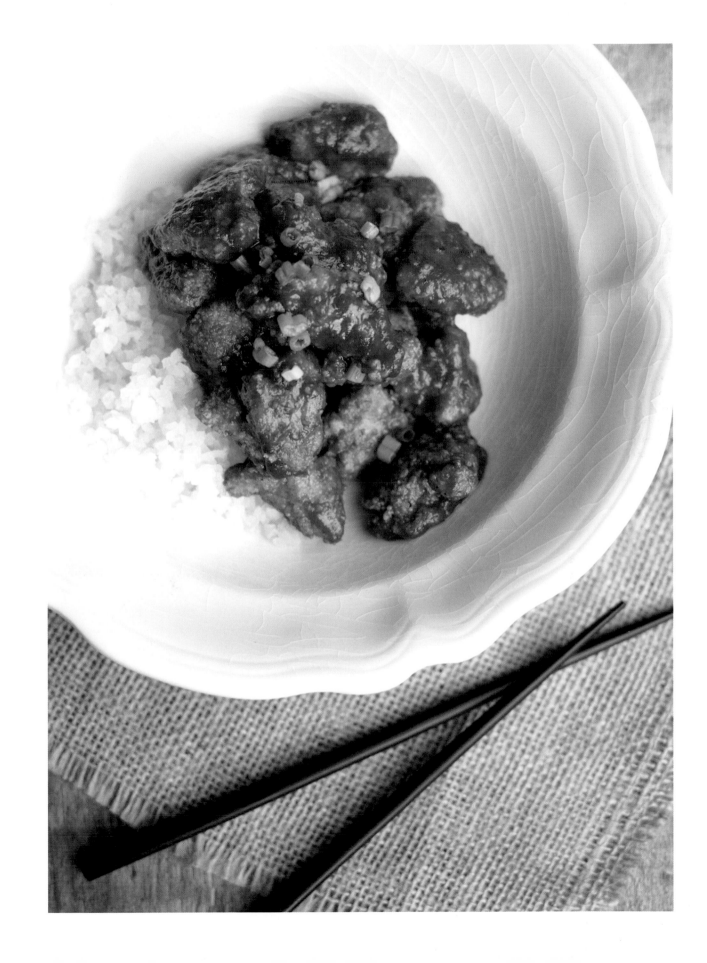

Chop Suey

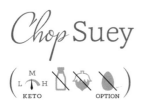

prep time: 8 minutes, plus time to marinate pork (not including time to make rice)
cook time: 5 minutes   yield: 4 servings

Chop suey literally means "assorted pieces." I don't know what "assorted pieces" went into my elementary school's version of chop suey, but I remember despising chop suey day! There was a rule at my school that you had to eat most of what was on your tray. Chop suey day was the only day I drank all of my milk so that I could hide the gross meal in my milk carton. But that version of chop suey was nothing like this one. The "assorted pieces" are vibrant and fresh compared to the pathetic-looking celery that dominated my school's version.

1 tablespoon plus 1 teaspoon fish sauce, divided

1½ teaspoons wheat-free tamari, or 2 tablespoons coconut aminos

4 cloves garlic, minced

1 teaspoon grated fresh ginger

1 teaspoon fine sea salt

1 pound pork tenderloin or pork belly, cut crosswise into ⅛-inch-thick strips

2 tablespoons avocado oil, divided, for frying

8 ounces bok choy, stems and leaves separated, then cut into ¼-inch-thick slices

4 ounces button or cremini mushrooms, thinly sliced

1 small onion, thinly sliced

1 green bell pepper, cut into ¼-inch-thick strips, then halved crosswise

2 stalks celery, cut on the diagonal into ¼-inch-wide pieces

½ cup thinly sliced cucumber

1 (5-ounce) can sliced bamboo shoots, drained

¼ cup chicken bone broth, homemade (page 356) or store-bought

3 tablespoons Swerve confectioners'-style sweetener or equivalent amount of liquid or powdered sweetener (see page 31)

¼ teaspoon guar gum (optional, for thickening)

Ground black pepper

Scallions, sliced on the diagonal, for garnish

Zero-Carb Fried "Rice" (page 44) or Cauliflower Fried Rice (page 46), for serving (omit for egg-free)

1. Combine 1 tablespoon of the fish sauce, the tamari, garlic, ginger, and salt in a medium-sized bowl. Add the pork and coat with the marinade. Allow to marinate in the refrigerator for 10 to 20 minutes or overnight.

2. Heat 1 tablespoon of the oil in a large cast-iron skillet or wok over high heat. Stir-fry the bok choy stems for 1 minute, then add the bok choy leaves, mushrooms, onion, bell pepper, celery, cucumber, and bamboo shoots. Season well with salt and stir-fry for 2 minutes more. Remove from the skillet and set aside.

3. In a medium-sized bowl, whisk together the broth, the remaining 1 teaspoon of fish sauce, and sweetener. Sift in the guar gum, if using, and whisk until well combined.

4. Heat the remaining 1 tablespoon of oil in the skillet. Remove the pork from the marinade; discard the marinade. Add the pork to the skillet and stir-fry for 2 minutes, or until it is cooked through. Add the reserved veggies and whisk in the broth mixture. Bring to a boil, then remove from the heat. Garnish with scallions. Serve over fried rice. Store in an airtight container in the refrigerator for up to 4 days. To reheat, place in a lightly greased skillet over medium heat for 5 minutes, stirring occasionally.

NUTRITIONAL INFO (per serving)				
calories	fat	protein	carbs	fiber
439	36g	22g	10g	4g

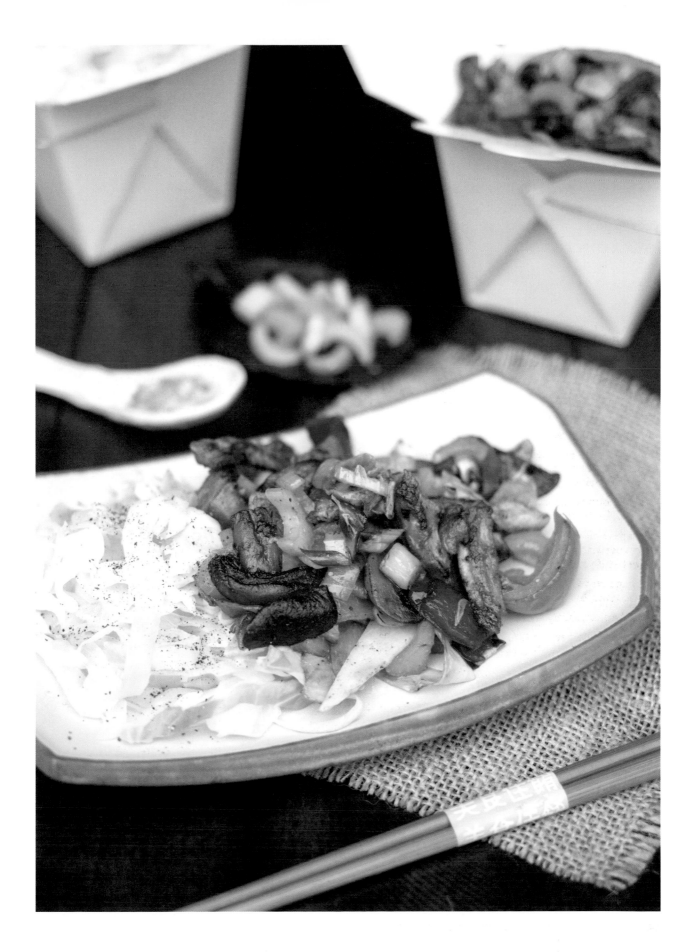

Singapore Noodles

(L ᴹ H KETO) prep time: 7 minutes   cook time: 19 minutes   yield: 4 servings

This is a twist on a classic dish you will see in most Chinese restaurants. Despite its name, it likely didn't originate in Singapore. Instead of traditional rice noodles, I use thinly shredded cabbage. Cabbage noodles don't get soggy like zucchini noodles often do, and the cabbage absorbs all the yummy curry flavor.

8 ounces medium shrimp, peeled and deveined

1 boneless, skinless chicken thigh, cut into ¼-inch strips

1 tablespoon wheat-free tamari, or ¼ cup coconut aminos

¼ teaspoon ground black pepper

1 tablespoon plus 1 teaspoon coconut oil or avocado oil, divided

2 cups thinly shredded green cabbage

2 teaspoons curry powder

¼ teaspoon fine sea salt

2 large eggs, lightly beaten

2 tablespoons thinly sliced scallions

2 cloves garlic, minced

1½ teaspoons grated fresh ginger

½ red bell pepper, thinly sliced

¼ small onion, thinly sliced

1. Place the shrimp and chicken in a medium-sized bowl. Add the tamari and black pepper and allow to marinate while you cook the cabbage pasta.

2. Heat 1 tablespoon of the oil in a large cast-iron skillet or wok over medium-low heat. Add the cabbage, curry powder, and salt. Cover and cook for 10 to 15 minutes, until the cabbage is very tender. Add the eggs and cook, stirring to break up the eggs with a spatula, for an additional 2 minutes, or until the eggs are set.

3. Remove the cabbage from the skillet and set aside. Heat the remaining 1 teaspoon of oil in the skillet over medium-high heat. Add the scallions, garlic, and ginger and stir-fry for 2 minutes. Add the shrimp and chicken and stir-fry for 1 minute, or until the shrimp is starting to turn pink and the chicken is starting to brown. Add the bell pepper and onion and stir-fry for another 2 minutes, or until the shrimp and chicken are cooked through. Stir in the cabbage until well combined. Serve immediately.

4. Store in an airtight container in the refrigerator for up to 3 days or in the freezer for up to 1 month. To reheat, place in a lightly greased skillet over medium heat for about 4 minutes, stirring occasionally.

NUTRITIONAL INFO (per serving)				
calories	fat	protein	carbs	fiber
203	9g	24g	6g	2g

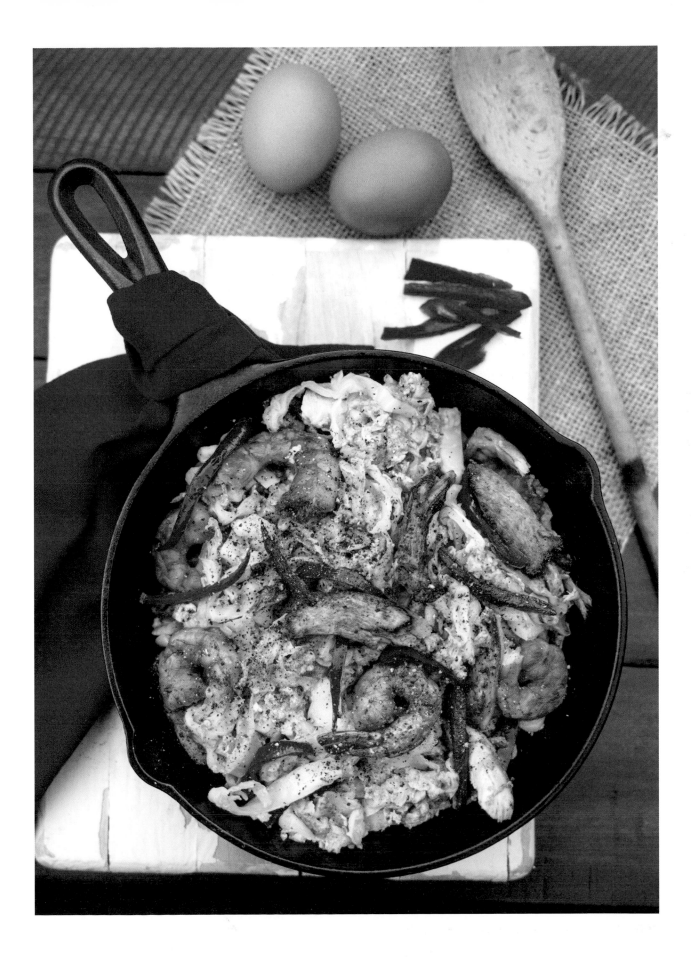

Szechuan Beef

(L M H KETO ⬦ ⬦ ⬦) prep time: 8 minutes, plus time to marinate beef   cook time: 8 minutes
yield: 2 servings

8 ounces boneless sirloin steak, sliced against the grain into ¼-inch-thick strips

—marinade

2 tablespoons beef bone broth, homemade (page 356) or store-bought

1½ teaspoons wheat-free tamari, or 2 tablespoons coconut aminos

2 cloves garlic, minced

—sauce

2 tablespoons beef bone broth

2 teaspoons Swerve confectioners'-style sweetener or equivalent amount of liquid or powdered sweetener (see page 31)

1½ teaspoons chili garlic sauce

1 teaspoon wheat-free tamari, or 1 tablespoon plus 1 teaspoon coconut aminos

½ teaspoon chili oil

⅛ teaspoon guar gum (optional, for thickening)

—stir-fry

2 tablespoons coconut oil, for frying

2 cloves garlic, minced

½ medium onion, thinly sliced

½ red bell pepper, thinly sliced

2 scallions, sliced on the diagonal, for garnish

1 teaspoon crushed red pepper, for garnish

1. Slice the beef against the grain into ¼-inch-thick strips.

2. Combine the ingredients for the marinade in a large bowl and stir well. Place the beef in the marinade and toss to coat. Cover and place in the refrigerator to marinate for at least 15 minutes or overnight.

3. Meanwhile, make the sauce: Place the broth, sweetener, chili garlic sauce, tamari, and chili oil in a large bowl. Sift in the guar gum, if using, and whisk until well combined. Set aside.

4. Heat 1 tablespoon of the coconut oil in a large cast-iron skillet or wok over medium-high heat. Remove the beef from the marinade; discard the marinade. Add the beef and stir-fry until browned on the edges, about 3 minutes. Remove from the skillet and set aside.

5. Heat the remaining 1 tablespoon of coconut oil in the skillet over medium-high heat. Add the garlic and stir-fry for 1 minute, or until fragrant. Add the onion and bell pepper and stir-fry until softened, about 3 minutes. Return the beef to the skillet and add the sauce. Stir well and allow to simmer until the sauce thickens. Place on a platter and garnish with scallions and crushed red pepper.

6. Store in an airtight container in the refrigerator for up to 4 days. To reheat, place in a lightly greased skillet over medium heat for about 5 minutes, stirring occasionally.

busy family tip: *To save time, make the sauce ahead. It will keep, stored in an airtight container in the refrigerator, for up to 3 days.*

NUTRITIONAL INFO (per serving)				
calories	fat	protein	carbs	fiber
443	28g	37g	11g	2g

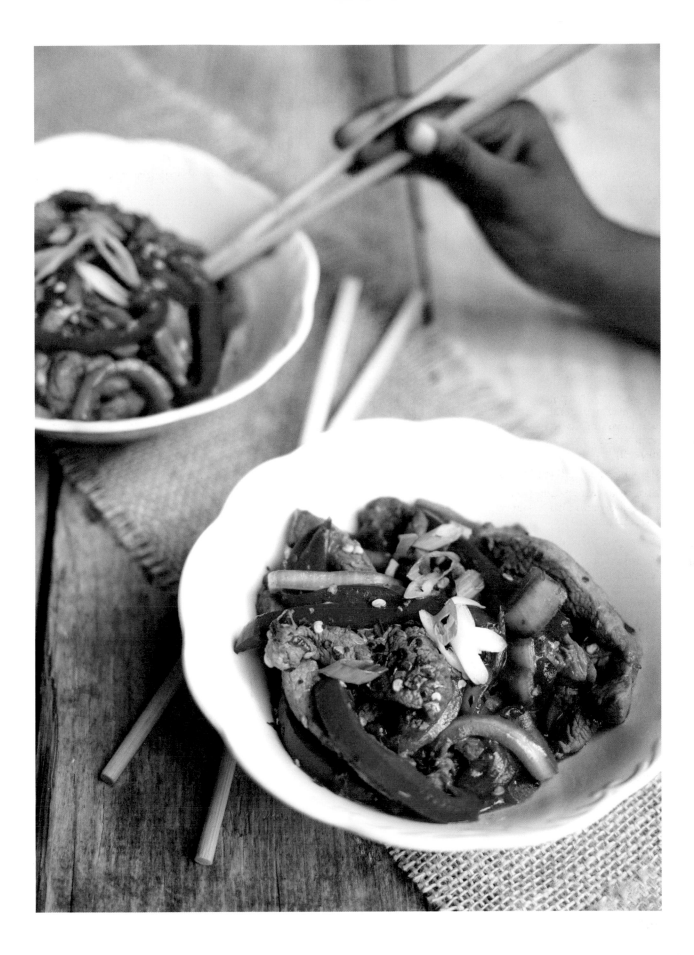

Bourbon Chicken

(L →M H KETO ⬜ 🚫 ⬤ OPTION)   prep time: 5 minutes (not including time to make fried rice)
cook time: 15 minutes   yield: 4 servings

When I first heard of bourbon chicken, I assumed it was made with bourbon, but the name has nothing to do with alcohol. It comes from the Chinese cook who created it while working in a restaurant on Bourbon Street in New Orleans!

2 tablespoons coconut oil

2 pounds boneless, skinless chicken thighs, cut into bite-sized pieces

½ teaspoon fine sea salt

½ cup chicken bone broth, homemade (page 356) or store-bought

⅓ cup Swerve confectioners'-style sweetener or equivalent amount of liquid or powdered sweetener (see page 31)

¼ cup tomato sauce

1 tablespoon plus 1 teaspoon wheat-free tamari, or ⅓ cup coconut aminos

1 tablespoon coconut vinegar or apple cider vinegar

¾ teaspoon crushed red pepper

1 clove garlic, smashed to a paste

¼ teaspoon grated fresh ginger

Scallions, sliced on the diagonal, for garnish

Sesame seeds, for garnish

1 batch Zero-Carb Fried "Rice" (page 44) or Cauliflower Fried Rice (page 46), for serving (optional; omit for egg-free)

1. Heat the oil in a wok or large cast-iron skillet over medium-high heat. Pat the chicken dry with a paper towel. Season well on all sides with the salt.

2. Place the chicken in the wok and stir-fry on all sides until light golden brown, about 4 minutes. Remove from the wok and set aside. Add the broth, sweetener, tomato sauce, tamari, vinegar, crushed red pepper, garlic, and ginger to the wok and whisk to combine. Simmer until reduced and thickened, about 10 minutes.

3. Return the chicken to the wok and simmer for 5 to 10 minutes, until the sauce has thickened and the chicken is warmed through. Garnish with scallions and sesame seeds and serve over fried rice, if desired.

4. Store in an airtight container in the refrigerator for up to 4 days. To reheat, place in a lightly greased skillet over medium heat for about 5 minutes, stirring occasionally.

NUTRITIONAL INFO (per serving)				
calories	fat	protein	carbs	fiber
495	32g	44g	8g	3g

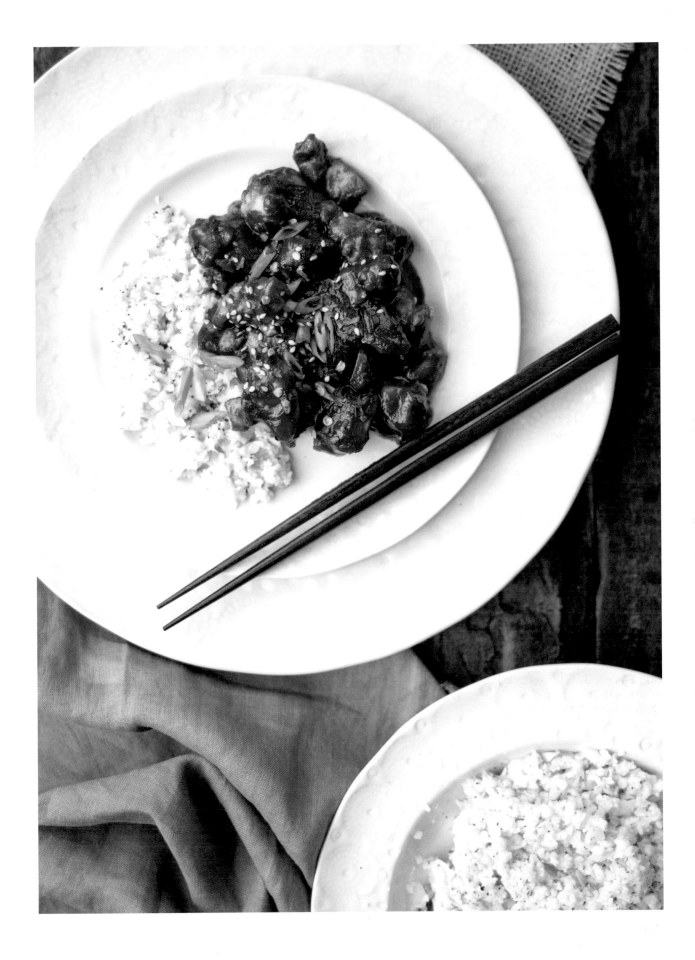

Char Siu

$\left(\begin{smallmatrix} & M & \\ L & \circlearrowright & H \\ & KETO & \end{smallmatrix} \quad \diagdown \quad \diagdown \quad \diagdown \right)$ prep time: 15 minutes, plus time to marinate   cook time: 20 minutes
yield: 4 servings

1 pound pork cheeks, or 1 (12-ounce) package fully cooked pork belly (see note)

½ cup tomato sauce

½ cup Swerve confectioners'-style sweetener or equivalent amount of liquid or powdered sweetener (see page 31)

¼ cup coconut vinegar or unseasoned rice vinegar

2 tablespoons wheat-free tamari, or ½ cup coconut aminos

2 cloves garlic, minced

1 teaspoon Chinese five-spice powder

1 teaspoon natural red food coloring (optional, for a traditional look)

Scallions, sliced on the diagonal, for garnish

1. Cut the pork cheeks with the grain into ½-inch-wide by 2-inch-long strips; place in an 8-inch square baking dish.

2. Combine the tomato sauce, sweetener, vinegar, tamari, garlic, five-spice powder, and food coloring, if using, in a small saucepan over medium-high heat. Cook, stirring, until bubbly and thick, about 3 minutes. Allow to cool slightly, then pour three-quarters of it over the pork and stir well to coat. Cover the dish, place in the refrigerator, and marinate for 2 hours or overnight. Store the rest of the sauce in a small sealed container in the refrigerator until ready to serve.

3. Preheat a grill to medium-high heat. Remove the pork from the marinade and discard the marinade.

4. Grill the pork cheeks for 10 minutes on each side, or until cooked through (an instant-read thermometer inserted in the center should read at least 145°F). If using pork belly, grill on each side for 2 minutes or until charred and heated through. Remove from the grill. Brush with the reserved sauce and garnish with scallions.

5. Store in an airtight container in the refrigerator for up to 4 days. To reheat, place in a lightly greased skillet over medium heat for about 5 minutes, stirring occasionally.

note: *Vacuum-sealed packages of fully cooked pork belly are available at Trader Joe's.*

NUTRITIONAL INFO (per serving)				
calories	fat	protein	carbs	fiber
323	20g	32g	3g	0.4g

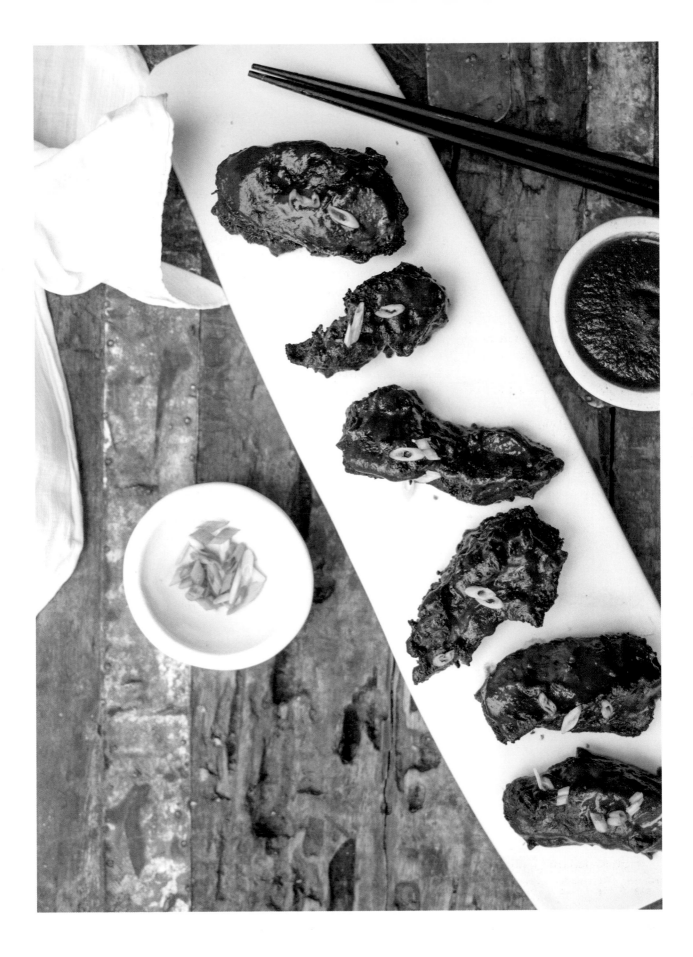

Moo Go Gai Pan

(L ⟶ H M KETO 🧂 🚫 🚫) **prep time:** 5 minutes **cook time:** 12 minutes **yield:** 2 servings

2 tablespoons coconut oil

2 cups sliced mushrooms (about 8 ounces)

2 cups sliced bok choy (about ¼ pound)

1 clove garlic, smashed to a paste or minced

1 teaspoon grated fresh ginger

½ pound boneless, skinless chicken thighs, sliced into ½-inch pieces

1 teaspoon fine sea salt

½ teaspoon ground black pepper

¼ cup plus 2 tablespoons chicken bone broth, homemade (page 356) or store-bought

1 teaspoon Swerve confectioners'-style sweetener or equivalent amount of liquid or powdered sweetener (see page 31)

1. Heat the oil in a large cast-iron skillet or wok over high heat. Add the mushrooms and stir-fry until golden brown, about 4 minutes. Add the bok choy and stir-fry for another 2 minutes, until softened. Transfer the mushrooms and bok choy to a plate and set aside.

2. Add the garlic and ginger to the skillet and stir-fry for 1 minute, until fragrant. Season the chicken on all sides with the salt and pepper, then add to the skillet. Stir-fry for 5 minutes, or until the chicken is golden brown and cooked through.

3. Add the broth and sweetener to the pan and bring to a boil, about 4 minutes. Remove from the heat and add the reserved mushrooms and bok choy. Stir to coat the vegetables with the sauce. Store in an airtight container in the refrigerator for up to 4 days. To reheat, place in a lightly greased skillet over medium heat for about 5 minutes, stirring occasionally.

NUTRITIONAL INFO (per serving)				
calories	fat	protein	carbs	fiber
469	32g	44g	6g	2g

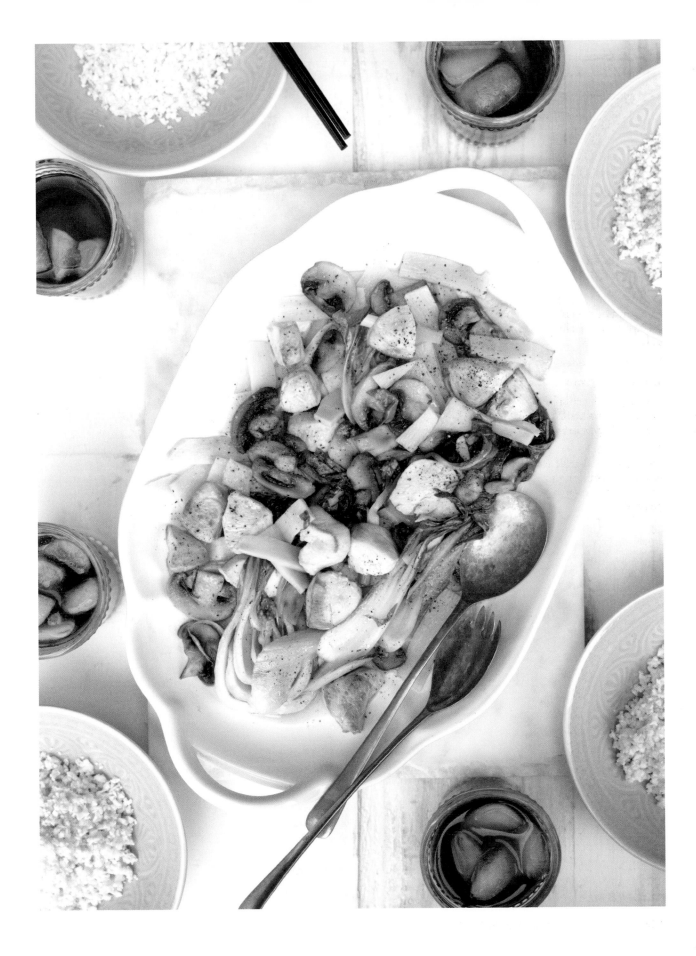

Kung Pow Shrimp

(L→H M KETO / OPTION) prep time: 4 minutes cook time: 9 minutes yield: 2 servings

¼ cup beef or chicken bone broth, homemade (page 356) or store-bought

1 tablespoon wheat-free tamari, or ¼ cup coconut aminos

1 teaspoon unseasoned rice vinegar or coconut vinegar

¼ teaspoon toasted (dark) sesame oil

¼ teaspoon grated fresh ginger

¼ teaspoon hot sauce, or more to desired heat

¼ teaspoon guar gum (optional, for thickening)

1 tablespoon coconut oil

¼ cup diced red bell peppers

¼ cup diced green bell peppers

12 ounces medium shrimp, peeled and deveined

2 cloves garlic, minced

Chopped pili nuts or sliced almonds, for garnish (omit for nut-free)

Chopped fresh chives or scallions

1. Make the sauce: Place the broth, tamari, vinegar, sesame oil, ginger, and hot sauce in a small bowl. Sift in the guar gum, if using, and whisk until well combined. Set aside.

2. Heat the oil in a wok or large cast-iron skillet over medium-high heat. Add the bell peppers and stir-fry for 2 minutes, or until tender. Add the shrimp and stir-fry until it is pink, about 3 minutes. Stir in the garlic and cook for 1 minute more. Reduce the heat to low, add the sauce, and simmer until the sauce thickens, about 4 minutes. Remove from the heat and place on a platter.

3. Garnish with chopped pili nuts, if using, and chives. Store in an airtight container in the refrigerator for up to 4 days. To reheat, place in a lightly greased skillet over medium heat for about 5 minutes, stirring occasionally.

NUTRITIONAL INFO (per serving)				
calories	fat	protein	carbs	fiber
282	10g	44g	4g	1g

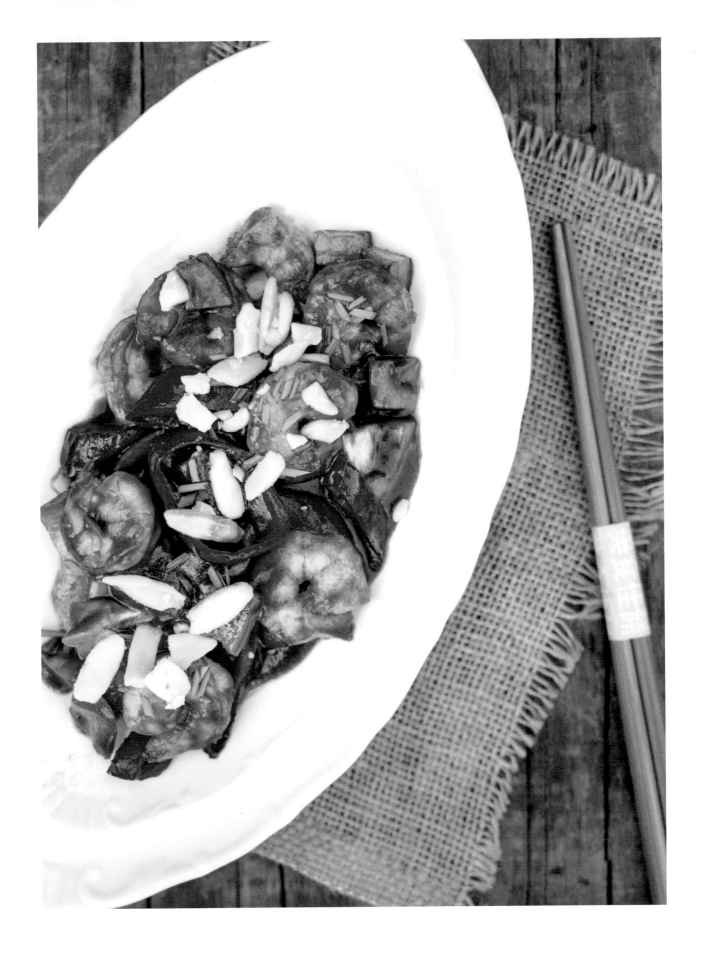

Chinese Lemon Chicken

(L → M → H / KETO)   prep time: 20 minutes   cook time: 10 minutes   yield: 4 servings

¾ cup chicken bone broth, homemade (page 356) or store-bought

¾ cup fresh lemon juice

2 tablespoons Swerve confectioners'-style sweetener or equivalent amount of liquid or powdered sweetener (see page 31)

1 tablespoon wheat-free tamari, or ¼ cup coconut aminos

¼ teaspoon fine sea salt

1 cup coconut oil or bacon fat, for frying

2 large eggs

1½ cups powdered Parmesan cheese (see page 363)

¼ teaspoon ground black pepper

1 pound boneless, skinless chicken thighs, cut into ¾-inch pieces

Black sesame seeds or toasted white sesame seeds, for garnish

Scallions, sliced on the diagonal, for garnish

1. Make the sauce: Bring the broth, lemon juice, sweetener, and tamari to a boil in a small saucepan over medium-high heat. Boil for 5 minutes, then add the salt and remove from the heat.

2. Make the chicken: Heat the oil in a 4-inch-deep (or deeper) cast-iron skillet over medium heat to 350°F. The oil should be 1 inch deep; add more oil if needed.

3. Crack the eggs into a shallow dish and beat lightly with a fork. In another shallow dish, combine the powdered Parmesan and pepper. Dip the chicken pieces into the eggs, then into the cheese mixture, coating the chicken well.

4. When the oil is hot, fry the chicken in batches for about 5 minutes, until golden brown and cooked through. Place the fried chicken in a serving dish and baste with the sauce. Garnish with sesame seeds and sliced scallions.

5. Store in an airtight container in the refrigerator for up to 4 days. To reheat, place in a lightly greased skillet over medium heat for about 5 minutes, stirring occasionally.

NUTRITIONAL INFO (per serving)				
calories	fat	protein	carbs	fiber
432	29g	43g	5g	0.4g

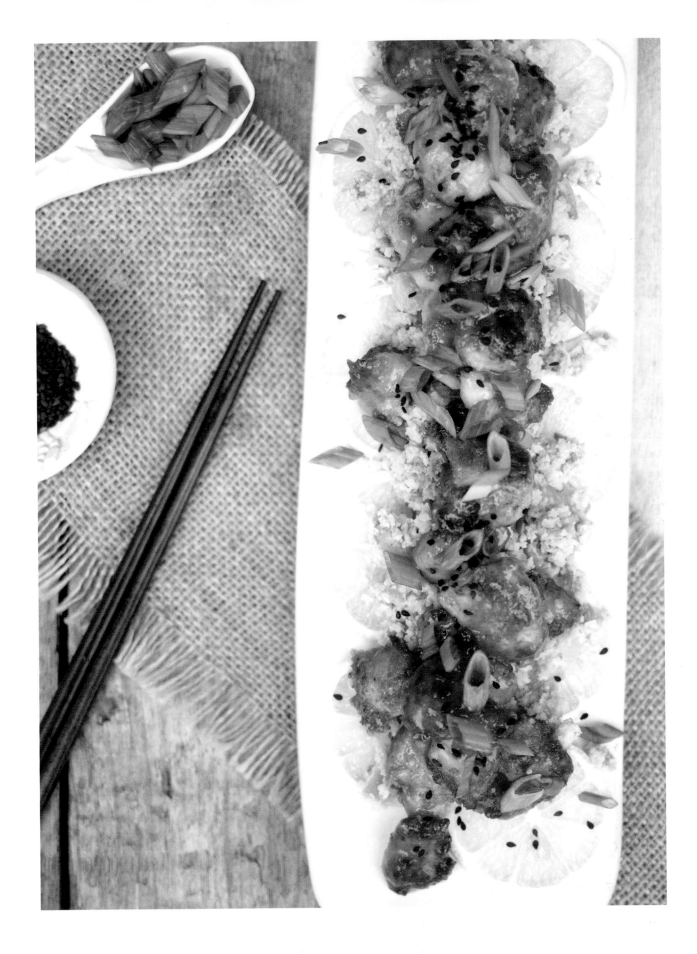

Sushi Rolls

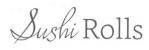 prep time: 20 minutes yield: 4 servings (four or five 1-inch pieces per serving)

Whenever I make sushi, I think of Anthony Bourdain. In his books, he often says he adores sushi, but he also gives tips on when not to order sushi. He jokingly says that he would never order sushi on a Tuesday because the fish is often five days old by then.

4 cups cooked riced cauliflower (see page 363)

1 ounce cream cheese (Kite Hill brand cream cheese style spread or coconut oil if dairy-free), at room temperature

1 avocado

1 cucumber

4 sheets nori

Black or white sesame seeds, for garnish

Wasabi paste, for serving

Pickled ginger, for serving

Wheat-free tamari or coconut aminos, for serving

—variation 1: california rolls

4 ounces canned crabmeat

—variation 2: smoked salmon rolls

4 ounces smoked salmon

4 ounces cream cheese (Kite Hill brand cream cheese style spread if dairy-free)

—variation 3: rainbow rolls

4 ounces sushi-grade fish (salmon, tuna, etc.)

1 tablespoon mayonnaise, homemade (page 357) or store-bought

1 teaspoon Sriracha sauce

1. In a large bowl, combine the cauliflower rice with the cream cheese.

2. Cut the avocado and cucumber into long strips, about ¼ inch thick or less.

3. To assemble the rolls, place a nori sheet on a cutting board or bamboo mat to help with the forming and rolling. Place 1 cup of the rice mixture on the nori. If making the California Roll or Smoked Salmon Roll, which are "normal" rolls (rice on the inside), leave a 1-inch border at the top of the nori sheet that is free of rice. If making the Rainbow Roll, which is an "inside-out roll" (rice on the outside), use your fingers to spread the rice mixture into a thin, even layer that covers the entire surface of the nori. Carefully flip it over so that the rice side is down. Repeat with the remaining nori sheets and rice mixture.

4. Follow the instructions on the opposite page to make one of the three sushi roll variations.

5. Using a very sharp knife, cut each roll into 1-inch pieces. Divide the pieces among 4 plates and sprinkle with sesame seeds. Serve with wasabi, pickled ginger, and tamari. If serving the Rainbow Roll, dollop some of the spicy mayo over the pieces.

6. Store the sushi in an airtight container in the refrigerator for up to 2 days.

California Roll

About ½ inch from the edge of the nori sheet closest to you, place a row of avocado, a row of cucumber, and a row of crabmeat. Carefully but tightly roll the sushi up to the 1-inch border at the top of the nori that has no rice on it. Wet this part of the nori with water and seal the roll shut. You can use the bamboo mat to help shape the roll.

NUTRITIONAL INFO (per serving)				
calories	fat	protein	carbs	fiber
166	10g	10g	12g	7g

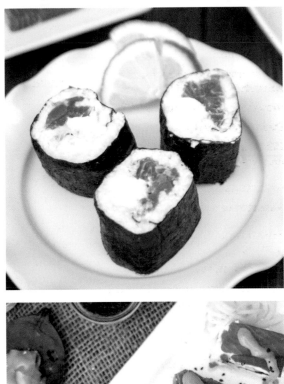

Smoked Salmon Roll

About ½ inch from the edge of the nori sheet closest to you, place a row of cucumber and a row of smoked salmon. Cut the cream cheese into 1-inch-long by ¼-inch-wide pieces and place a row along the salmon. Carefully but tightly roll the sushi up to the 1-inch border at the top of the nori that has no rice on it. Wet this part of the nori with water and seal the roll shut. You can use the bamboo mat to help shape the roll.

NUTRITIONAL INFO (per serving)				
calories	fat	protein	carbs	fiber
276	20g	12g	13g	7g

Rainbow Roll

About ½ inch from the edge of the nori sheet closest to you, place a row of cucumber, a row of fish, and a row of avocado. Carefully roll the sushi with the bamboo mat to make an even-shaped roll. (Alternatively, place 1-inch slices of fish and avocado on the outside of the roll and press them in place with the bamboo mat.) To make the spicy mayo, stir the mayo and hot sauce together until blended.

NUTRITIONAL INFO (per serving)				
calories	fat	protein	carbs	fiber
198	13g	11g	12g	7g

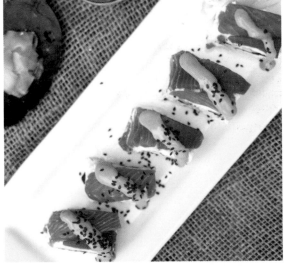

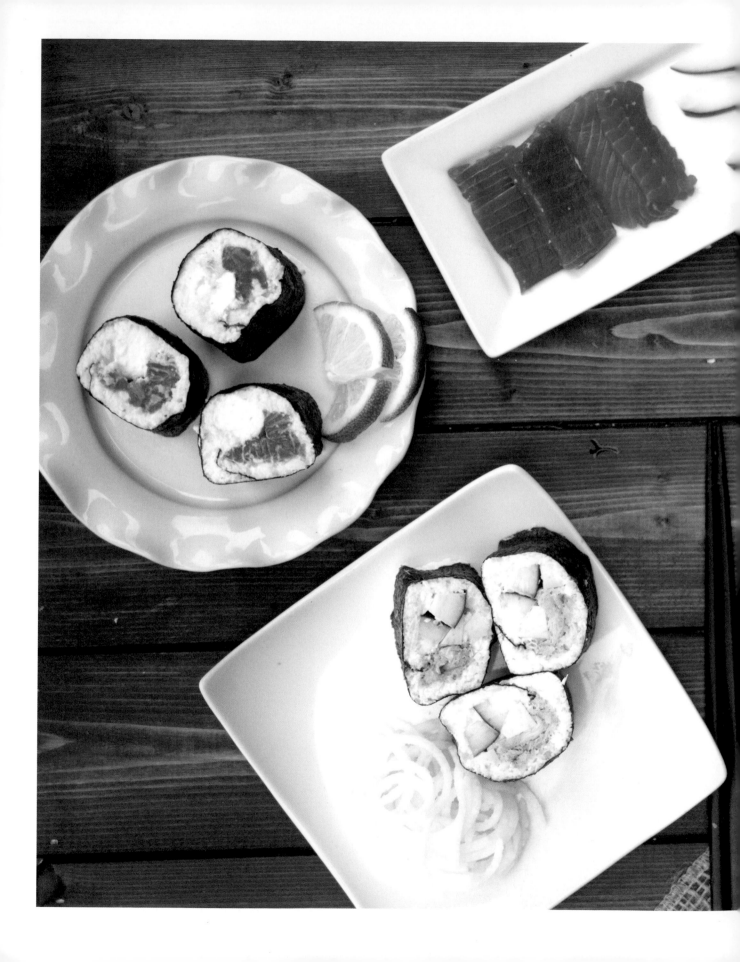

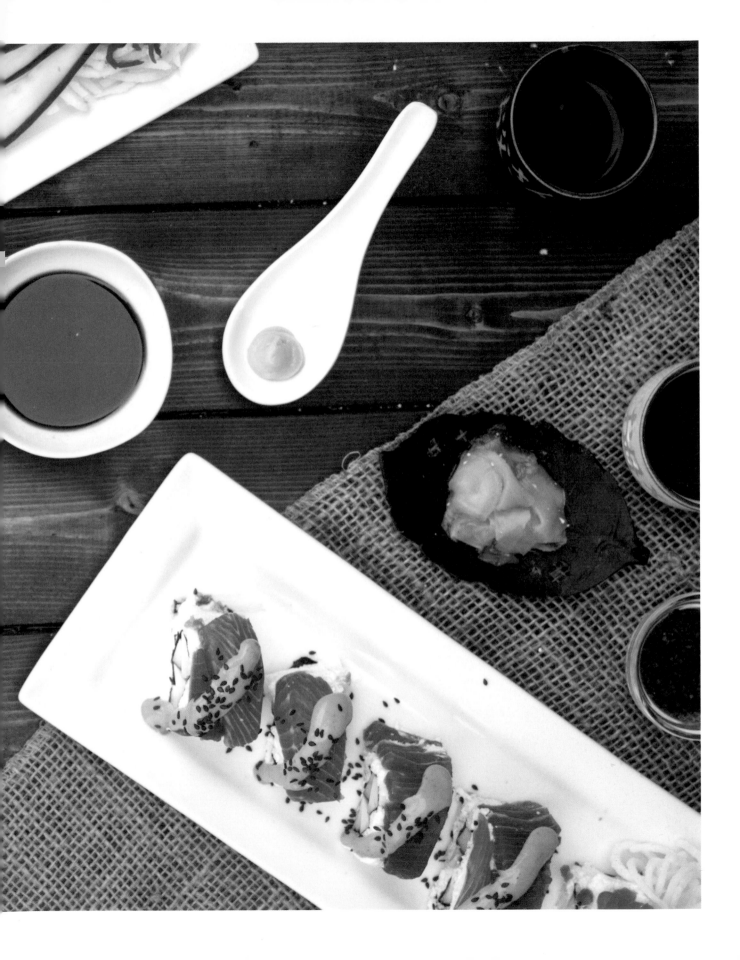

Deconstructed Pot Sticker Bowl

(L →H M KETO ⬜ ⬛) prep time: 6 minutes cook time: 17 minutes yield: 6 servings

4 cups finely shredded cabbage (about 1 pound)

½ cup sliced scallions (about 1 bunch), plus extra for garnish

¼ cup chicken bone broth, homemade (page 356) or store-bought

2 tablespoons wheat-free tamari, or ½ cup coconut aminos

2 tablespoons fresh lime juice

2 teaspoons coconut vinegar or unseasoned rice vinegar

2 cloves garlic, minced

½ teaspoon grated fresh ginger

⅛ teaspoon crushed red pepper

1 pound ground pork

Ground white pepper

2 large eggs, lightly beaten

Diced red bell peppers, for garnish (optional)

1. Place the cabbage, scallions, broth, tamari, lime juice, vinegar, garlic, ginger, and crushed red pepper in a medium-sized bowl. Stir well.

2. Transfer the mixture to a wok or large cast-iron skillet over medium heat. Stir-fry for 10 minutes, until the vegetables are softened.

3. Add the ground pork, season with white pepper, and stir-fry, breaking up the pork with a spatula, until the pork is cooked through, about 5 minutes.

4. Make a well in the center of the pork mixture, add the eggs, and scramble for 2 minutes, or until the eggs are set. Stir the eggs into the pork mixture until well combined. Serve garnished with scallions and red bell peppers, if desired.

5. Store in an airtight container in the refrigerator for up to 4 days. To reheat, place in a lightly greased skillet over medium heat for about 5 minutes, stirring occasionally.

NUTRITIONAL INFO (per serving)				
calories	fat	protein	carbs	fiber
242	18g	17g	4g	1g

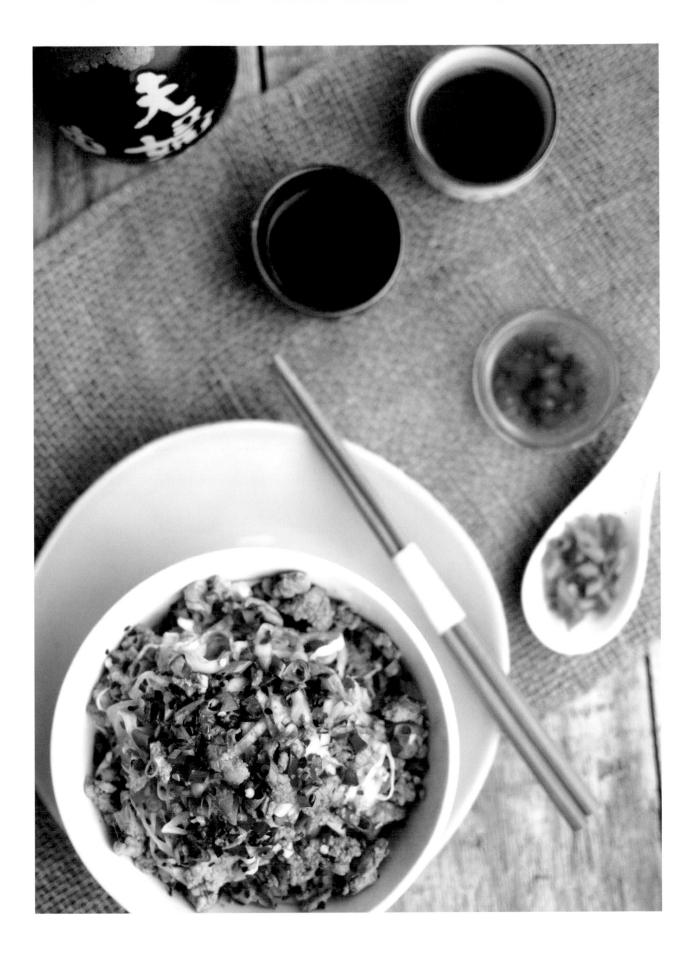

Green Tea Ice Cream

(L ⟶ H KETO   OPTION   OPTION)   prep time: 5 minutes, plus time to churn   yield: 2¾ cups (¼ cup per serving)

This ice cream is incredibly easy to make. Just be sure to use MCT oil, which is needed to create a smooth ice cream. And don't skip the salt: it does more than add flavor; it also helps keep the ice cream soft.

½ cup unsweetened cashew milk (or hemp milk if nut-free)

¼ cup Swerve confectioners'-style sweetener or equivalent amount of liquid or powdered sweetener (see page 31)

4 large eggs

4 large egg yolks

1 teaspoon pure vanilla extract, or seeds scraped from 1 vanilla bean (about 8 inches long)

¾ cup plus 2 tablespoons coconut oil (or unsalted butter if not dairy-sensitive)

¼ cup MCT oil

1 tablespoon matcha powder

½ teaspoon fine sea salt

—special equipment

Ice cream maker

1. Place the ingredients in a blender and puree until smooth.

2. Pour into an ice cream maker and churn according to the manufacturer's instructions, generally 15 to 30 minutes depending on the machine. Serve immediately or transfer to a container and freeze for up to 1 month.

variation: green tea ice pops. *If you don't have an ice cream maker, pour the mixture into 8 ice pop molds and freeze for at least 3 hours, until set.*

NUTRITIONAL INFO (per serving)				
calories	fat	protein	carbs	fiber
247	26g	3g	2g	0g

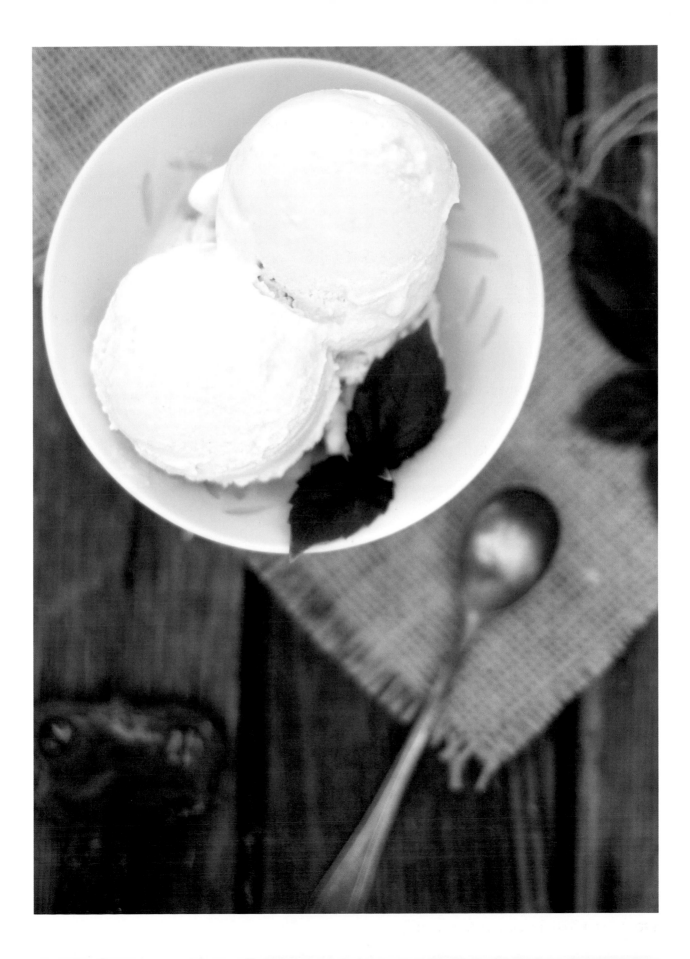

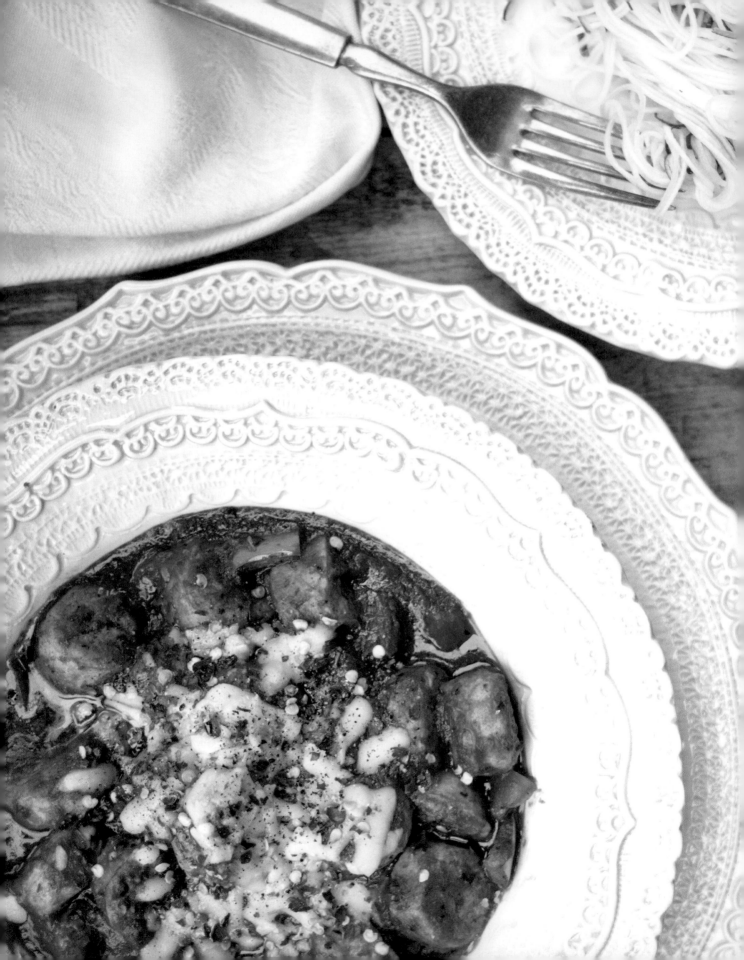

Italian Classics

I could just as easily have named this chapter Bambinos because that is the name I would give my own Italian restaurant. In Italian, *bambino* means "baby" or "young child." Since I have two amazing children, you would probably think that I named it after them, but the real reason is that there is a special place in my heart: my parents' cabin in north-central Wisconsin. When we visit them there, it seems as if the world stops: no traffic, no noise, no internet or cell service—we spend all day swimming, kayaking, fishing, and enjoying each other's company.

One of our family traditions is to drive into the town of Tomahawk and enjoy a meal at Bambinos, a tiny restaurant on Main Street. You would never guess that it has some of the best food you'll ever taste: pizzas ranging from classic pepperoni to exotic flavors such as Reuben, along with favorites such as Italian wedding soup, chicken parmigiana, and the most amazing tiramisu. Since my family is keto now, we haven't been there in years, but Bambinos has been an inspiration to me. I would love to own a little Italian pizzeria on a lake where I can make mouthwatering keto pizzas, Italian specialties, and, of course, tiramisu!

Italian Dressing

(L M H KETO OPTION)   **prep time:** 5 minutes   **yield:** 1¼ cups (2 tablespoons per serving)

Olive Garden's Italian dressing is so beloved that you can now find bottles of it in grocery stores, but those are filled with inflammatory canola oil and sugar. My version tastes very similar, but leaves out all the junk.

½ cup mayonnaise, homemade (page 357) or store-bought

⅓ cup coconut vinegar or apple cider vinegar

¼ cup grated Parmesan cheese (about 1 ounce)

2 tablespoons Swerve confectioners'-style sweetener or equivalent amount of liquid or powdered sweetener (see page 31)

1 tablespoon avocado oil or extra-virgin olive oil

1 tablespoon fresh lemon juice

1½ teaspoons Italian seasoning

1 clove garlic, minced

Fine sea salt

1. Place the mayonnaise, vinegar, Parmesan, sweetener, oil, lemon juice, Italian seasoning, and garlic in a blender and pulse until well combined. Taste and adjust the seasoning to your liking, adding salt and more lemon juice or sweetener if desired.

2. Store in an airtight container in the refrigerator for up to 2 weeks.

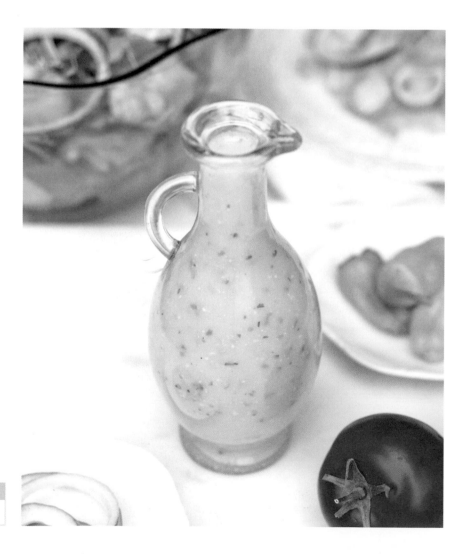

NUTRITIONAL INFO (per serving)				
calories	fat	protein	carbs	fiber
97	10g	1g	0.2g	0g

Alfredo Sauce

prep time: 5 minutes   cook time: 17 minutes   yield: 1 cup (¼ cup per serving)

I use this sauce in several ways, but one of my favorites is to serve it over Zoodles (page 360) with seafood. Below it is pictured with Gnocchi (page 146).

½ cup (1 stick) unsalted butter or ghee

2 cloves garlic, smashed to a paste or minced

2 ounces cream cheese

⅓ cup beef bone broth, homemade (page 356) or store-bought

½ cup grated Parmesan cheese (about 2 ounces)

1. Heat the butter and garlic in a small saucepan over medium heat. Cook until light golden brown, about 2 minutes, stirring constantly or the butter and garlic will burn. Reduce the heat to low and stir in the cream cheese, broth, and Parmesan. Simmer for at least 15 minutes. The longer the sauce simmers, the more the flavors will open up.

2. Store in the refrigerator for up to 4 days. To reheat, place in a saucepan over medium heat for about 3 minutes, stirring often.

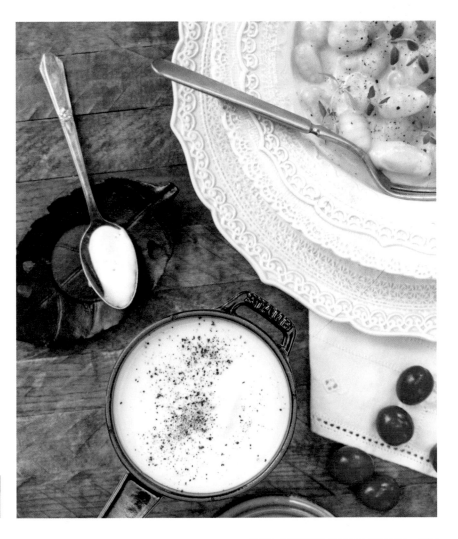

NUTRITIONAL INFO (per serving)				
calories	fat	protein	carbs	fiber
313	31g	7g	1g	0.1g

Mama Maria's Marinara

(KETO · OPTION) prep time: 7 minutes   cook time: at least 40 minutes
yield: 4 cups (½ cup per serving)

¼ cup unsalted butter (or avocado oil if dairy-free)

¼ cup grated onions (about 1 small)

4 cloves garlic, minced

3½ pounds garden-ripe tomatoes, or 2 (28-ounce) cans whole tomatoes

2 tablespoons chopped fresh basil leaves, plus extra for garnish

2 tablespoons chopped fresh oregano leaves, plus extra for garnish

1 teaspoon fine sea salt

2 tablespoons extra-virgin olive oil, for drizzling

1. Heat the butter in a large saucepan over medium heat. Add the onions and sauté for 5 to 8 minutes, until light golden. (This helps open up the sweetness of the onions, a trick I learned from an Italian chef.) Add the garlic and sauté for an additional 3 minutes.

2. If using fresh tomatoes, remove the skins by slicing an "X" in the bottom of each tomato and blanching them in boiling water for 30 seconds; rinse in cold water and remove the skins, which will slide right off. Using your fingers, crush the tomatoes.

3. Add the crushed tomatoes, basil, oregano, and salt to the saucepan. Reduce the heat and simmer, uncovered, for 30 minutes to 2 hours. The longer the sauce simmers, the more the flavors will open up.

4. When ready to serve, drizzle the sauce with the oil. Garnish with fresh herbs for an additional flavor profile (another trick from the Italian chef!). Store in an airtight container in the refrigerator for up to 8 days or in the freezer for up to 2 months. To reheat, place in a saucepan over medium heat for about 3 minutes, stirring often.

NUTRITIONAL INFO (per serving)				
calories	fat	protein	carbs	fiber
134	11g	2g	8g	2g

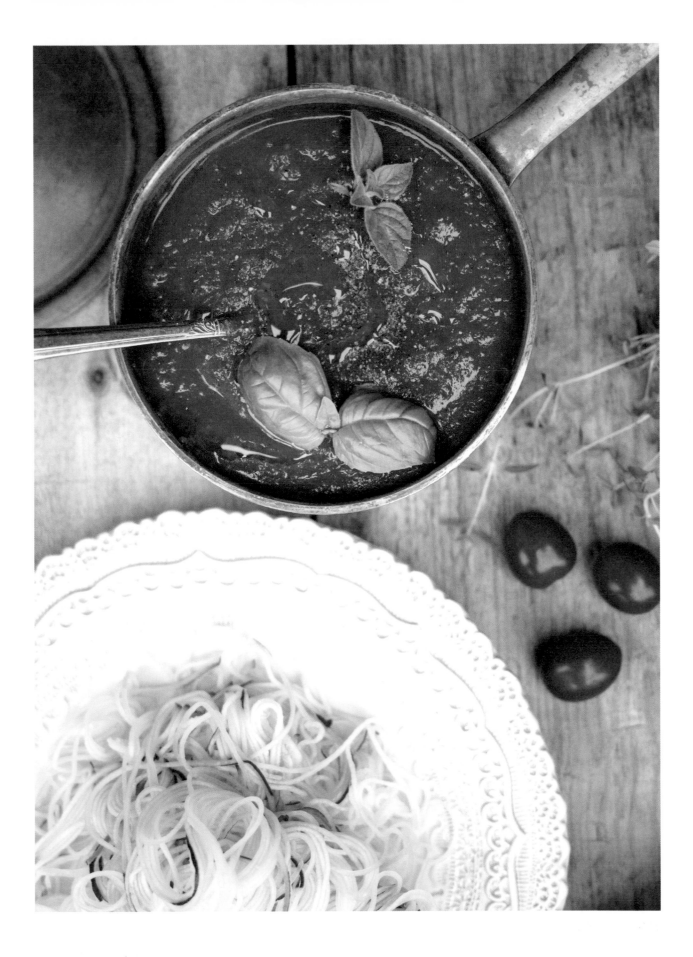

Mama Maria's Pizza Sauce

(L M H KETO · OPTION · 🚫 · 🚫) **prep time:** 5 minutes   **yield:** 1¼ cups (¼ cup per serving)

1 cup tomato sauce

3 tablespoons grated Parmesan cheese (or nutritional yeast if dairy-free)

2 tablespoons Swerve confectioners'-style sweetener or equivalent amount of liquid or powdered sweetener (see page 31) (optional)

2 teaspoons Italian seasoning

1 teaspoon garlic powder

¾ teaspoon onion powder

¼ teaspoon ground black pepper

Place the ingredients in a small bowl and mix until smooth. Cover and refrigerate for up to 3 days until ready to use. Stir or shake before using.

note: *This sauce tastes great on keto pizza (see pages 182 and 186).*

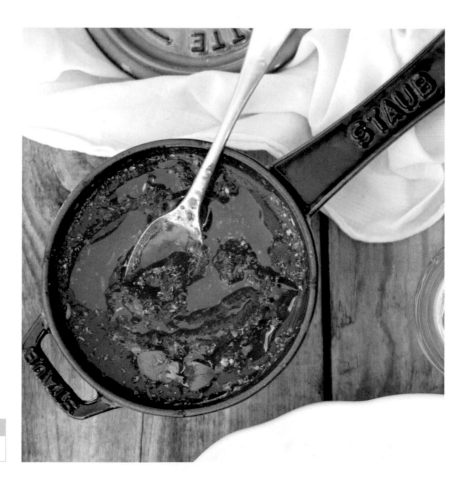

NUTRITIONAL INFO (per serving)				
calories	fat	protein	carbs	fiber
34	2g	2g	3g	0.5g

Italian Wedding Soup

(L M H KETO OPTION)   **prep time:** 10 minutes   **cook time:** 15 minutes   **yield:** 4 servings

1 pound ground beef

¾ cup chopped onions (about 1 medium), divided

1 cup finely chopped mushrooms (about 8 ounces)

¼ cup finely grated Parmesan cheese (or nutritional yeast if dairy-free)

1 large egg

1 teaspoon dried basil leaves

1 teaspoon dried oregano leaves

1 teaspoon fine sea salt

1½ teaspoons coconut oil or avocado oil

1 small zucchini, chopped into ¼-inch pieces (about ¾ cup)

¼ cup chopped celery

1 head escarole, chopped into bite-sized pieces

6 cups chicken bone broth, homemade (page 356) or store-bought

Coarsely grated or shredded Parmesan cheese, for garnish (optional)

1. Place the ground beef, ¼ cup of the onions, the mushrooms, Parmesan, egg, basil, oregano, and salt in a large bowl and mix until well combined. Form the mixture into ½-inch meatballs.

2. Heat the oil in a large pot over medium-high heat. Add the zucchini, remaining ½ cup of onions, and celery and sauté until the vegetables have softened, about 5 minutes. Add the escarole and broth and bring to a boil over high heat.

3. Lower the heat to medium and add the meatballs. Simmer for 10 minutes, or until the meatballs are cooked through. Taste and season the soup with additional salt, if desired. Serve with Parmesan cheese sprinkled on top, if desired. Store in an airtight container in the refrigerator for up to 4 days or in the freezer for up to 2 months. To reheat, place in a saucepan over medium heat for about 3 minutes.

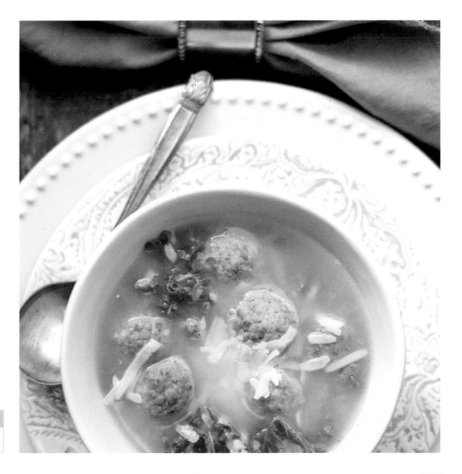

NUTRITIONAL INFO (per serving)				
calories	fat	protein	carbs	fiber
353	26g	25g	4g	1g

Zuppa Toscana

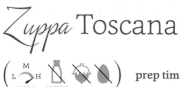

prep time: 5 minutes   **cook time:** 25 minutes   **yield:** 8 servings

1 tablespoon avocado oil (or unsalted butter if not dairy-sensitive)

½ cup chopped onions (about 1 medium)

8 ounces mushrooms, sliced

3 strips bacon, diced

3 cloves garlic, minced

1 pound bulk Italian sausage

1 teaspoon crushed red pepper

½ teaspoon fine sea salt

½ teaspoon ground black pepper

10 cups chicken bone broth, homemade (page 356) or store-bought

1 medium zucchini, cut into ½-inch dice

2 ounces fresh kale, stems removed, leaves torn into bite-sized pieces (about 1 cup)

1 cup heavy cream (or coconut milk if dairy-free)

½ cup grated Parmesan cheese (omit for dairy-free)

1. Heat the oil in a large pot over medium heat. Add the onions, mushrooms, and bacon and cook until the bacon is slightly crisp, about 3 minutes. Add the garlic and cook for an additional 3 minutes, or until fragrant. Add the sausage, crushed red pepper, salt, and black pepper. Sauté, breaking up the sausage with a spatula, until the sausage is cooked through, about 4 minutes. Add the broth and stir, scraping up the browned bits from the bottom of the pot. Bring to a boil.

2. Add the zucchini to the pot and cook for 8 minutes, or until the zucchini is tender. Stir in the kale and allow the leaves to wilt slightly, about 2 minutes. Lower the heat to a bare simmer and stir in the heavy cream until well combined.

3. Ladle the soup into bowls and top each bowl with 1 tablespoon of Parmesan cheese. Store in an airtight container in the refrigerator for up to 3 days. To reheat, place in a saucepan over medium-high heat for about 4 minutes.

NUTRITIONAL INFO (per serving)				
calories	fat	protein	carbs	fiber
398	29g	25g	6g	2g

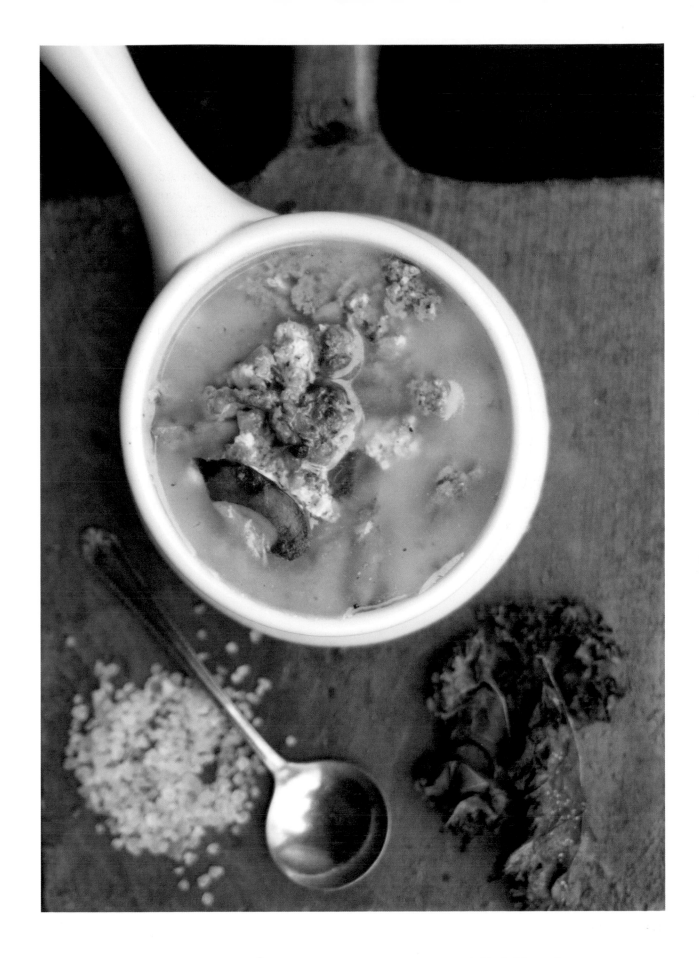

Italian Restaurant Salad

(L M H KETO ⬦ OPTION) **prep time:** 3 minutes (not including time to make dressing)   **cook time:** 1 minute
yield: 4 servings

If you've ever been to Olive Garden, you are familiar with this salad, served right when you arrive. When I was little, my brother and I would dare each other to eat the "hot" pepperoncini served in the salad and would act as though we had eaten ghost peppers! Even though pepperoncini are mild, they were the hottest things our little German palates had ever tried.

The croutons for this salad are made with the rinds of hard cheese, such as Parmesan or aged Gouda. It's a great way to make use of something you might otherwise discard! When I'm done with a chunk of Parmesan, I store the rind in the freezer until I want to make these tasty, cheesy croutons.

—croutons

1 aged Gouda or Parmesan cheese rind, about 3½ inches wide and ½ inch thick

4 cups chopped romaine lettuce

1 cup pitted black olives

¼ red onion, thinly sliced

4 mild pepperoncini peppers

1 medium tomato, diced

Grated Parmesan cheese, for garnish

Fine sea salt and ground black pepper

½ batch Italian Dressing (page 124)

1. Make the croutons: Cut the cheese rind into ¼-inch squares. Place the squares on a microwavable plate about 2 inches apart. Microwave on high for 1 minute or until the squares puff up to about twice their size. Allow to cool completely. Store extras in an airtight container in the fridge for up to 4 days.

2. Place the lettuce in a large serving bowl. Top with the black olives, red onion slices, pepperoncini, diced tomato, and keto croutons. Garnish with grated Parmesan and season with salt and pepper to taste, keeping in mind that the Parmesan will add saltiness. Serve with the dressing.

NUTRITIONAL INFO (per serving)				
calories	fat	protein	carbs	fiber
221	20g	5g	6g	1g

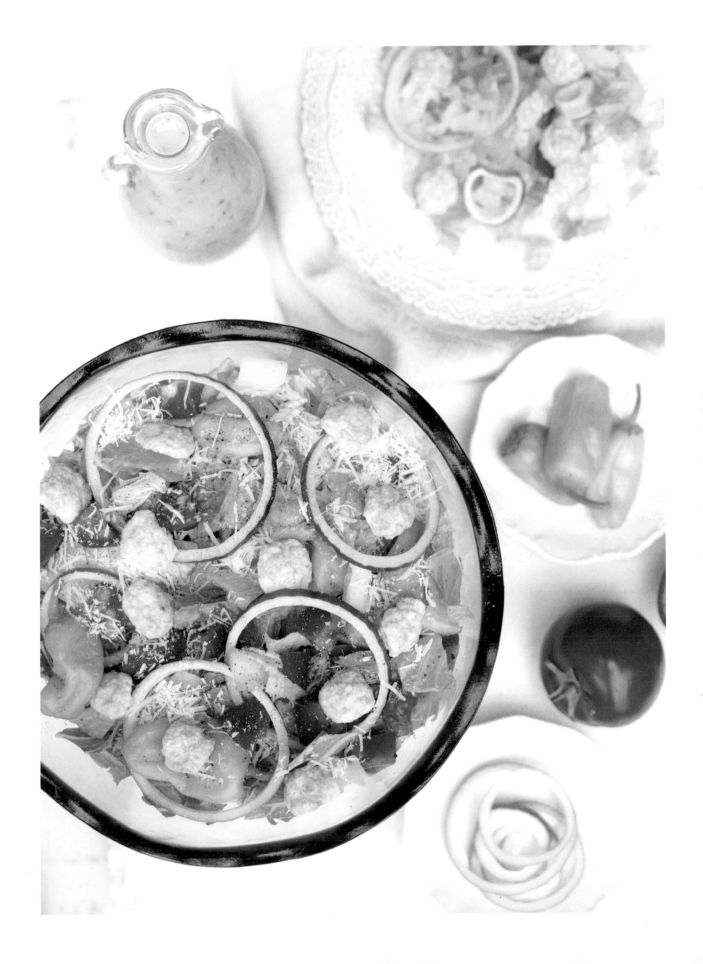

Garlic Bread

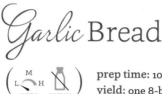

prep time: 10 minutes   **cook time:** 75 minutes

yield: one 8-by-4-inch loaf (20 slices, 1 slice per serving)

To make a garlic bread that is closer to what you would get at an Italian restaurant, I developed an almond flour–based bread just for this recipe. It is higher in carbohydrates than my Keto Bread (page 362) but is more like a traditional bread and very easy to make, with one caveat: make sure to grind the psyllium husks to a very fine powder and weigh all the ingredients. This will ensure that the dough rises properly and the bread doesn't get hollow and gummy. I use Jay Robb's whole psyllium husks and grind them in a blender until they're fine and powdery and half their original volume. (*Note:* If you use a different brand, you may not get the same results.) If you weigh all the ingredients and grind the psyllium husks to a powder and the bread still doesn't rise properly or has a gummy texture, try grinding the husks a second time when you make the bread again.

Because this bread is higher in carbs, please consume it in moderation. If you need a low-carb garlic bread, you can use a loaf of my Keto Bread instead.

—bread

3 cups (280 g) blanched almond flour

½ cup plus 2 tablespoons (90 g) psyllium husk powder (no substitutes)

1 tablespoon baking powder

1 teaspoon fine sea salt

6 large egg whites (180 g)

5 tablespoons (90 g) apple cider vinegar

1½ cups (340 g) boiling water

4 cloves garlic, minced

½ cup melted unsalted butter, ghee, or extra-virgin olive oil

Chopped fresh basil or parsley leaves, for garnish

1. Preheat the oven to 350°F. Grease an 8 by 4-inch loaf pan.

2. Place the almond flour, psyllium husk powder, baking powder, and salt in a medium-sized bowl and mix well to combine. Stir in the egg whites and vinegar and mix until a thick dough forms. Add the water and mix until the dough firms up.

3. Form the dough into a loaf and place it in the greased pan. Bake for 60 to 75 minutes, until the bread is firm to the touch and golden brown. Remove from the oven and allow to cool completely in the pan.

4. When the bread is cool, place an oven rack in the top position and turn the broiler to high. Cut the cooled bread into 20 slices. Place the slices on 2 rimmed baking sheets.

5. In a small bowl, mix the garlic with the melted butter. Brush the mixture onto the slices of bread, about 2 teaspoons per slice, and place under the broiler for 2 minutes, or until the bread is golden brown. Remove from the oven and garnish with parsley. Slice into triangles and serve immediately.

variation: cheesy garlic bread. *Before garnishing the garlic bread and cutting it into triangles, sprinkle each piece with a tablespoon of shredded mozzarella or grated Parmesan and set under the broiler for a minute or two to melt the cheese.*

NUTRITIONAL INFO (per serving)				
calories	fat	protein	carbs	fiber
177	15g	6g	8g	5g

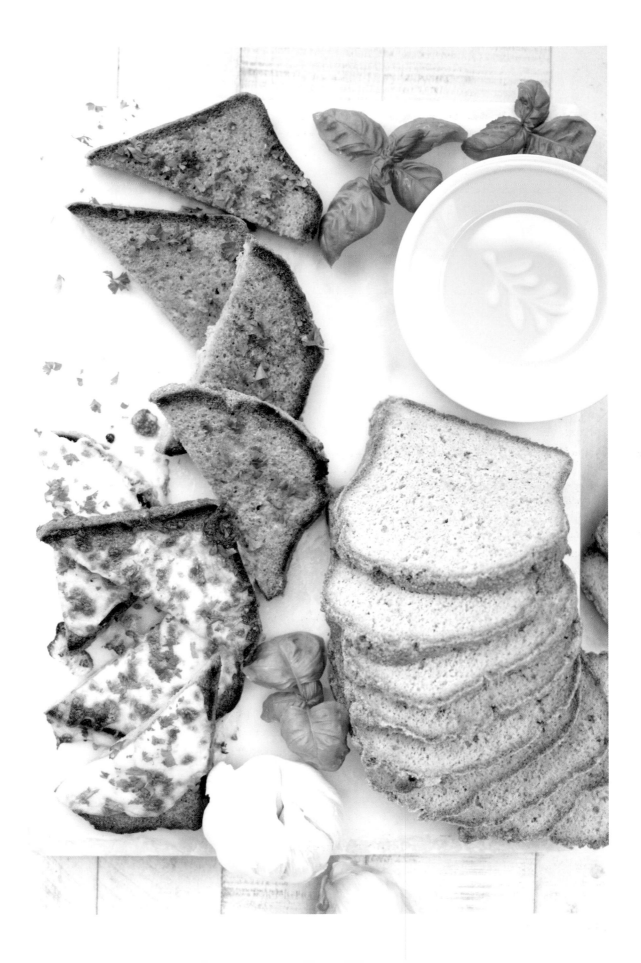

Mama Maria's Stuffed Mushrooms

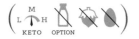

prep time: 5 minutes **cook time:** 25 minutes
yield: 20 large mushrooms (5 per serving)

This dish is a classic appetizer at many Italian restaurants. I call these Mama Maria's Stuffed Mushrooms because my dad absolutely loved these at our local Italian restaurant, Mama Maria's. I knew the mushrooms were stuffed with breadcrumbs, so I remade them. Now, when my dad comes to visit, I make him his favorite Italian dishes from Mama Maria's—with *this* Mama Maria running the kitchen!

20 large button mushrooms

1 tablespoon unsalted butter or coconut oil

¼ cup diced onions (about 1 small)

2 cloves garlic, minced

8 ounces bulk Italian sausage

½ teaspoon fine sea salt

½ teaspoon ground black pepper

4 ounces cream cheese (Kite Hill brand cream cheese style spread if dairy-free), at room temperature

¼ cup grated Parmesan cheese (or nutritional yeast if dairy-free), plus extra Parmesan for the topping

1 cup marinara, homemade (page 126) or store-bought

Fresh oregano, for garnish

1. Preheat the oven to 350°F.

2. Wash the mushrooms and remove the stems. Set the caps aside to dry on a paper towel. Finely chop the stems.

3. Melt the butter in a skillet over medium heat, then add the onions, garlic, and chopped mushroom stems. Cook for 2 to 3 minutes, until the onions begin to soften. Add the sausage, season with the salt and pepper, and cook, breaking up the sausage with a spatula, until the sausage is lightly browned and cooked through, about 5 minutes.

4. Transfer the sausage mixture to a medium-sized bowl. Stir in the cream cheese and Parmesan until well combined. Stuff 1 tablespoon of the cheese mixture into each mushroom cap.

5. Pour the marinara into two 8-inch square baking dishes or two pie pans and set the mushrooms on top, then sprinkle them with a few tablespoons of Parmesan cheese. Bake for 25 minutes, or until the mushrooms are soft and the cheese is melted.

6. Serve garnished with oregano. Store in an airtight container in the refrigerator for up to 4 days. To reheat, place on a rimmed baking sheet in a 375°F oven for about 3 minutes.

NUTRITIONAL INFO (per serving)				
calories	fat	protein	carbs	fiber
455	37g	18g	11g	2g

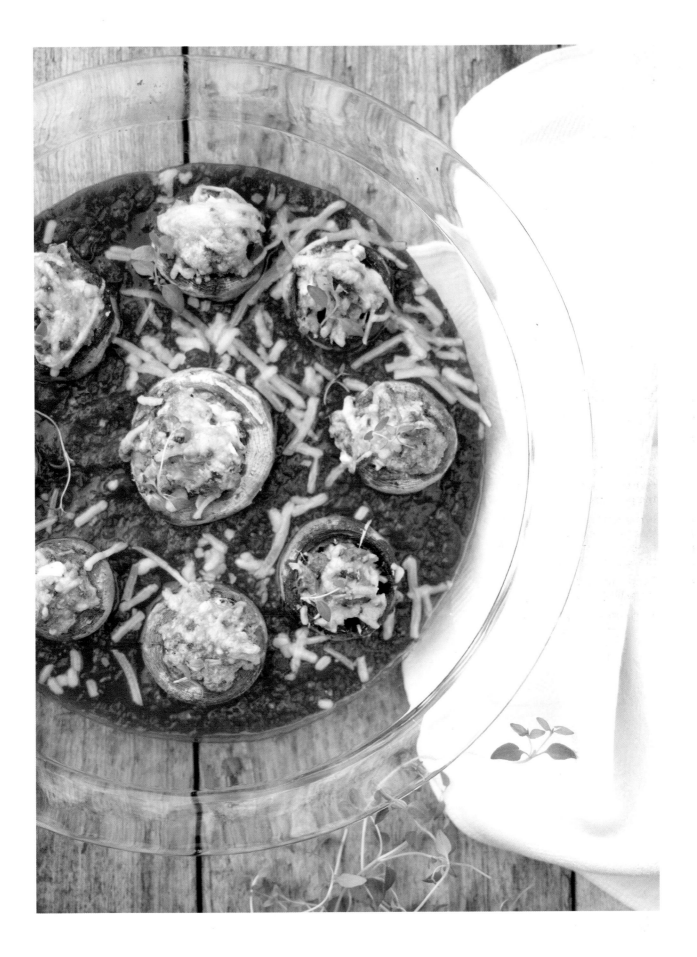

Mama Maria's Meatballs

(L M T H) prep time: 8 minutes   cook time: 35 minutes   yield: 8 servings
KETO OPTION

I know what you're thinking: I call these Mama Maria's Meatballs because my name is Maria and I am a mama. That's partly true, and I do love meatballs! But these are also named for the wonderful Italian restaurant where Craig and I used to eat in our pre-keto days.

2 pounds ground beef

¼ cup chopped onions (about 1 small)

2 cloves garlic, minced

2 large eggs

1 cup grated Romano cheese (or nutritional yeast if dairy-sensitive), plus extra Romano for garnish

1½ tablespoons Italian seasoning

2 teaspoons fine sea salt

½ teaspoon ground black pepper

2 cups mushrooms (about 1 pound), finely chopped

1 cup beef broth, homemade (page 356) or store-bought, or marinara, homemade (page 126) or store-bought

2 cups marinara, homemade (page 126) or store-bought, for serving

1. Preheat the oven to 350°F.

2. In a large bowl, combine the ground beef, onions, garlic, eggs, Romano cheese, Italian seasoning, salt, and pepper. Add the mushrooms to the meat mixture. Slowly stir in the broth, ½ cup at a time. The mixture should be very moist but still able to hold its shape when rolled into meatballs. Form the mixture into 2-inch meatballs. Arrange the meatballs in a single layer on a rimmed baking sheet. Bake for 30 to 35 minutes, turning occasionally, until evenly browned.

3. Serve with marinara. Garnish with extra Romano cheese, if desired. Store the meatballs in an airtight container in the refrigerator for up to 4 days or in the freezer for up to 2 months. To reheat, place on a rimmed baking sheet in a preheated 350°F oven for about 3 minutes.

NUTRITIONAL INFO (per serving)				
calories	fat	protein	carbs	fiber
449	34g	29g	6g	1g

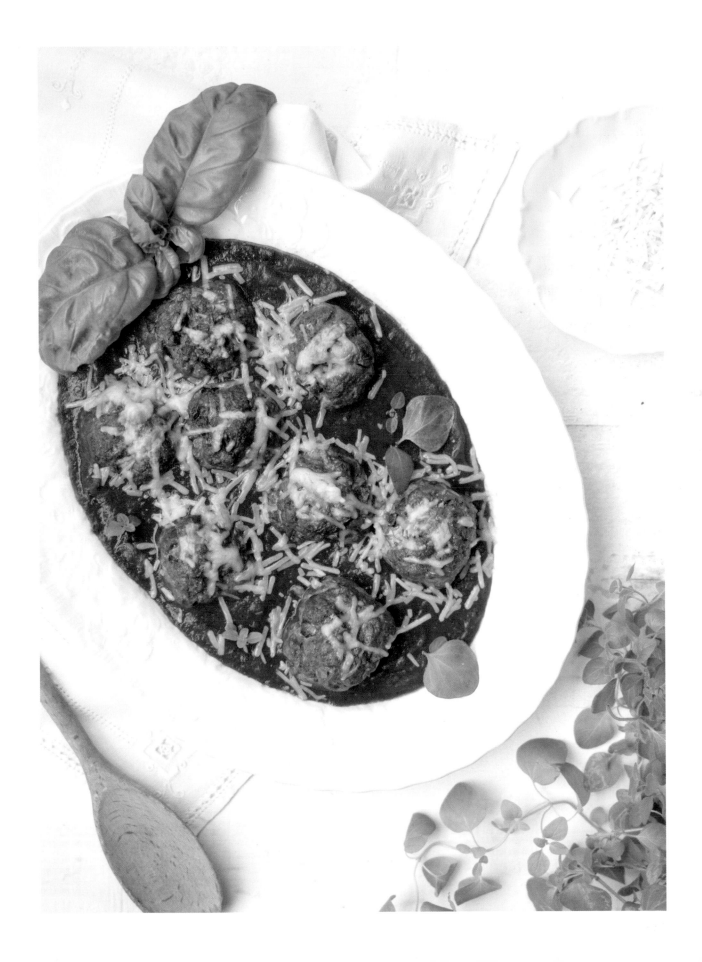

Cheesy Zucchini Agnolotti

prep time: 7 minutes   cook time: 10 minutes (see tip)
yield: 4 servings (2 agnolotti per serving)

1 medium zucchini, about 8 inches long by 1½ inches in diameter

2 teaspoons fine sea salt

2 ounces cream cheese or mascarpone cheese (Kite Hill brand cream cheese style spread if dairy-free), at room temperature

¼ cup grated Parmesan cheese (or nutritional yeast if dairy-free)

1 teaspoon Italian seasoning

1 cup marinara, homemade (page 126) or store-bought, warmed

Shredded mozzarella cheese, for topping (optional; omit for dairy-free)

1. Preheat the oven to 350°F.

2. Trim the ends off the zucchini. Using a mandoline, slice the zucchini lengthwise into very thin planks, about $\frac{1}{16}$ inch thick. You will need 16 slices.

3. Place the slices of zucchini in a colander in the sink. Sprinkle evenly with the salt and allow the excess water to drain from the zucchini for 5 minutes. Squeeze the zucchini slices gently to release the remaining excess moisture.

4. To make each agnolotto, place 2 slices of zucchini on a work surface in a cross shape so that they overlap in the center.

5. In a medium-sized bowl, mix together the cream cheese, Parmesan, and Italian seasoning until well combined.

6. Place 1 tablespoon of the cream cheese mixture in the center of the cross of zucchini slices. Fold the edges over to make a tight agnolotto-shaped "pocket." Repeat with the remaining zucchini slices. Place the agnolotti with the zucchini ends down in a 13 by 9-inch baking dish. Bake for 10 minutes, or until the zucchini is soft and the cheese is melted.

7. Place ¼ cup of marinara on each plate. Top with 2 agnolotti. If desired, sprinkle with mozzarella and set under the broiler for a minute or two to melt the cheese (make sure your plates are oven-safe!). Store in an airtight container in the refrigerator for up to 4 days. To reheat, place on a rimmed baking sheet in a preheated 350°F oven for about 3 minutes.

busy family tip: *To make this recipe even easier, you can skip the oven and use the microwave instead. Heat the assembled agnolotti for 1 minute, or until the cheese is melted and the agnolotti are heated to your liking.*

NUTRITIONAL INFO (per serving)				
calories	fat	protein	carbs	fiber
222	18g	7g	10g	3g

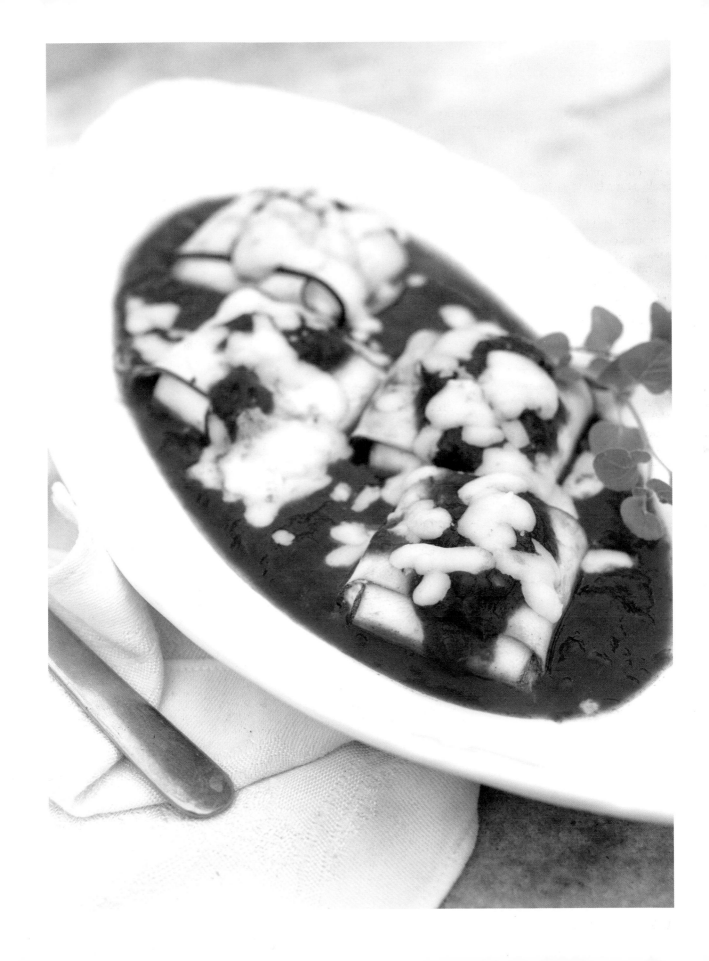

Five-Cheese "Ziti"

(L M H KETO OPTION) prep time: 10 minutes (not including time to make Alfredo sauce)
cook time: 30 minutes   yield: 8 servings

—sauce

4 cups tomato sauce

2 cups Alfredo Sauce (page 125)

½ cup ricotta cheese

¼ cup shredded mozzarella cheese (about 1 ounce)

3 tablespoons shredded fontina cheese

1 clove garlic, minced

—topping

3 cups shredded mozzarella cheese (about 12 ounces)

½ cup pork dust (see page 363) or blanched almond flour

3 tablespoons grated Romano cheese

3 tablespoons grated Parmesan cheese

2 large cloves garlic, minced

3 tablespoons melted butter or macadamia nut oil

3 tablespoons chopped fresh parsley

6 (7-ounce) packages fettuccini Miracle Noodles, or 2 large zucchini, spiral-sliced into noodles, for serving

1 cup shredded mozzarella cheese (about 4 ounces)

1. Make the sauce: Combine the tomato sauce, Alfredo sauce, ricotta, mozzarella, fontina, and garlic in a large bowl. Cover the bowl and refrigerate until ready to use.

2. Make the topping: Place the mozzarella, pork dust, Romano, and Parmesan in a medium-sized bowl. Stir well, then add the garlic, melted butter, and parsley and mix until well combined. Cover the bowl and refrigerate until ready to use.

3. When ready to serve, preheat the oven to 375°F. Rinse and drain the Miracle Noodles. (Or, if using zucchini noodles, place the zucchini noodles in a colander in the sink. Sprinkle with 1 teaspoon of salt and let sit for 5 minutes to drain. Gently squeeze the zucchini noodles to release any excess moisture.)

4. Spread ½ cup of the sauce in the bottom of a 13 by 9-inch baking dish. Place the noodles over the sauce, then top with the remaining sauce. Mix thoroughly. Spread the 1 cup of mozzarella over the noodles and sauce mixture. Top the mozzarella with the prepared topping, spreading it evenly. Bake for 30 minutes, or until the topping is golden brown and the cheese is melted. Store in an airtight container in the refrigerator for up to 4 days. To reheat, place in a baking dish in a preheated 350°F oven for about 6 minutes.

NUTRITIONAL INFO (per serving)				
calories	fat	protein	carbs	fiber
552	48g	26g	8g	1g

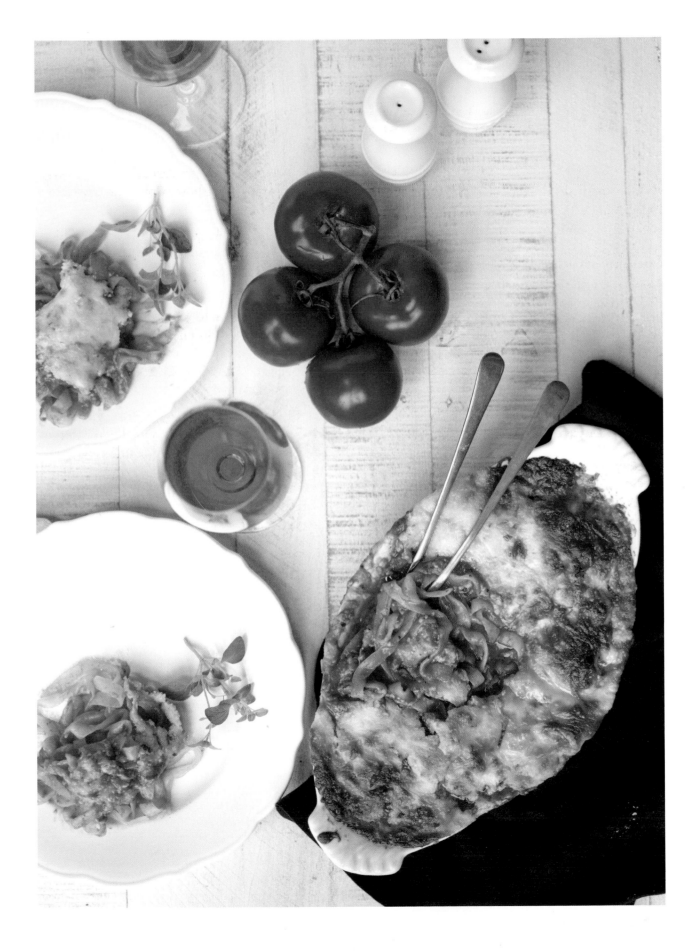

Chicken Scaloppine

(L →H M KETO 🧴 OPTION 🚫 🥚)   **prep time:** 5 minutes   **cook time:** 10 minutes   **yield:** 4 servings

4 boneless, skinless chicken thighs

½ teaspoon fine sea salt

1 teaspoon ground black pepper

2 tablespoons ghee or unsalted butter (or nondairy Paleo fat if dairy-sensitive)

1 pound button mushrooms, sliced (about 2 cups)

1 clove garlic, minced

¼ cup chicken bone broth, homemade (page 356) or store-bought

¼ cup heavy cream (or coconut cream if dairy-sensitive)

2 tablespoons capers, drained, for garnish

Chopped fresh parsley, for garnish

1. Pat the chicken thighs dry with paper towels. Using a cast-iron skillet, rolling pin, or mallet, gently pound the thighs to an even thickness of about ½ inch. Season the chicken on both sides with the salt and pepper.

2. Heat the ghee in a large cast-iron skillet over medium-high heat. Sear the chicken for 5 minutes per side, or until cooked through. Transfer the chicken to a platter.

3. Add the mushrooms and garlic to the skillet, adding more ghee if needed. Sauté until the mushrooms are golden brown on both sides, about 5 minutes. Add the broth and deglaze the pan, using a whisk to scrape up any bits from the bottom of the skillet. Reduce the heat, stir in the heavy cream, and simmer for 2 minutes.

4. Serve the chicken with the sauce from the skillet. Garnish with the capers and parsley. Store in an airtight container in the refrigerator for up to 4 days. To reheat, place on a rimmed baking sheet in a preheated 350°F oven for about 3 minutes.

busy family tip: *Have your butcher pound the chicken for you.*

NUTRITIONAL INFO (per serving)				
calories	fat	protein	carbs	fiber
301	21g	26g	5g	1g

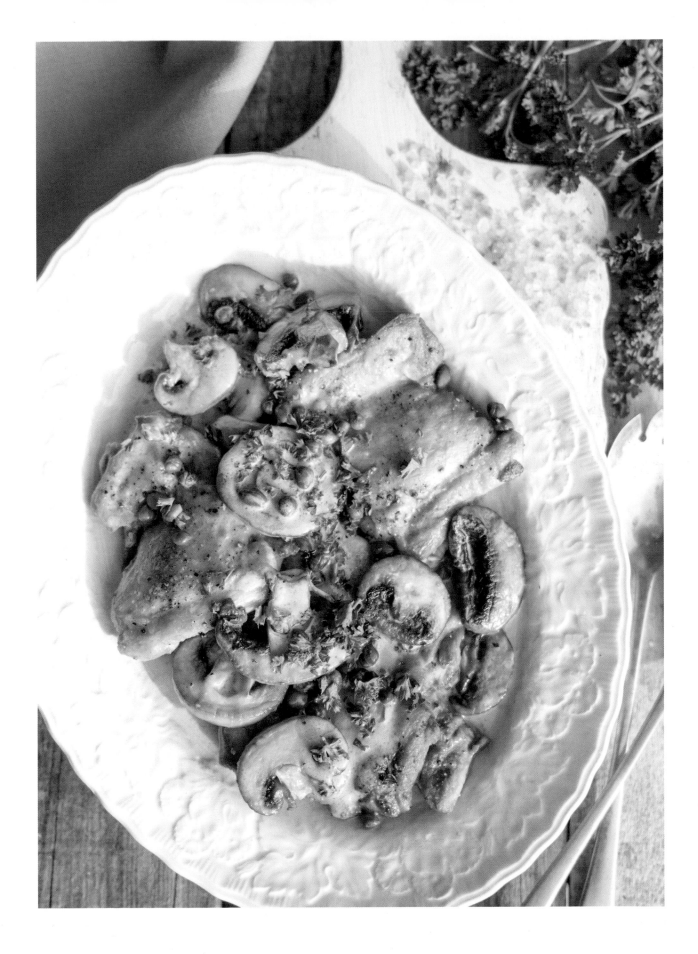

Gnocchi—Three Ways

(L M H KETO ⊗) prep time: 10 minutes (not including time to make marinara or Alfredo sauce)
cook time: 15 minutes   yield: 4 servings

—gnocchi

1 cup shredded mozzarella cheese (about 4 ounces)

1 cup powdered Parmesan cheese (see page 363)

1 teaspoon Italian seasoning

1 teaspoon garlic powder

3 large egg yolks

4 cups chicken bone broth, homemade (page 356) or store-bought, or water

—brown butter sauce (option 1)

¼ cup (½ stick) unsalted butter

1 teaspoon chopped fresh oregano or sage leaves

½ teaspoon fine sea salt

—marinara (option 2)

2 cups Mama Maria's Marinara (page 126), warmed

—alfredo sauce (option 3)

1 batch Alfredo Sauce (page 125), warmed

1. Preheat the oven to 350°F.

2. In a large heatproof bowl, combine the mozzarella, Parmesan, Italian seasoning, and garlic powder. Bake for 10 minutes (or microwave for 1 to 2 minutes), until the cheese is completely melted. Stir well to combine. Stir in the egg yolks and mix with a hand mixer until smooth.

3. Separate the dough into 3 balls. On a clean work surface, use your hands to roll each ball into a log that is about ¾ inch thick and 2 feet long. Use a knife to cut the dough into ¾-inch pieces.

4. Bring the broth to a boil in a large pot. Meanwhile, use a fork to make indentations on each piece of dough to resemble traditional gnocchi. Gently drop the gnocchi into the boiling broth and cook for about 1 minute, until they float. Remove the gnocchi from the pot with a slotted spoon and place them on a plate lined with a paper towel to drain briefly.

5. To make the brown butter sauce, heat the butter, oregano, and salt in a small skillet over medium-high heat, stirring, until brown flecks appear, about 4 minutes.

6. To serve, transfer the drained gnocchi to a platter and top with the sauce of your choice.

NUTRITIONAL INFO (per serving)				
calories	fat	protein	carbs	fiber
396	34g	24g	2g	0.4g

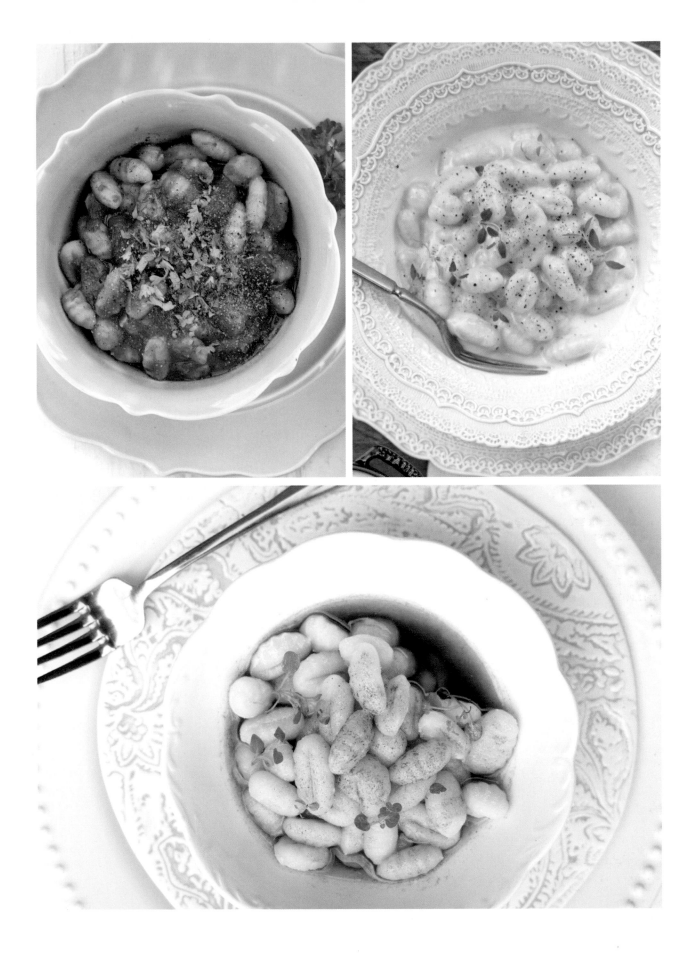

Spaghetti and Meatballs

(M L↷H KETO OPTION) **prep time:** 5 minutes (not including time to make meatballs)
cook time: 20 minutes   **yield:** 8 servings

One of the reasons I prefer cabbage pasta over zucchini noodles is that cabbage pasta does not get soggy when sauced. Cabbage pasta can be stored with the sauce; not only will it hold up well, it will also grab onto flavors and taste even better as leftovers!

1 tablespoon avocado oil

1 small head green cabbage, thinly shredded

2 cloves garlic, minced

1 batch Mama Maria's Meatballs (page 138), warmed

Grated Parmesan cheese, for garnish (omit for dairy-free)

Fresh basil leaves, for garnish

1. Heat the oil in a large cast-iron skillet over medium-low heat. Add the cabbage and garlic, cover, and braise for 20 minutes, or until the cabbage is very soft.

2. Place the cabbage pasta on a platter. Top with the baked meatballs and marinara. Garnish with Parmesan cheese and basil. Store in an airtight container in the refrigerator for up to 4 days or in the freezer for up to 1 month. To reheat, place in a lightly greased skillet over medium heat for about 3 minutes.

busy family tip: *You can also cook the cabbage pasta in a slow cooker. Place the oil, garlic, and cabbage in a 4-quart slow cooker, cover, and cook on low for 2 hours or on high for 1 hour.*

NUTRITIONAL INFO (per serving)				
calories	fat	protein	carbs	fiber
552	40g	37g	13g	4g

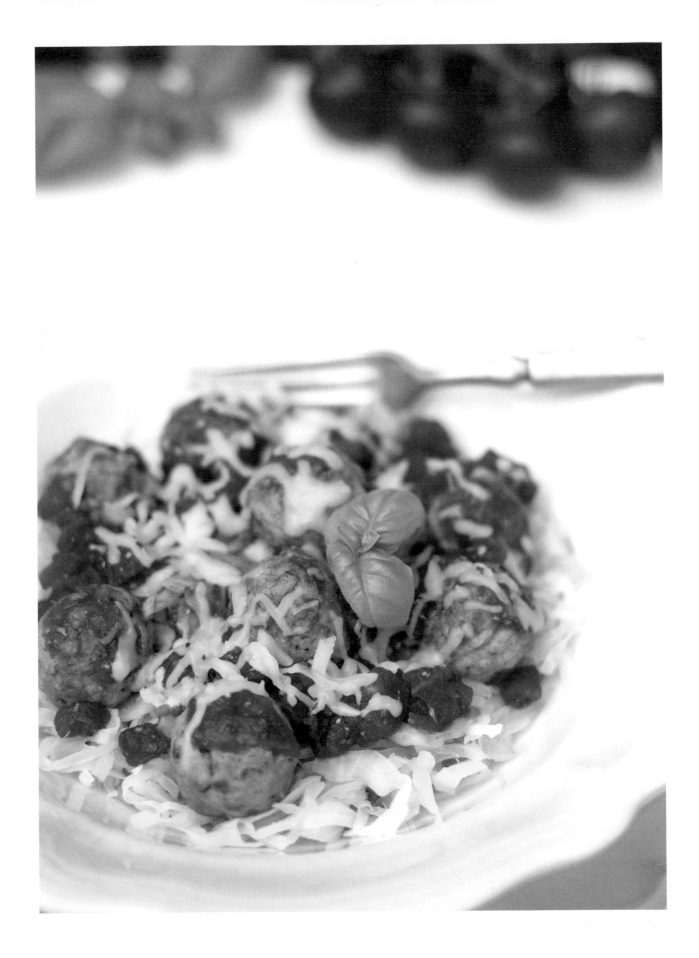

Chicken Parmigiana

(L ⊤ H ⬦) **prep time:** 10 minutes (not including time to make zoodles) **cook time:** 10 minutes
KETO **yield:** 4 servings

4 boneless, skinless chicken thighs

Fine sea salt and ground black pepper

2 large eggs

1 cup powdered Parmesan cheese (see page 363)

2 teaspoons Italian seasoning

3 tablespoons avocado oil or coconut oil, for frying

1 cup marinara, homemade (page 126) or store-bought

4 ounces fresh mozzarella cheese, thinly sliced

Finely chopped fresh basil, for garnish

1 batch Zoodles (page 360), for serving (optional)

1. Preheat the oven to 400°F.

2. Place the chicken thighs between 2 pieces of parchment paper and, using a cast-iron skillet, rolling pin, or mallet, gently pound the thighs until they are about ¼ inch thick. Season the chicken well on both sides with salt and pepper.

3. Crack the eggs into a shallow baking dish. Beat in 1 tablespoon of water and season with a pinch each of salt and pepper. Place the powdered Parmesan and Italian seasoning in another shallow baking dish and mix until well combined.

4. Dredge each chicken thigh in the eggs and let any excess drip off, then dip both sides of the chicken in the Parmesan mixture.

5. Heat the oil in a large cast-iron skillet over medium-high heat. Place the chicken in the skillet and sear until golden brown, about 2 minutes per side.

6. Pour the marinara into a 13 by 9-inch baking dish. Place the chicken on top of the marinara. Top each thigh with 1 ounce of mozzarella. Bake for 5 minutes, or until the chicken is cooked through and the cheese is melted. Remove from the oven and garnish with basil. Serve over zoodles, if desired. Store in an airtight container in the refrigerator for up to 4 days. To reheat, place in a lightly greased skillet over medium heat for about 3 minutes.

busy family tip: *Ask your butcher to pound the chicken for you.*

NUTRITIONAL INFO (per serving)				
calories	fat	protein	carbs	fiber
619	46g	46g	10g	3g

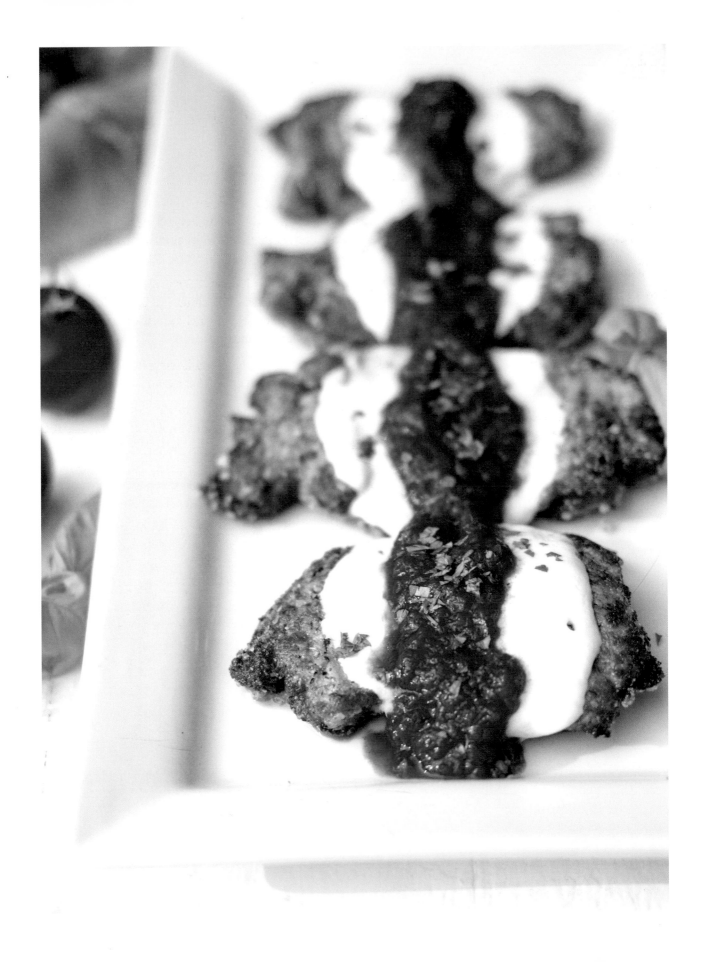

Shrimp Caprese Pasta

(L →M H KETO) **prep time:** 10 minutes, plus 1 hour to marinate   **cook time:** 7 minutes
yield: 4 servings

2 cups chopped fresh round or plum tomatoes or quartered cherry tomatoes

½ cup chopped fresh basil leaves, plus extra for garnish

2 tablespoons avocado oil or extra-virgin olive oil

3 cloves garlic, minced

1 teaspoon Italian seasoning

1½ teaspoons fine sea salt, divided

1¼ teaspoons ground black pepper, divided

2 tablespoons unsalted butter

½ cup chicken bone broth, homemade (page 356) or store-bought

1½ cups heavy cream

1 cup grated Parmesan cheese (about 4 ounces), plus extra for garnish

1 batch Zoodles (page 360) or Cabbage Pasta (page 361)

1 pound medium shrimp, peeled and deveined

½ cup shredded mozzarella cheese (about 2 ounces)

1. Place the tomatoes in a large bowl. Stir in the basil, oil, garlic, Italian seasoning, ½ teaspoon of the salt, and ¼ teaspoon of the pepper. Cover the bowl, place in the refrigerator, and marinate for 1 hour.

2. Melt the butter in a large cast-iron skillet over medium heat. Add the broth, increase the heat, and bring to a boil. Reduce the heat to low and stir in the heavy cream and Parmesan. Simmer until the sauce has reduced a bit, about 5 minutes. Preheat the broiler to high.

3. Remove the tomatoes from the marinade with a slotted spoon and add to the skillet; discard the marinade. Place the zoodles on a platter. Top with the sauce, which will heat the zoodles.

4. Place the shrimp on a rimmed baking sheet and season with the remaining 1 teaspoon each of salt and pepper. Broil for 4 minutes, or until the shrimp turns pink. Top the shrimp with the mozzarella and broil for 1 minute more.

5. Transfer the shrimp to the platter with the sauced zoodles. Garnish with basil and Parmesan cheese. Store in an airtight container in the refrigerator for up to 4 days. To reheat, place in a lightly greased skillet over medium heat for about 3 minutes.

NUTRITIONAL INFO (per serving)				
calories	fat	protein	carbs	fiber
734	62g	45g	7g	2g

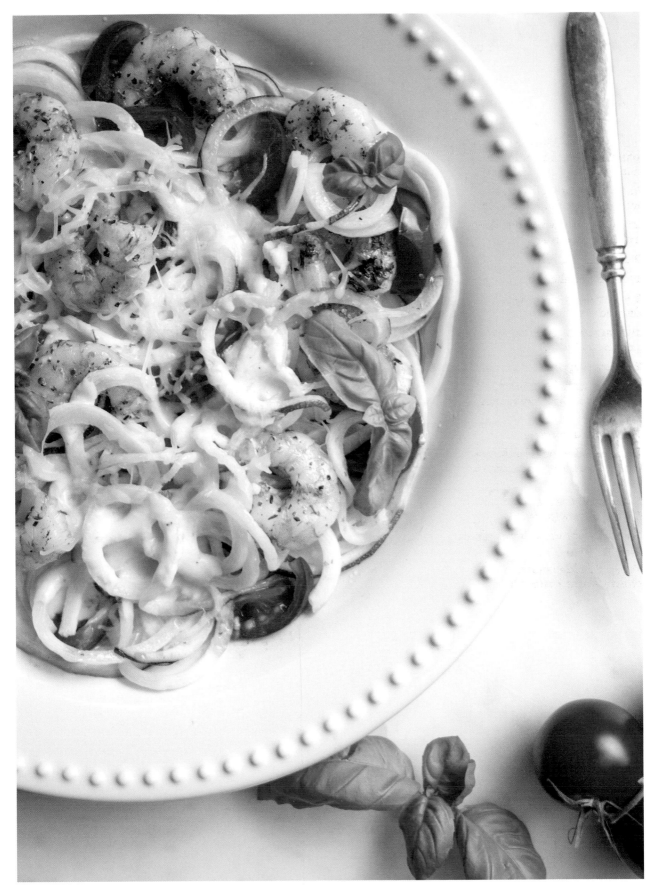

Sausage and Pepper Rustica

(L ⊤ H KETO OPTION) **prep time:** 10 minutes   **cook time:** 20 minutes   **yield:** 4 servings

2 tablespoons coconut oil or avocado oil

2 bell peppers, any color, chopped

½ cup diced onions (about 1 medium)

½ teaspoon fine sea salt

1 pound Italian sausages, sliced into ½-inch pieces

2 cups marinara, homemade (page 126) or store-bought

¼ teaspoon crushed red pepper

½ cup shredded mozzarella cheese (about 2 ounces) (optional; omit for dairy-free)

1 batch Cabbage Pasta (page 361) or Zoodles (page 360), for serving

1. Heat the oil in a large cast-iron skillet over medium-high heat. Add the bell peppers and onions and cook for 4 minutes, or until the onions are translucent and the peppers are soft. Season with the salt.

2. Place the sausage in the skillet and cook for 5 minutes, stirring occasionally, or until the sausage is cooked through. Add the marinara and crushed red pepper and continue to cook until the marinara is hot. Top with the mozzarella, if desired.

3. Serve the sausage mixture over the cabbage pasta. Store in an airtight container in the refrigerator for up to 4 days. To reheat, place in a lightly greased skillet over medium heat for about 3 minutes.

NUTRITIONAL INFO (per serving)				
calories	fat	protein	carbs	fiber
555	45g	26g	14g	4g

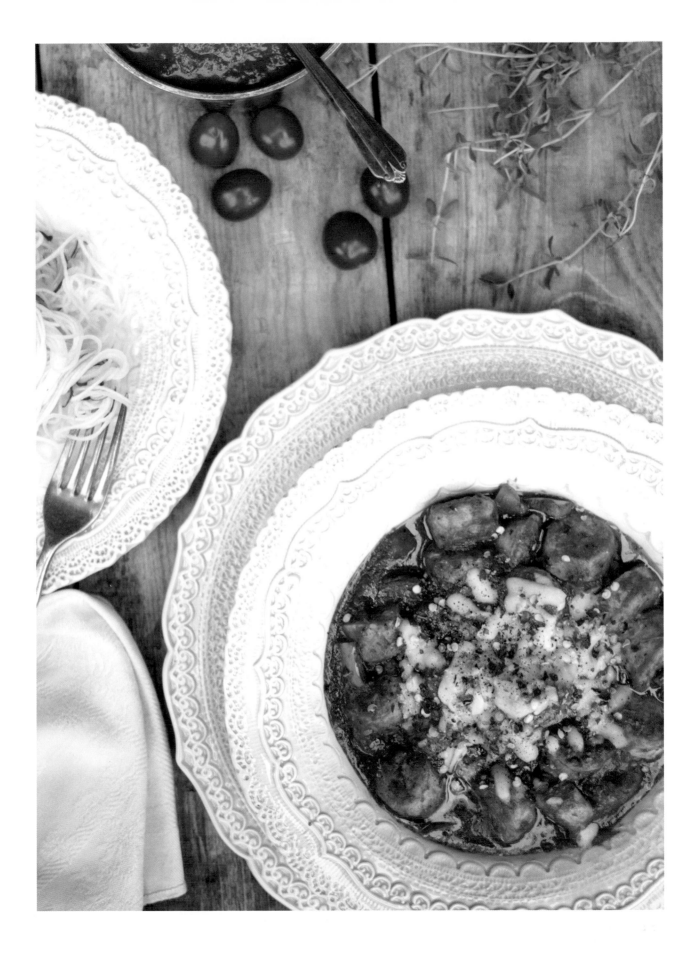

Stuffed Manicotti

prep time: 10 minutes   **cook time:** about 40 minutes
yield: 4 servings (2 manicotti per serving)

—filling

1 cup shredded mozzarella cheese (about 4 ounces)

1 cup grated Parmesan cheese (about 4 ounces), plus extra for garnish

8 ounces cream cheese, at room temperature

2 ounces fresh spinach (about 1 cup)

2 large eggs

1/8 teaspoon ground nutmeg

—crepes

2 large raw eggs

2 hard-boiled eggs

4 ounces cream cheese, at room temperature

Pinch of fine sea salt

Coconut oil, for frying

Marinara, homemade (page 126) or store-bought, for serving

1. Make the filling: In a small bowl, combine the mozzarella, Parmesan, cream cheese, spinach, eggs, and nutmeg. Set aside.

2. Make the crepes: Place the raw eggs, hard-boiled eggs, cream cheese, and salt in a blender and blend until very smooth.

3. Heat some oil in a 9-inch nonstick skillet over medium-high heat. Place 1/4 cup of the crepe batter in the skillet and swirl to spread it to the edges. Cook until golden brown, about 2 minutes per side. Remove from the skillet and repeat with the remaining batter to make a total of 8 crepes.

4. Preheat the oven to 400°F. Spread 2 heaping tablespoons of the filling in the center of each crepe. Fold the side over the filling, like a soft taco.

5. Place the manicotti in a 13 by 9-inch baking dish. Bake for 10 minutes, or until the cheese filling is heated through. Serve over marinara. Garnish with extra Parmesan cheese, if desired. Store in an airtight container in the refrigerator for up to 4 days. To reheat, place in a baking dish in a preheated 350°F oven for about 3 minutes.

busy family tip: _I make the crepe batter the night before and store the blender jar in the refrigerator for an easy dinner the next day._

NUTRITIONAL INFO (per serving)				
calories	fat	protein	carbs	fiber
592	48g	34g	4g	0.2g

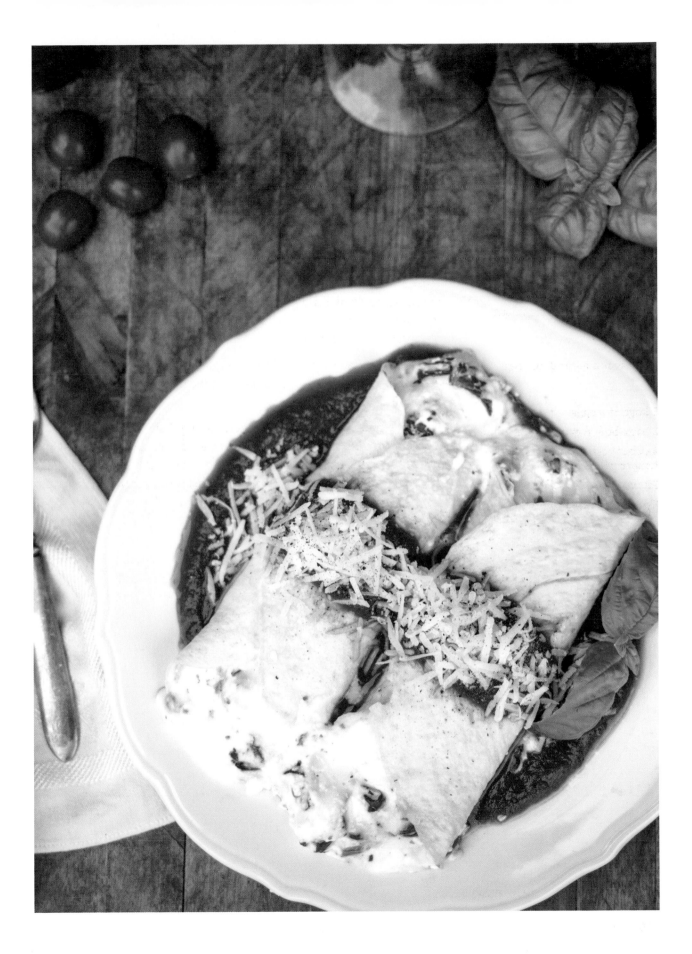

Steak Gorgonzola Alfredo

(L M H KETO ⬚ ⬚) prep time: 10 minutes, plus time to marinate (not including time to make zoodles or Alfredo sauce) cook time: 20 minutes yield: 4 servings

This is a very popular dish served at Olive Garden. It has an intense depth of flavor. The marinade in this recipe adds undertones of citrus and a touch of rosemary, replicating the flavors of the restaurant dish. If you are in a rush or you forget to marinate the steak, this dish will still be delicious!

—marinade

¼ cup avocado oil

¼ cup fresh lemon juice

2 cloves garlic, smashed to a paste

½ teaspoon dried ground rosemary

1 pound boneless sirloin steak, sliced into ¼-inch medallions

1 teaspoon fine sea salt

1 teaspoon ground black pepper

2 teaspoons coconut oil

1 batch Zoodles (page 360) or Cabbage Pasta (page 361)

1 cup fresh spinach

1 batch Alfredo Sauce (page 125), warmed

1 cup sliced cherry tomatoes

2 ounces Gorgonzola cheese, crumbled

1. Marinate the steak: Combine the avocado oil, lemon juice, garlic, and rosemary in a shallow bowl. Add the steak and turn to coat on both sides. Cover the bowl, place in the refrigerator, and marinate for at least 1 hour or overnight.

2. Remove the steak from the marinade and pat dry; discard the marinade. Season the steak on all sides with the salt and pepper. Heat the coconut oil in a large cast-iron skillet over medium-high heat. Add the steak and cook for 2 minutes per side for medium-done steak, or until done to your liking.

3. Place the zoodles in a serving dish, add the spinach, and toss to combine. Add the Alfredo sauce and toss to coat. Place the steak in the serving dish. Top with the tomatoes and Gorgonzola and serve.

4. Store in an airtight container in the refrigerator for up to 4 days. To reheat, place in a lightly greased skillet over medium heat for about 3 minutes.

busy family tip: *The Alfredo sauce can be made up to 4 days ahead and stored in an airtight container in the refrigerator.*

NUTRITIONAL INFO (per serving)				
calories	fat	protein	carbs	fiber
710	64g	29g	7g	2g

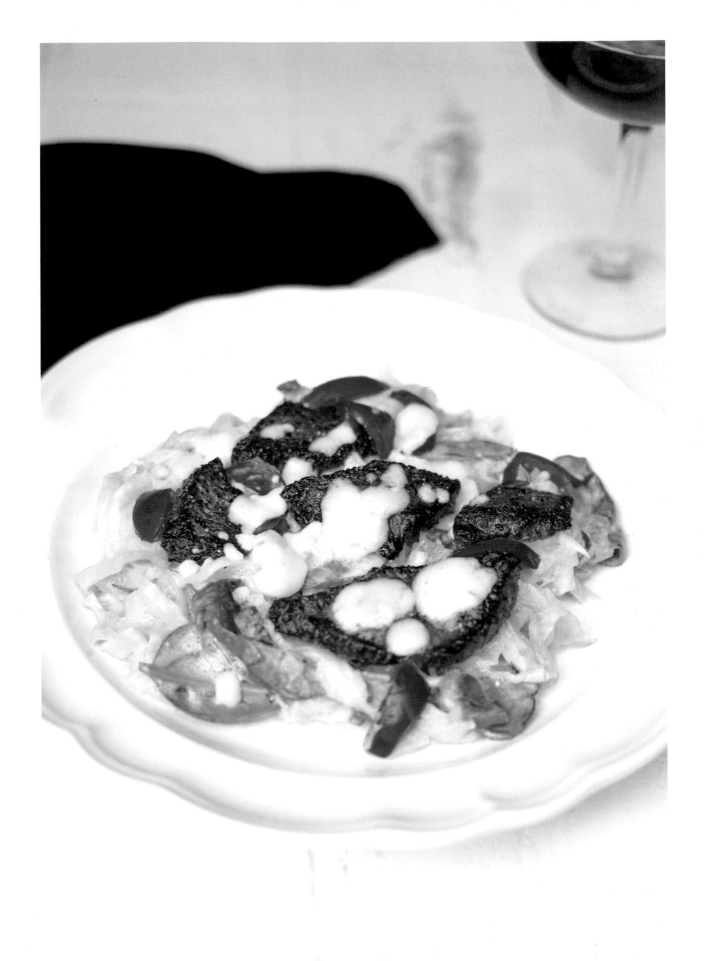

Chicken Piccata

L M H KETO OPTION   **prep time:** 5 minutes   **cook time:** 9 minutes   **yield:** 2 servings

2 boneless, skinless chicken thighs

1 teaspoon Italian seasoning

½ teaspoon fine sea salt

2 tablespoons unsalted butter or coconut oil

½ cup chicken bone broth, homemade (page 356) or store-bought

2 tablespoons fresh lemon juice

2 tablespoons capers, drained

1 lemon, thinly sliced, for garnish

2 tablespoons chopped fresh parsley leaves, for garnish

1. Place the chicken thighs between 2 pieces of parchment paper. Using a cast-iron skillet, rolling pin, or mallet, gently pound the thighs until they are about ¼ inch thick. Remove the parchment and season the chicken on all sides with the Italian seasoning and salt.

2. Heat the butter in a large cast-iron skillet over medium-high heat. Add the chicken and cook for 3 to 5 minutes per side, until golden brown and cooked through. Place the chicken on a platter; leave the drippings in the skillet.

3. Add the broth, lemon juice, and capers to the skillet and deglaze the pan, using a whisk to scrape up the bits from the bottom of the skillet. Bring the sauce to a boil and cook for 4 minutes. Pour the sauce over the chicken. Garnish with lemon slices and parsley.

4. Store in an airtight container in the refrigerator for up to 4 days. To reheat, place in a lightly greased skillet over medium heat for about 3 minutes.

busy family tip: *Ask your butcher to pound the chicken for you.*

NUTRITIONAL INFO (per serving)				
calories	fat	protein	carbs	fiber
299	22g	24g	3g	1g

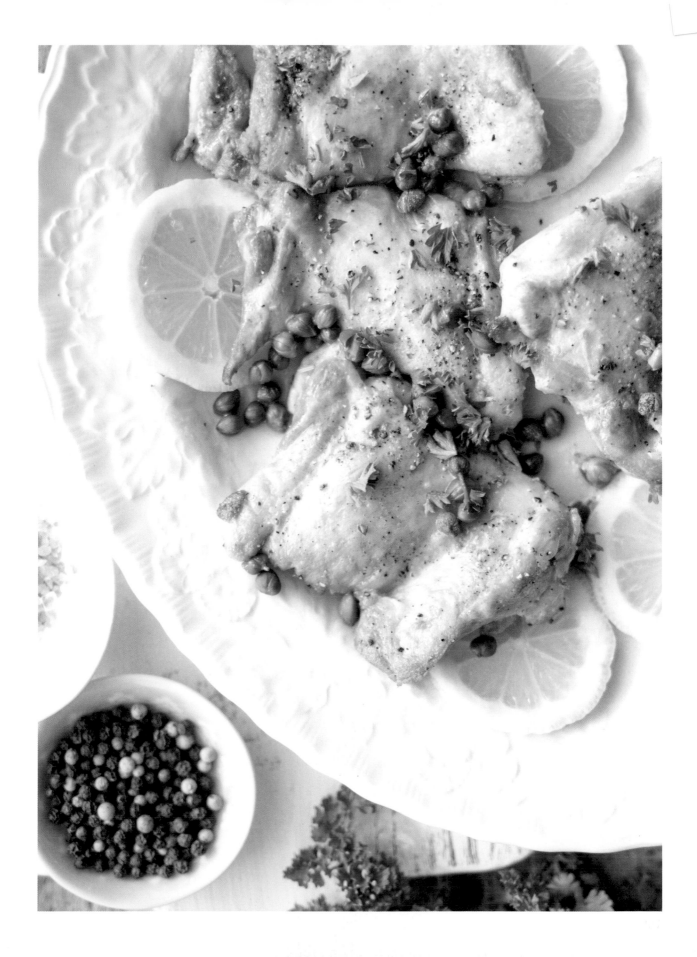

Sugo Bianco

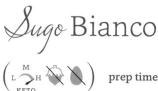

prep time: 5 minutes   cook time: 25 minutes   yield: 8 servings

Sugo bianco, Italian for "white chicken," is a popular dish at restaurants like Romano's Macaroni Grill. It is made with grilled chicken and a white Asiago sauce, and usually served over pasta. Here, it is served over a ketogenic pasta!

¾ cup unsalted butter, divided

⅓ cup chicken bone broth, homemade (page 356) or store-bought

½ cup grated Asiago or Parmesan cheese (about 2 ounces)

2 ounces cream cheese, at room temperature

1 pound boneless, skinless chicken breasts, sliced into ½-inch-thick strips

1 teaspoon fine sea salt

½ teaspoon ground black pepper

½ cup diced red onions (about 1 medium)

4 ounces pancetta or bacon, diced (about ½ cup)

2 large cloves garlic, minced

1 cup heavy cream

¾ cup sliced scallions (about 1 bunch)

1 batch Cabbage Pasta (page 361) or Zoodles (page 360), for serving

1 small tomato, diced

1 tablespoon chopped fresh parsley

1. Make the sauce: Place ½ cup of the butter in a small saucepan over medium-high heat. Cook until light golden brown, stirring constantly to prevent burning, about 4 minutes. Reduce the heat to a simmer and whisk in the broth, Asiago, and cream cheese. Simmer for at least 15 minutes. The longer the sauce simmers, the more the flavors will open up.

2. Meanwhile, heat a grill to high heat. Season the chicken on all sides with the salt and pepper. Grill the chicken for about 5 minutes per side, until browned. Remove from the heat and set aside.

3. Heat the remaining ¼ cup of butter in a large skillet over medium heat. Add the onions and sauté for 2 minutes, until soft. Add the pancetta and garlic and sauté for another 4 minutes, or until the pancetta is crisp. Whisk in the heavy cream to deglaze the pan, scraping up the browned bits from the bottom of the skillet.

4. Add the grilled chicken and scallions to the skillet and cook for 4 minutes, or until the chicken is cooked through. Stir in the cheese sauce until well combined. Serve over cabbage pasta or zoodles. Garnish with diced tomatoes and chopped parsley.

5. Store in an airtight container in the refrigerator for up to 4 days. To reheat, place in a lightly greased skillet over medium heat for about 3 minutes.

NUTRITIONAL INFO (per serving)				
calories	fat	protein	carbs	fiber
513	45g	26g	3g	1g

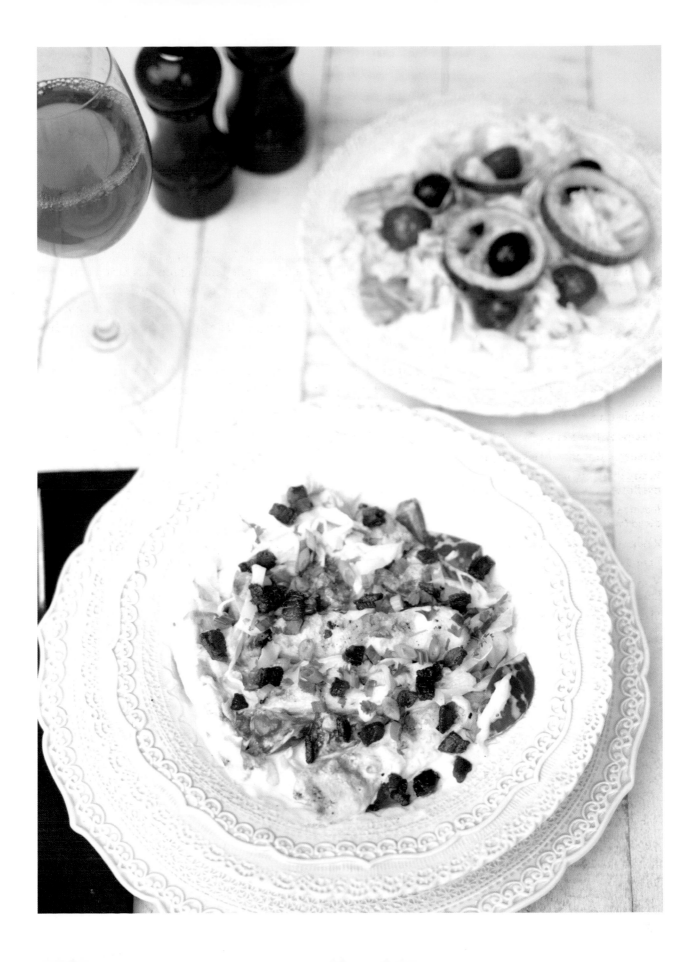

Protein Noodle Lasagna

(L ⟩ H M / KETO) **prep time:** 10 minutes, plus 15 minutes to cool   **cook time:** 50 minutes   **yield:** 8 servings

1 pound bulk Italian sausage

12 ounces ground beef

3 tablespoons chopped onions

2 cloves garlic, minced

4 cups marinara, homemade (page 126) or store-bought

1 pound ricotta cheese

1 large egg

½ teaspoon fine sea salt

16 thin slices deli chicken breast (about 8 ounces)

12 ounces mozzarella cheese, sliced

¾ cup grated Parmesan cheese (about 6 ounces)

1. Preheat the oven to 425°F.

2. Put the sausage, ground beef, onions, and garlic in a Dutch oven over medium heat. Cook until the sausage and beef are well browned, about 5 minutes, stirring often to crumble the meat. Stir in the marinara and remove from the heat.

3. In a medium-sized bowl, combine the ricotta, egg, and salt.

4. To assemble the lasagna, spread 1½ cups of the meat sauce in a 13 by 9-inch baking dish. Arrange half of the chicken slices over the meat sauce. Spread half of the ricotta mixture over the chicken. Top with one-third of the mozzarella. Spoon 1½ cups of the meat sauce over the mozzarella and sprinkle with ¼ cup of the Parmesan. Repeat the layers, using the rest of the meat sauce, chicken, ricotta, mozzarella, and Parmesan.

5. Cover and bake for 25 minutes. Uncover and bake for an additional 25 minutes, until the cheese is melted. Let cool for 15 minutes before serving. Store in an airtight container in the refrigerator for up to 4 days or in the freezer for up to 1 month. To reheat, place in a preheated 375°F oven for about 8 minutes.

tip: *If you use part-skim mozzarella, there will be excess moisture in the dish after baking; you may have to drain some of the moisture.*

NUTRITIONAL INFO (per serving)				
calories	fat	protein	carbs	fiber
561	42g	42g	4g	0.3g

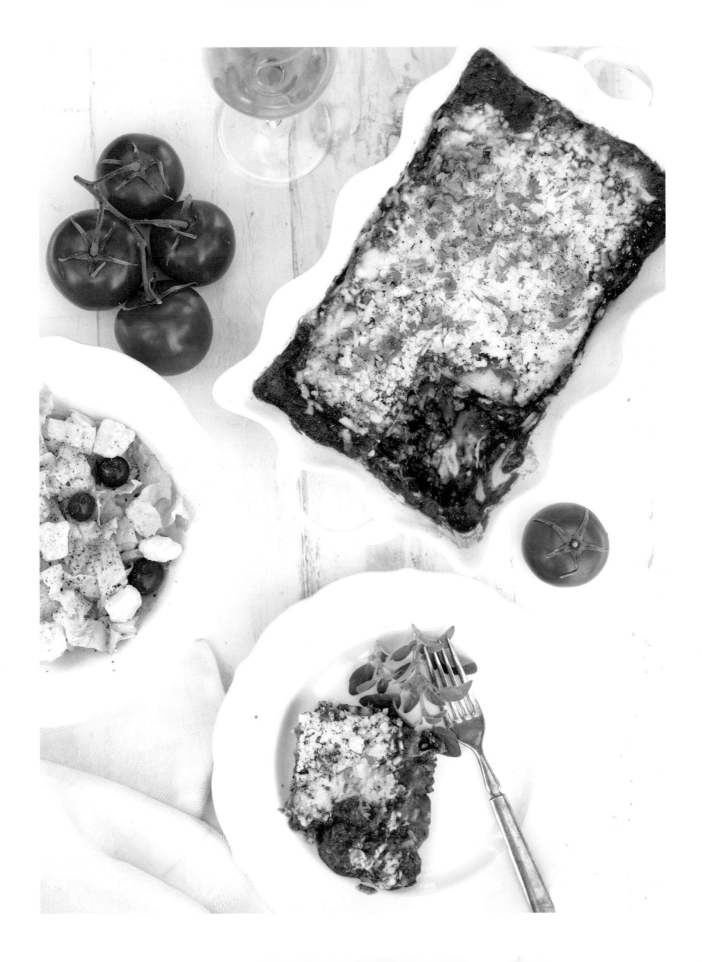

Chicken Milanese

(L—H KETO M) **prep time:** 10 minutes (not including time to make dressing)   **cook time:** 4 minutes
yield: 4 servings

4 boneless, skinless chicken thighs

1 teaspoon fine sea salt

1 teaspoon ground black pepper

2 large eggs

½ cup powdered Parmesan cheese (see page 363)

2 teaspoons Italian seasoning

3 tablespoons avocado oil or coconut oil, for frying

2 cups coarsely chopped leaf lettuce

1 tomato, diced

¼ cup Italian Dressing (page 124)

1 lemon, quartered

1. Preheat the oven to 400°F.

2. Place the chicken thighs between 2 pieces of parchment paper. Using a cast-iron skillet, rolling pin, or mallet, gently pound the thighs until they are about ¼ inch thick. Season the chicken on both sides with the salt and pepper.

3. Crack the eggs into a shallow baking dish, add 1 tablespoon of water, and stir well to combine. Place the powdered Parmesan and Italian seasoning in another shallow baking dish and stir to combine.

4. Dip each chicken thigh in the eggs just to coat, then dip both sides of the chicken in the Parmesan mixture.

5. Heat the oil in a large cast-iron skillet over medium-high heat. When the oil is hot, sear each thigh until golden brown, 2 to 3 minutes per side, or until the chicken is cooked through.

6. Meanwhile, make the salad: Place the lettuce and tomatoes in a medium-sized bowl, drizzle with the dressing, and toss to combine.

7. Place the fried chicken thighs on 4 serving plates and divide the salad among the plates. Squirt some lemon juice over each piece of chicken and salad. Store in separate airtight containers in the refrigerator for up to 4 days. To reheat the chicken, place in a lightly greased skillet over medium heat for about 3 minutes.

busy family tip: *Ask your butcher to pound the chicken for you.*

NUTRITIONAL INFO (per serving)				
calories	fat	protein	carbs	fiber
480	36g	38g	3g	1g

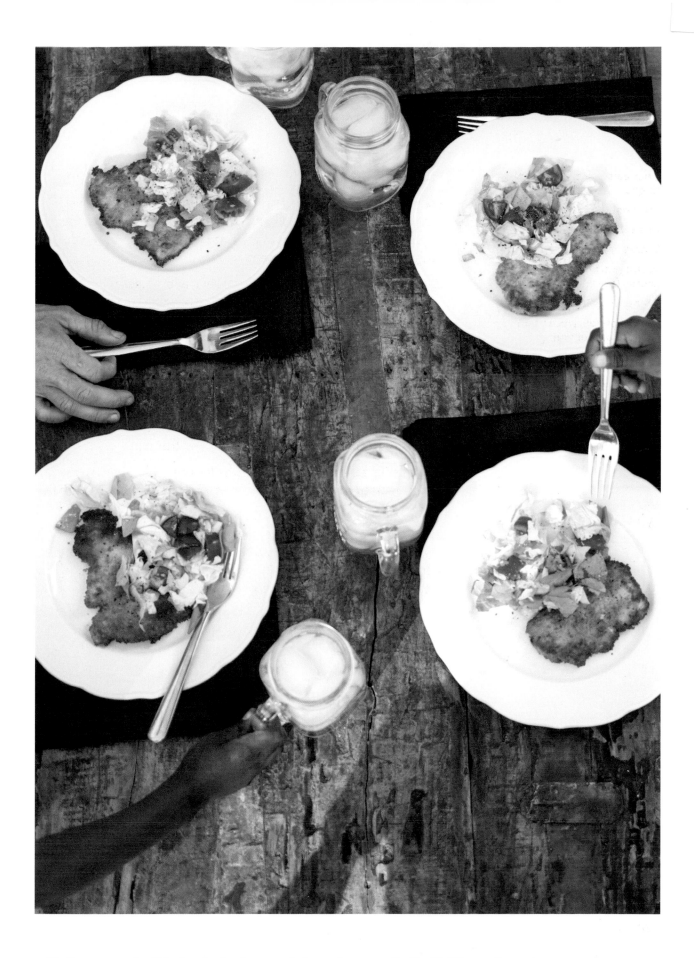

Chicken Cacciatore

$\left(\begin{smallmatrix} & M & \\ L & \curvearrowright & H \\ & KETO & \end{smallmatrix} \right.$ 🧂 🚫 🚫 $\left. \right)$ **prep time:** 7 minutes   **cook time:** about 1 hour   **yield:** 6 servings

I love this dish not only for the intense flavors but also because the Italian word *caccia-tore* means "hunter." I grew up bowhunting and still love it to this day. This flavorful dish is typically made with tomatoes, bell peppers, onions, and plenty of herbs. It also can include wine, but since I am not an advocate of consuming alcohol, this version leaves out the wine.

6 bone-in, skin-on chicken thighs

2 teaspoons fine sea salt

1 teaspoon ground black pepper

3 tablespoons avocado oil, coconut oil, or lard, for frying

1 pound button mushrooms, sliced

¼ cup diced onions (about 1 small)

¼ cup diced red bell peppers

3 cloves garlic

1 (28-ounce) can crushed tomatoes

1 cup chicken bone broth, homemade (page 356) or store-bought

2 tablespoons chopped fresh basil leaves, or 1 teaspoon dried basil

2 tablespoons chopped fresh oregano leaves, or 1 teaspoon dried

Capers, drained, for garnish

Chopped fresh thyme leaves, for garnish

1. Preheat the oven to 350°F.

2. Pat the chicken dry and season well on both sides with the salt and pepper. Heat the oil in a Dutch oven or large cast-iron skillet over medium heat. Place the chicken in the pot and sear until golden brown on both sides, about 4 minutes per side. Remove the chicken from the pot and set aside.

3. Place the mushrooms, onions, bell peppers, and garlic in the pot and sauté for 5 minutes, or until the onions are translucent. Add the tomatoes, broth, basil, and oregano, bring to a light boil, and boil, stirring occasionally, for 10 minutes, until the sauce has reduced and thickened a bit.

4. Return the chicken to the pot. Cover, transfer the pot to the oven, and bake for 45 minutes. Remove from the oven and serve garnished with capers and thyme. Store in an airtight container in the refrigerator for up to 4 days. To reheat, place in a lightly greased skillet over medium heat for about 3 minutes.

NUTRITIONAL INFO (per serving)				
calories	fat	protein	carbs	fiber
275	18g	20g	10g	2g

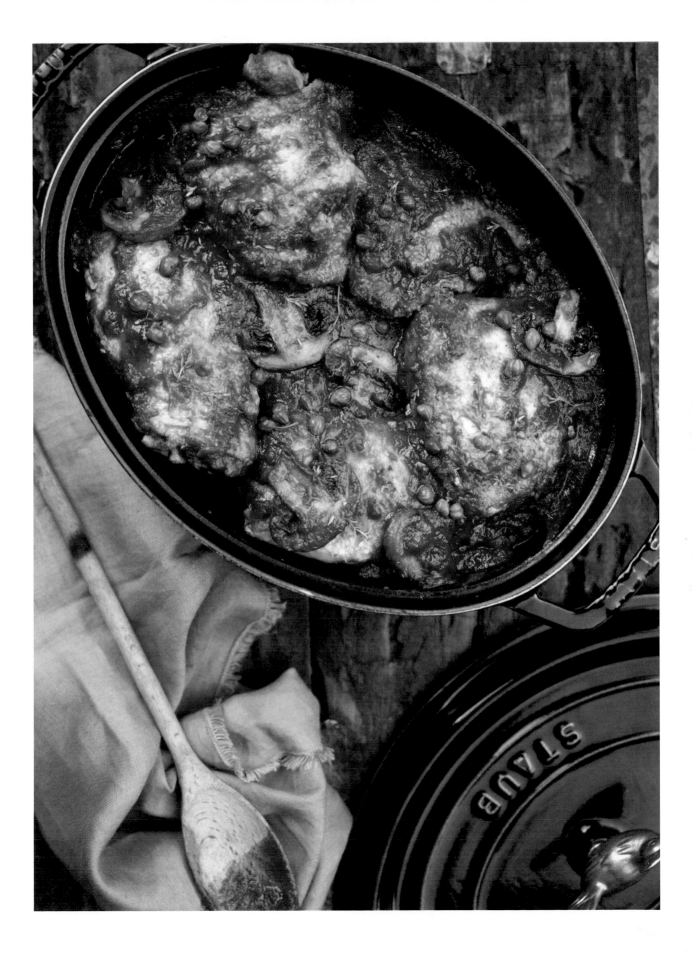

Shrimp Portofino

prep time: 5 minutes (not including time to make cabbage pasta)
cook time: 12 minutes   **yield:** 4 servings

This recipe was inspired by Romano's Macaroni Grill's Grilled Shrimp Portofino dish. If you miss a tasty, buttery shrimp pasta, you must try this keto version!

3 tablespoons unsalted butter or ghee (or avocado oil if dairy-free)

1 cup white mushrooms, sliced (about 8 ounces)

4 large cloves garlic, finely chopped

20 large shrimp, peeled, deveined, and tails removed

2 teaspoons fine sea salt

1½ teaspoons ground black pepper

3 cups fresh spinach

½ cup fresh lemon juice (2 to 3 lemons)

½ cup chicken bone broth, homemade (page 356) or store-bought

2 cups heavy cream (or 1¼ cups chicken bone broth blended with ¾ cup Kite Hill brand cream cheese style spread if dairy-free)

1 batch Cabbage Pasta (page 361) or Zoodles (page 360), for serving

1. Heat the butter in a large cast-iron skillet over medium heat. Add the mushrooms and garlic and sauté for 4 minutes, or until the mushrooms are golden brown. Add the shrimp, season with the salt and pepper, and sauté for 4 minutes, or until the shrimp turns pink. Add the spinach, lemon juice, and broth, stir, and cook for 1 minute, or until the spinach has just wilted.

2. Stir in the heavy cream, increase the heat to medium-high, and simmer, stirring frequently, for 3 minutes. Remove from the heat, add the cabbage pasta, and stir until the cabbage is hot and all the ingredients are well mixed.

3. Store in an airtight container in the refrigerator for up to 4 days. To reheat, place in a lightly greased skillet over medium heat for about 3 minutes, stirring occasionally.

NUTRITIONAL INFO (per serving)				
calories	fat	protein	carbs	fiber
587	58g	17g	7g	2g

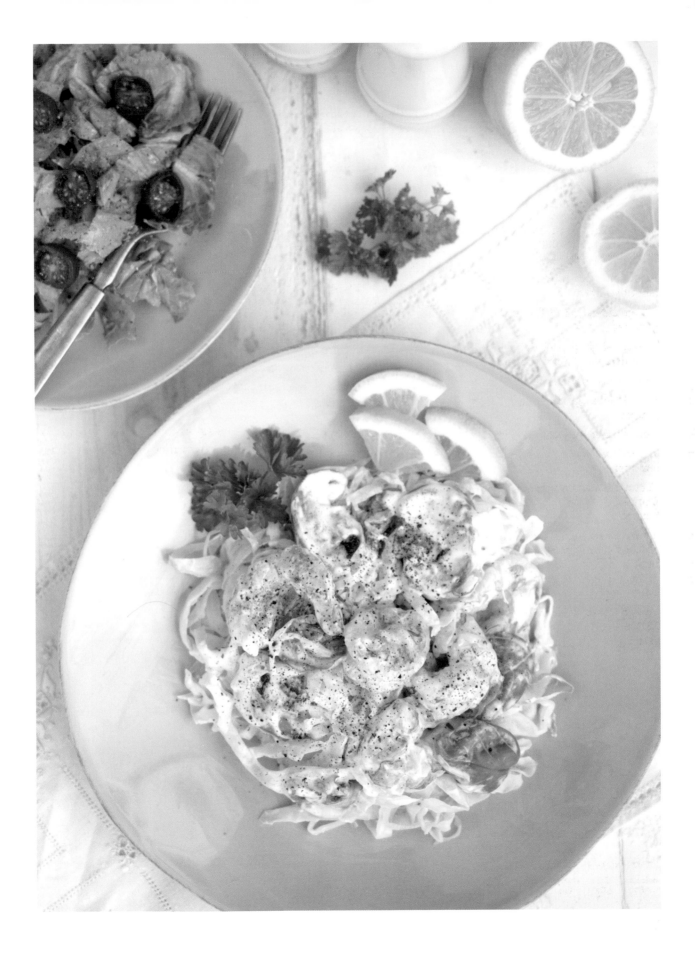

Toscana Paglia e Fieno

prep time: 5 minutes (not including time to make cabbage pasta)
cook time: 9 minutes   yield: 4 servings

I often ordered this fantastic Italian dish when Craig and I first started dating. *Paglia e fieno* translates to "straw and hay" and refers to the two pastas, a yellow one made with eggs and a green one made with spinach, traditionally used in this dish. A cream sauce is the typical topping. Here, cabbage pasta stands in for the "straw" and vibrant green asparagus for the "hay." Green peas are traditionally included as well, but because peas are a starch, I let the asparagus provide that fresh flavor of spring. You will never miss the peas!

¼ cup diced asparagus (about 4 spears)

1 cup heavy cream

2 tablespoons unsalted butter

½ cup diced cooked ham

1 batch Cabbage Pasta (page 361)

½ cup grated Parmesan cheese (about 2 ounces)

2 large egg yolks, lightly beaten

1. Bring a small saucepan of water to a boil. Add the asparagus and cook for 2 minutes. Drain and rinse under cold running water to preserve the green color.

2. In a large saucepan, combine the heavy cream, butter, ham, and asparagus. Cook until the butter is melted, about 1 minute. Stir in the cabbage pasta. Cook for 4 minutes, or until the cabbage is well coated. Stir in the Parmesan cheese and egg yolks and cook for 1 minute more, or until the sauce has thickened a bit. Serve immediately.

3. Store in an airtight container in the refrigerator for up to 4 days. To reheat, place in a lightly greased skillet over medium heat for about 3 minutes.

NUTRITIONAL INFO (per serving)				
calories	fat	protein	carbs	fiber
408	39g	13g	6g	2g

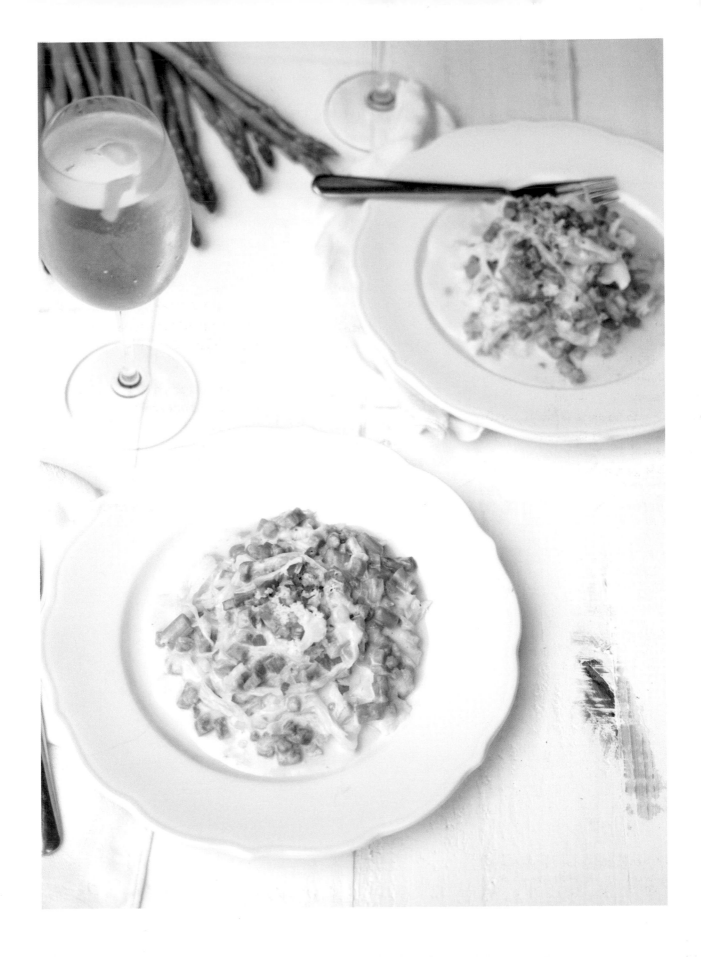

Salmon Sorrento

L M H KETO OPTION · prep time: 7 minutes · cook time: about 20 minutes · yield: 4 servings

As soon as you walk into Buca di Beppo, a fun Italian chain restaurant, the smell of garlic and the sound of classic Frank Sinatra tunes immediately hit your senses. One of their classic entrées is Salmon Sorrento, which is prepared with lemon, garlic, and capers. If you miss eating out at your favorite Italian restaurant, break out the garlic and crank up the Sinatra at home!

3 tablespoons avocado oil (replace 1 tablespoon with unsalted butter if not dairy-sensitive)

3 cloves garlic, minced

1¼ cups diced fresh or canned tomatoes

¼ cup fresh lemon juice

2 tablespoons capers, rinsed and drained

1 tablespoon chopped fresh parsley leaves, plus extra for garnish

¼ teaspoon ground black pepper

4 (6-ounce) skinless salmon fillets

1 teaspoon fine sea salt

1. Heat the oil in a large cast-iron skillet over medium-high heat. Add the garlic and sauté for 1 minute, until fragrant. Add the tomatoes, lemon juice, capers, parsley, and pepper. Cook for 5 minutes, stirring often, until the liquid has reduced a bit.

2. While the sauce is simmering, rinse the salmon and pat dry with paper towels. Season on all sides with the salt. Reduce the heat to medium. Use a spatula to push the sauce to one side and place the salmon in the skillet. Spoon the sauce over the salmon.

3. Cover the skillet and cook for 15 minutes, or until the salmon flakes easily with a fork. The exact timing will depend on the thickness of the fillets. Remove from the skillet and place on a platter. Serve with the sauce and garnish with parsley. Store in an airtight container in the refrigerator for up to 4 days. To reheat, place in a lightly greased skillet over medium heat for about 3 minutes.

NUTRITIONAL INFO (per serving)				
calories	fat	protein	carbs	fiber
309	16g	34g	5g	1g

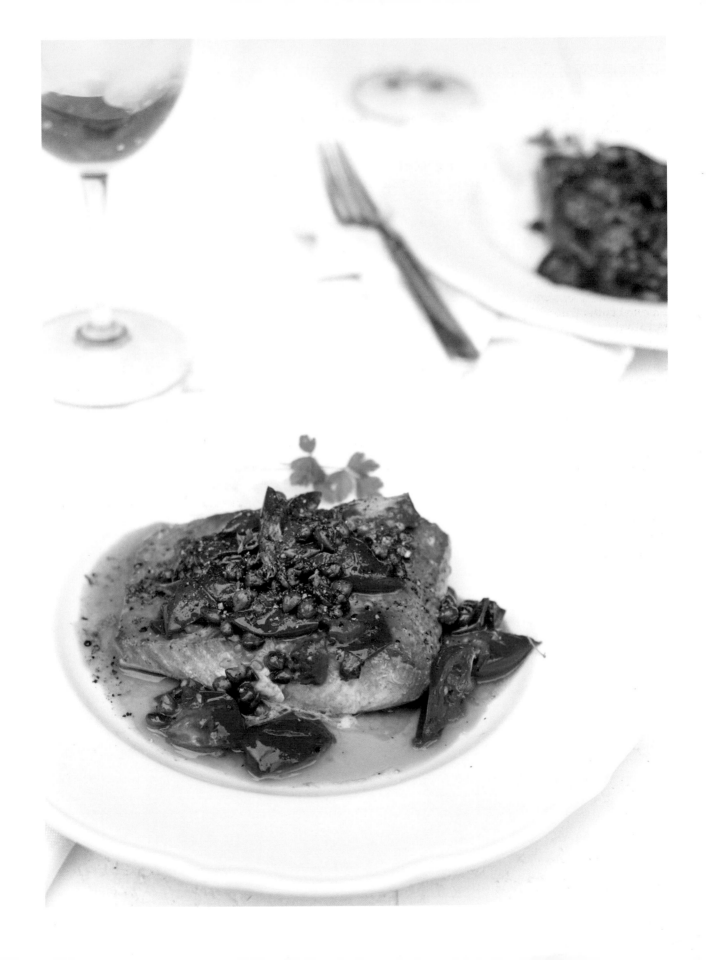

Prosciutto – Stuffed Chicken

 prep time: 15 minutes   cook time: 30 minutes   yield: 4 servings

Buca di Beppo serves a stuffed chicken dish that is to die for! The chicken is stuffed with mozzarella and prosciutto and served with homemade marinara and pesto cream sauces. I think my ketogenic version is even better.

4 boneless, skinless chicken thighs

4 thin slices prosciutto

4 (1-ounce) slices mozzarella or fontina cheese

1 tablespoon plus 1 teaspoon Dijon mustard

1 cup powdered Parmesan cheese or pork dust (see page 363)

—creamy pesto

2 cups loosely packed fresh basil leaves

¼ cup walnuts or pine nuts

2 tablespoons fresh lemon juice

1 clove garlic, minced

1 teaspoon fine sea salt

½ teaspoon ground black pepper

½ cup avocado oil or extra-virgin olive oil

¼ cup heavy cream

1 cup marinara, homemade (page 126) or store-bought, warmed, for serving

Fresh basil leaves, for garnish

Grated Parmesan cheese, for garnish

1. Preheat the oven to 375°F.

2. Place the chicken thighs between 2 pieces of parchment paper. Using a cast-iron skillet, rolling pin, or mallet, gently pound the thighs until they are about ¼ inch thick.

3. Remove the top piece of parchment and place a slice of prosciutto on the chicken. Top the prosciutto with a slice of mozzarella. Roll up the chicken tightly and use toothpicks to secure the ends. Spread a thin layer of mustard over the chicken and sprinkle with the Parmesan. Repeat with the remaining chicken, prosciutto, mozzarella, mustard, and Parmesan.

4. Place the stuffed chicken on a rimmed baking sheet. Bake for 27 to 30 minutes, until the chicken is cooked through.

5. Meanwhile, make the pesto: Place the basil, walnuts, lemon juice, garlic, salt, and pepper in a food processor or blender and puree until smooth. Add the oil slowly with the food processor or blender running on low speed, scraping down the sides occasionally. Once the oil is well blended, slowly add the cream. Taste and add more salt or lemon juice, if desired. Divide the pesto among 4 plates.

6. Place a stuffed chicken thigh on top of the pesto on each plate. Dollop ¼ cup of marinara onto each chicken thigh and garnish with basil and Parmesan cheese. Store in an airtight container in the refrigerator for up to 4 days. To reheat, place on a rimmed baking sheet in a preheated 350°F oven for about 3 minutes.

busy family tip: *Ask your butcher to pound the chicken for you.*

NUTRITIONAL INFO (per serving)				
calories	fat	protein	carbs	fiber
755	64g	45g	3g	1g

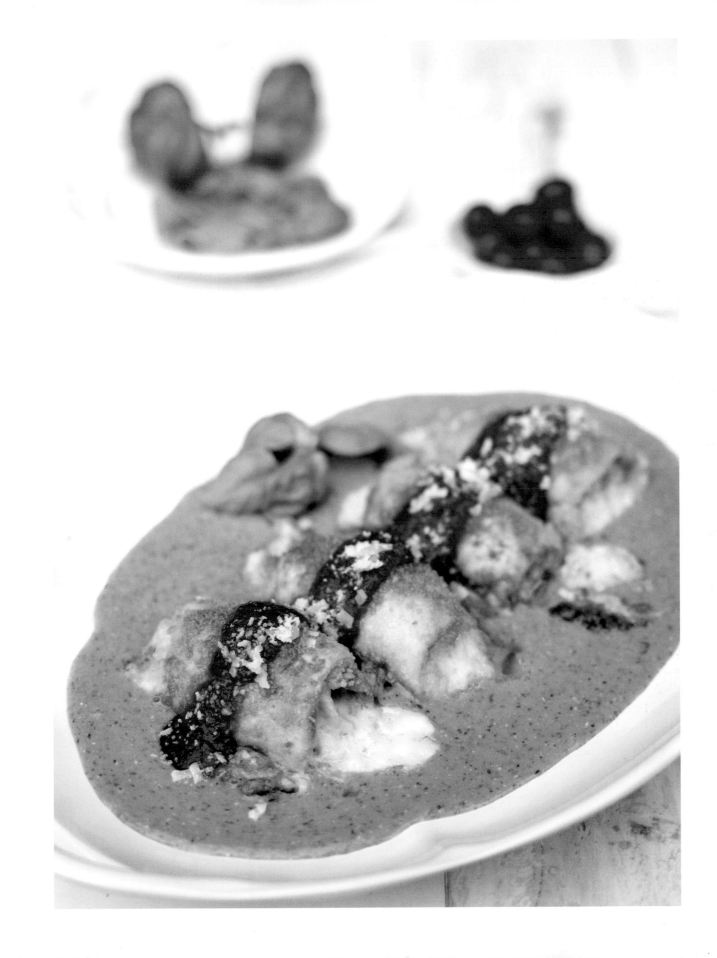

Chicken Scarpariello

prep time: 10 minutes   cook time: 30 minutes   yield: 4 servings

2 tablespoons coconut oil or ghee

2 Italian sausages, cut into 1-inch pieces

4 bone-in, skin-on chicken thighs

1½ teaspoons fine sea salt, divided

¾ teaspoon ground black pepper, divided

1 cup sliced mushrooms (about 8 ounces)

4 jarred cherry peppers, sliced in half

½ red bell pepper, cut into 1-inch strips

1 small onion, sliced

4 cloves garlic, minced

¾ cup chicken bone broth, homemade (page 356) or store-bought

1 tablespoon fresh lemon juice

2 teaspoons dried oregano leaves

Chopped fresh basil, for garnish

Chopped fresh parsley, for garnish

1. Preheat the oven to 400°F.

2. Heat the oil in a Dutch oven over medium heat. Add the sausage pieces and cook for 3 minutes, or until seared on both sides. Transfer the sausage to a plate, leaving the drippings in the pot.

3. Pat the chicken thighs dry and season well with 1 teaspoon of the salt and ½ teaspoon of the black pepper. Increase the heat to medium-high, add the chicken, skin side down, and cook for 3 minutes per side, or until the chicken is seared. Remove the chicken and set aside, leaving the drippings in the pot.

4. Add the mushrooms to the pot and sauté for 3 minutes, or until golden brown.

5. Add the cherry peppers, bell pepper, and onion and sauté for 4 minutes, or until the onion is translucent. Add the garlic and sauté for another minute. Stir in the broth, lemon juice, oregano, the remaining ½ teaspoon of salt, and the remaining ¼ teaspoon of black pepper until well combined.

6. Place the chicken and sausage on top of the vegetables. Transfer the Dutch oven to the oven and bake, uncovered, for 25 minutes, or until the chicken is cooked through. Serve garnished with basil and parsley.

7. Store in an airtight container in the refrigerator for up to 4 days. To reheat, place in a lightly greased skillet over medium heat for about 3 minutes.

NUTRITIONAL INFO (per serving)				
calories	fat	protein	carbs	fiber
353	25g	24g	8g	2g

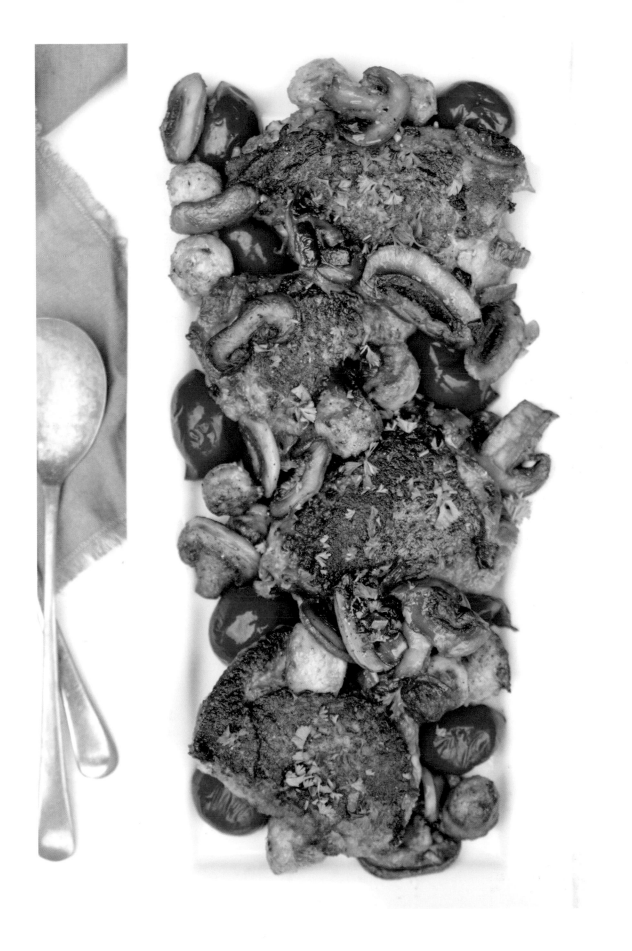

Pasta Carbonara

(L—M—H 🚫 KETO)   **prep time:** 6 minutes   **cook time:** 10 minutes   **yield:** 4 servings

4 strips bacon, diced

4 cups thinly shredded green cabbage (about 1 pound)

¼ cup chopped onions (about 1 small)

1 clove garlic, minced

4 large egg yolks, lightly beaten

¼ cup grated Parmesan cheese (about 1 ounce), plus extra for garnish

Fine sea salt and ground black pepper

2 tablespoons chopped fresh parsley leaves, for garnish

1. Place the bacon in a medium-sized cast-iron skillet over medium-high heat. Cook for 3 minutes, or until the bacon is crisp. Remove the bacon, leaving the fat in the skillet. Add the cabbage, onions, and garlic, reduce the heat to medium, and cook until the cabbage is very soft, about 8 minutes. Return the bacon to the skillet.

2. Add the eggs and cook, stirring constantly with tongs or a large fork, until the eggs are barely set, about 2 minutes. Stir in the Parmesan cheese until well combined. Season with salt and pepper to taste. Garnish with additional Parmesan and the parsley. Store in an airtight container in the refrigerator for up to 4 days. To reheat, place in a lightly greased skillet over medium heat for about 3 minutes.

NUTRITIONAL INFO (per serving)				
calories	fat	protein	carbs	fiber
207	13g	15g	8g	3g

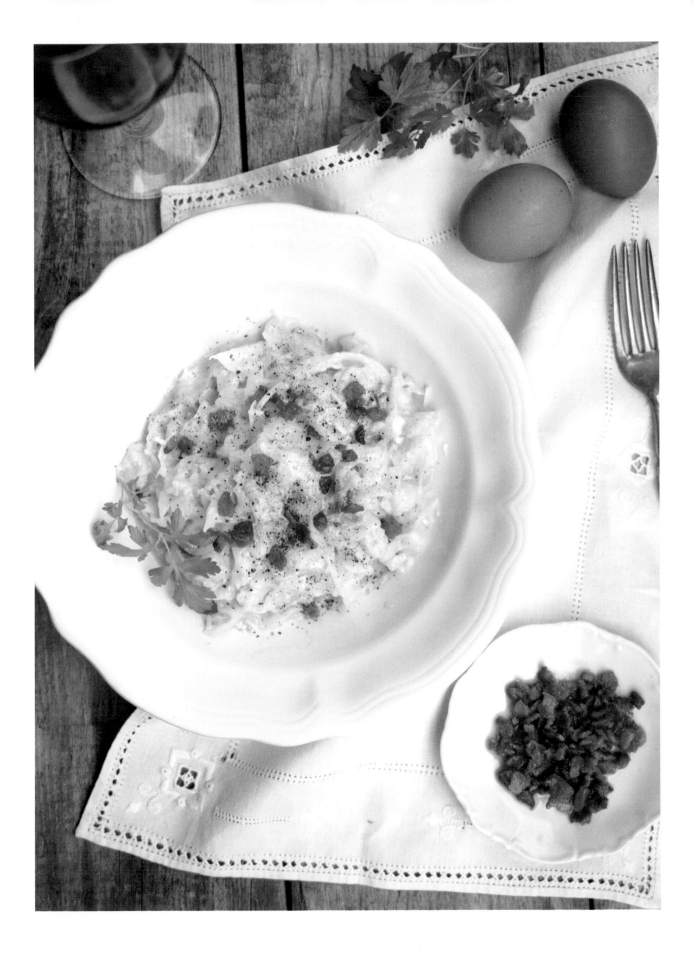

Craig's Special Pizza

$$\left(\begin{smallmatrix} & M & \\ L & \circlearrowright & H \\ & \text{KETO} & \end{smallmatrix}\right)$$ **prep time:** 10 minutes, plus 1 hour to chill the dough if needed (not including time to make pizza sauce) **cook time:** 10 minutes **yield:** 4 servings

Craig and I had the opportunity to visit Germany together when he took a trip there for work. We went out to a restaurant and ordered pepperoni pizza (yeah, we were typical Americans at the time . . . I was only twenty!). The waiter came out with a piece of pepperoni and a hot pepper. He pointed to the pepper and said, "This is pepperoni pizza; are you sure you want this?"

I call this dish Craig's Special because Craig always has to have bacon on his pizza! Even in Hawaii, where we were surrounded by fresh fish, Craig wanted me to make pizza with bacon. Of course, you can use any toppings you like and make this your own "special."

This recipe may seem daunting, but you can make multiple batches of the dough and store it in airtight containers in the freezer for up to 2 months. You can also bake the pizza and freeze it for later, although it is much better fresh!

—pizza dough

1¾ cups shredded mozzarella cheese (about 7 ounces)

2 tablespoons unsalted butter

1 large egg

¾ cup blanched almond flour

⅛ teaspoon fine sea salt

—toppings

½ cup Mama Maria's Pizza Sauce (page 128)

1 cup diced cooked bacon

½ cup diced fresh tomatoes

½ cup sliced olives

¼ cup shredded mozzarella cheese (about 1 ounce)

¼ cup shredded Parmesan cheese (about 1 ounce)

—for garnish

Fresh basil leaves

Crushed red pepper

1. Place a pizza stone in the oven and preheat the oven to 425°F. (You can use a baking sheet, but a pizza stone will bake the bottom better.) Grease a piece of parchment paper.

2. Make the dough: Place the mozzarella and butter in a medium-sized heatproof bowl and microwave for 1 to 2 minutes, until the cheese is entirely melted. Stir well.

3. Add the egg and mix with your hands or a hand mixer on medium speed until well combined. Add the almond flour and salt and combine well with the butter. Use your hands and work it like a traditional dough, kneading for about 3 minutes. If the dough is too sticky, chill in the refrigerator for 1 hour or overnight.

4. Place the dough on the greased parchment and pat it out with your hands to form a large circle (about 10 inches in diameter) or oval (about 12 inches long). Spread the pizza sauce over the dough, then add the toppings. Slide the pizza on the parchment onto the hot pizza stone.

5. Bake for 10 minutes, or until the crust is golden brown and fully cooked. Remove from the oven and garnish with basil and crushed red pepper. Store in an airtight container in the refrigerator for up to 4 days. To reheat, place on a rimmed baking sheet in a preheated 400°F oven or toaster oven for about 5 minutes.

NUTRITIONAL INFO (per serving)				
calories	fat	protein	carbs	fiber
425	36g	23g	8g	3g

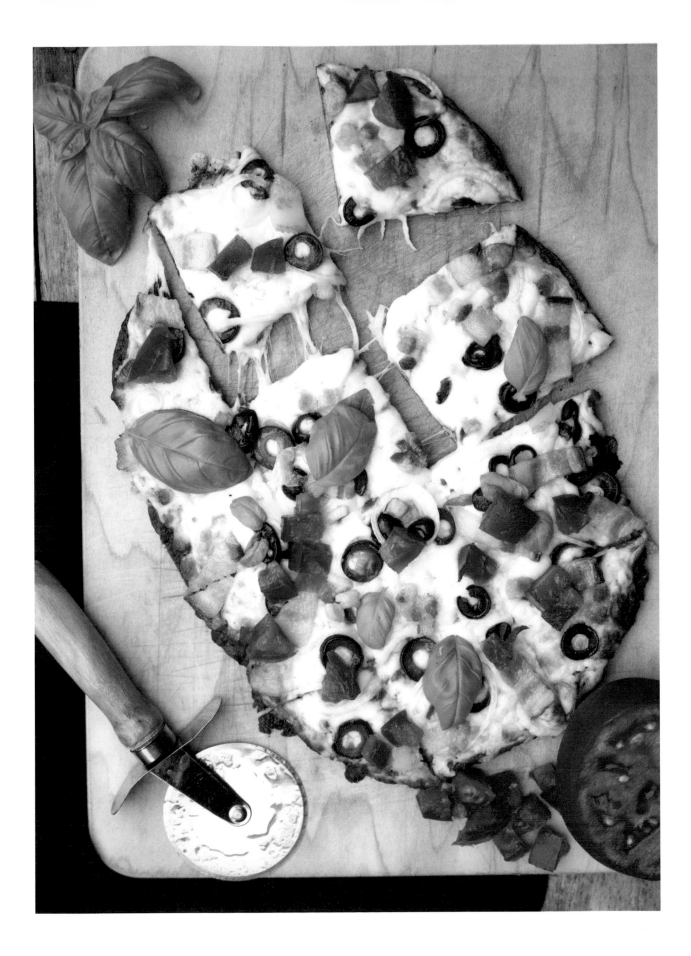

Calzones

(L M > H KETO) prep time: 8 minutes, plus 1 hour to chill the dough if needed   cook time: 10 minutes   yield: 4 servings

I remember visiting my Grandma Rosemary in Connecticut when I was sixteen. Just before I traveled, my aunt had me watch a movie called *Mystic Pizza,* which was one of Julia Roberts' first movie roles. Grandma took me to Mystic, Connecticut, just to eat at the restaurant depicted in the movie. I had my first calzone that day. It was dense and chewy, but more than anything, I remember how beautiful the ocean was.

1 batch pizza dough (from Craig's Special Pizza, page 182)

—fillings

1½ cups shredded mozzarella cheese (about 6 ounces)

½ cup diced marinated red peppers

½ cup sliced black olives

1 cup fresh basil leaves

Marinara, homemade (page 126) or store-bought, for serving

1. Place a pizza stone in the oven and preheat the oven to 425°F. (You can use a baking sheet, but a pizza stone will bake the bottom better.) Grease a piece of parchment paper.

2. Place one-quarter of the dough on the parchment and pat it out with your hands to form a small circle (about 4 inches in diameter). Repeat with the remaining dough to make a total of 4 circles. Place one-quarter of the fillings in the center of each circle. Fold each circle in half and pinch the edges with your fingers to seal. Slide the calzones on the parchment onto the hot pizza stone.

3. Bake for 10 minutes, or until the crust is golden brown and fully cooked. Serve with marinara. Store in an airtight container in the refrigerator for up to 4 days. To reheat, place on a rimmed baking sheet in a preheated 400°F oven or toaster oven for about 5 minutes.

NUTRITIONAL INFO (per serving)				
calories	fat	protein	carbs	fiber
412	34g	26g	6g	3g

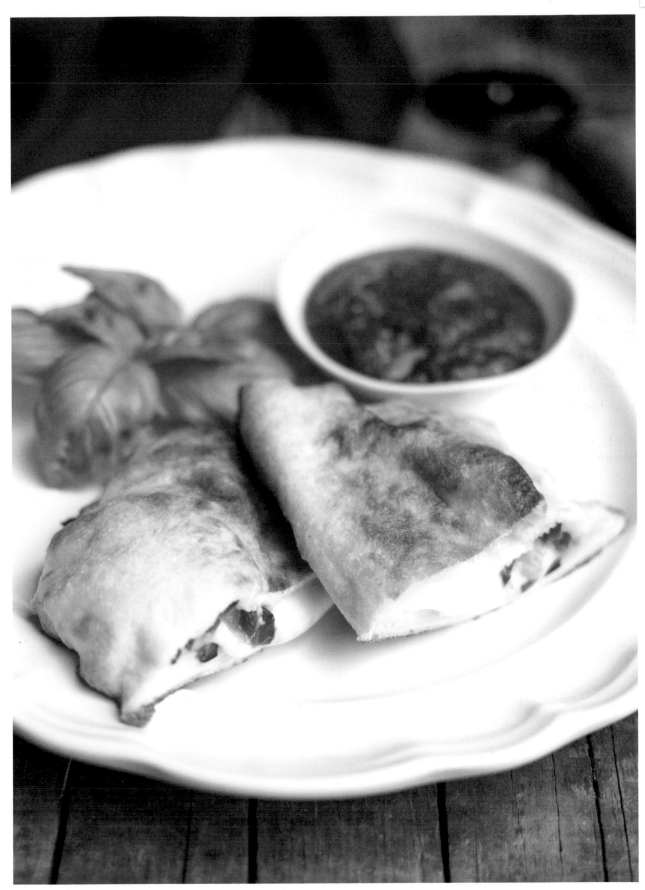

Deconstructed Chicken Parm Pizza

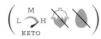

prep time: 5 minutes (not including time to make pizza sauce)   **cook time:** 19 minutes
yield: 4 servings

—crust

1 pound ground chicken

½ teaspoon fine sea salt

2 cups powdered Parmesan cheese (see page 363)

—toppings

½ cup Mama Maria's Pizza Sauce (page 128) or Mama Maria's Marinara (page 126)

1 (8-ounce) ball fresh mozzarella, thinly sliced

¼ cup fresh basil leaves, for garnish

1. Place a pizza stone in the oven and preheat the oven to 425°F. (You can use a baking sheet, but a pizza stone will bake the bottom better.)

2. Place the ground chicken in a large bowl. Add the salt and Parmesan and use your hands to combine well.

3. Grease a sheet of parchment paper and set it on an unrimmed baking sheet or pizza peel for easy transfer to the oven. Place the crust mixture on the parchment and use your hands to form it into a 12-inch circle or 10-inch square. Slide the piece of parchment with the crust onto the hot pizza stone in the oven. Bake for 12 to 15 minutes, until the crust is turning light golden brown and the chicken is cooked through.

4. Meanwhile, prepare your desired toppings.

5. Remove the crust from the oven and top with sauce and mozzarella slices. Place back in the oven for 7 minutes or until the cheese is melted. Serve garnished with fresh basil.

variation: chicken alfredo pizza. *Complete Steps 1 through 3. Spread ½ cup Alfredo Sauce (page 125) over the baked crust. Top with ¼ cup chopped basil leaves, 3 sliced cherry tomatoes, and ½ cup shredded mozzarella. Return to the oven and bake for 4 minutes, or until the cheese is melted. Garnish with ½ teaspoon crushed red pepper before serving.*

variation: taco pizza. *Complete Steps 1 through 3. While the crust is baking, place ½ cup (2 ounces) ground beef in a cast-iron skillet over medium heat. Season with ½ teaspoon chili powder, ½ teaspoon ground cumin, ½ teaspoon fine sea salt, and ½ teaspoon ground black pepper. Cook, while crumbling, until the beef is cooked through. Spread ½ cup Easy Blender Enchilada Sauce (page 196) or store-bought sugar-free salsa over the baked crust. Top the sauce with the cooked ground beef, ½ cup shredded cheddar cheese, and ¼ cup sliced black olives. Bake for 7 minutes, or until the cheese is melted. Garnish with ½ cup shredded romaine lettuce and 4 quartered cherry tomatoes before serving.*

NUTRITIONAL INFO (per serving)				
calories	fat	protein	carbs	fiber
651	43g	68g	2g	0.3g

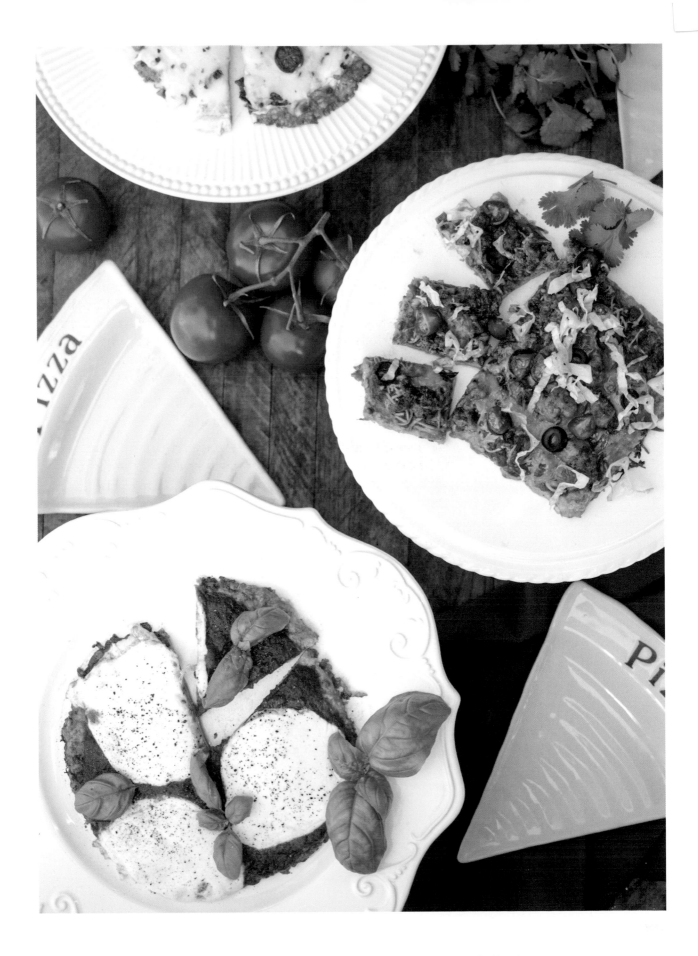

Keto Cannoli

(L →M H KETO) 🌰 prep time: 10 minutes, plus 1 hour to chill the filling   cook time: 20 minutes
yield: 6 cannoli (1 per serving)

Cannoli is usually garnished with chopped pistachios on the ends, but because pistachios are high in starch, I suggest using pili nuts instead, which have only 1 gram of carbohydrate per serving. Or you are welcome to use crushed macadamia nuts.

6 strips bacon

—filling

1 cup heavy cream, very cold

4 ounces mascarpone cheese, at room temperature

¼ cup Swerve confectioners'-style sweetener or equivalent amount of liquid or powdered sweetener (see page 31)

½ teaspoon almond extract or pistachio extract

Chopped pili nuts or macadamia nuts, for garnish

—special equipment

6 cannoli tubes (1 inch in diameter and 3 inches long)

1. Preheat the oven to 375°F. Line a rimmed baking sheet with parchment paper.

2. Tightly wrap 1 strip of bacon around each cannoli tube, overlapping the edges so the bacon totally covers the tube. Bake for 20 minutes, or until the bacon is crisp. Remove from the oven and allow to cool completely on the cannoli tubes.

3. Make the filling: Using a hand mixer, whip the heavy cream until soft peaks form. Fold in the mascarpone, sweetener, and extract. Place the filling in an airtight container and refrigerate for 1 hour before using.

4. Carefully wiggle the bacon to release it from the cannoli tubes while maintaining its shape.

5. Assemble the cannoli: Place the filling in a pastry bag or in a zip-top bag with a corner cut off. Fill each cannoli, leaving some extra filling sticking out of each end. Sprinkle the ends with pili nuts and enjoy! These are best served fresh so the bacon is crisp, but extras can be stored in an airtight container in the refrigerator for up to 4 days.

busy family tip: *The cannoli filling can be made up to 1 week ahead and stored in an airtight container in the refrigerator.*

NUTRITIONAL INFO (per serving)				
calories	fat	protein	carbs	fiber
288	31g	2g	0g	0g

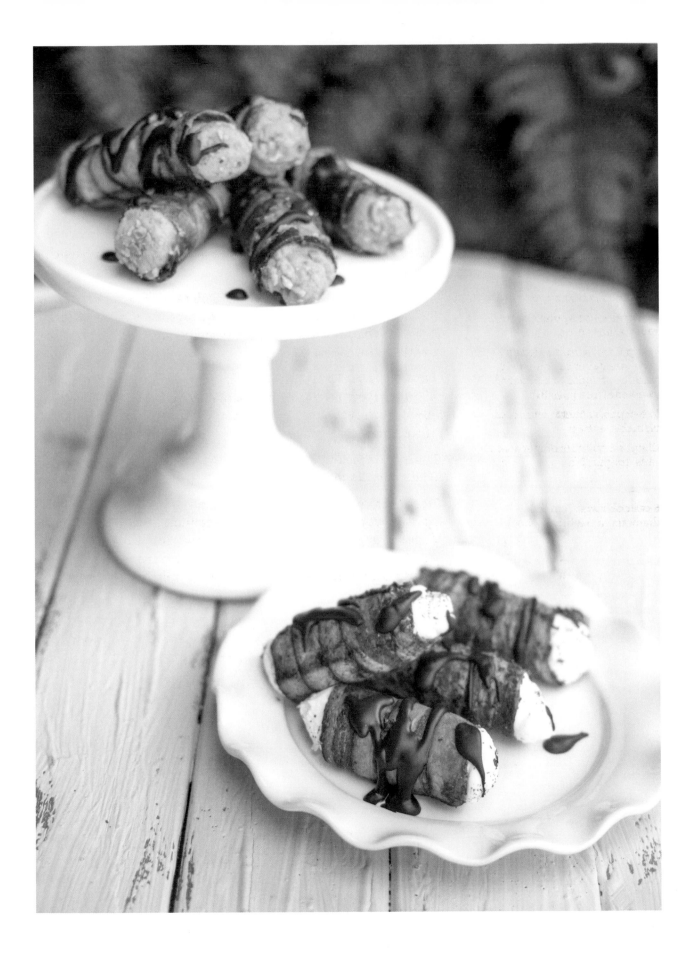

Dessert Pizza

(L $\circlearrowright$ H) — M / KETO   prep time: 10 minutes   cook time: 10 minutes   yield: 4 servings

Bambinos' pizza buffet always included a dessert pizza.

—crust

1 batch pizza dough (from Craig's Special Pizza, page 182)

¼ cup Swerve confectioners'-style sweetener or equivalent amount of liquid or powdered sweetener (see page 31)

—cream cheese topping

1 (8-ounce) package cream cheese or mascarpone cheese, at room temperature

¼ cup Swerve confectioners'-style sweetener or equivalent amount of powdered sweetener

Seeds scraped from 1 vanilla bean (about 8 inches long), or 1 teaspoon vanilla extract

—chocolate drizzle

¾ cup heavy cream

2 ounces unsweetened chocolate, finely chopped

⅓ cup Swerve confectioners'-style sweetener or equivalent amount of powdered sweetener

—strawberry glaze

1½ ounces cream cheese, at room temperature

2 tablespoons unsweetened cashew milk, warmed

2 tablespoons Swerve confectioners'-style sweetener or equivalent amount of powdered sweetener

½ teaspoon strawberry extract

Fresh mint leaves, for garnish

1. Place a pizza stone in the oven and preheat the oven to 400°F. (You can use a baking sheet, but a pizza stone will bake the bottom better.) Grease a piece of parchment paper.

2. Make the dough: Follow the directions for making the pizza dough from Craig's Special Pizza, but add ¼ cup Swerve confectioners'-style sweetener (or equivalent) when you mix in the almond flour and salt. Place the dough on the parchment and pat it out with your hands to form a large circle (about 10 inches in diameter). Slide the pizza on the parchment onto the hot pizza stone.

3. Bake for 10 minutes, or until the crust is golden brown and fully cooked. Allow to cool for 5 minutes.

4. While the pizza is baking, make the cream cheese topping: Combine the cream cheese, sweetener, and vanilla bean seeds in a small bowl and mix with a spatula until smooth. Set aside.

5. Make the chocolate drizzle: Place the heavy cream in a saucepan and heat on medium until simmering. Remove from the heat, add the chocolate, and stir until the chocolate is melted. Stir in the sweetener. Set the drizzle aside.

6. Make the glaze: In a small bowl, whisk the 1½ ounces of cream cheese, cashew milk, sweetener, and strawberry extract until well combined. Taste and adjust the sweetness and flavor, adding more sweetener and/or extract, if desired.

7. Spread the cream cheese topping over the crust. Drizzle with the chocolate and the glaze. Garnish with mint. This is best served fresh, but extras can be stored in an airtight container in the refrigerator for up to 4 days.

NUTRITIONAL INFO (per serving)				
calories	fat	protein	carbs	fiber
532	47g	21g	7g	2g

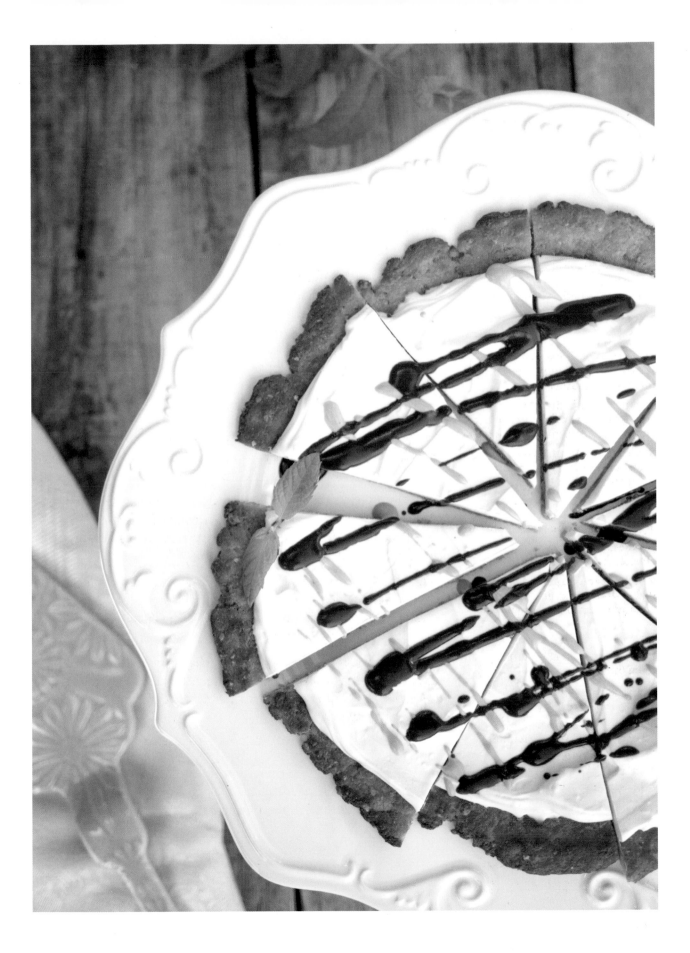

Traditional Tiramisu

$\left(\begin{smallmatrix} & M & \\ L & \searrow & H \\ & \text{KETO} & \end{smallmatrix}\right)$ **prep time:** 15 minutes, plus at least 1 hour to set   **cook time:** 25 minutes   **yield:** 8 servings

Our old favorite restaurant, Bambinos, made one of the best tiramisus I have ever tasted. It seems like such a complex dish with all the deep flavors, but in reality it is quite simple to make!

—ladyfingers (makes about 20)

3 large eggs, separated

¼ cup Swerve confectioners'-style sweetener or equivalent amount of liquid or powdered sweetener (see page 31)

1 teaspoon vanilla extract

½ cup blanched almond flour

¼ teaspoon baking powder

—coffee dip

¾ cup brewed decaf espresso or strong brewed decaf coffee

¼ cup Swerve confectioners'-style sweetener or equivalent amount of liquid or powdered sweetener

1 teaspoon rum extract

½ teaspoon vanilla extract

—"zabaglione" filling

4 large egg yolks

¾ cup Swerve confectioners'-style sweetener or equivalent amount of liquid or powdered sweetener

½ teaspoon rum extract

¾ cup heavy cream

1 (8-ounce) package mascarpone or cream cheese, at room temperature

Unsweetened cocoa powder, for dusting

1. Preheat the oven to 375°F. Line 2 rimmed baking sheets with parchment paper.

2. Make the ladyfingers: Put the egg whites in a medium-sized bowl and the yolks in a larger bowl. Using a hand mixer, beat the yolks with the sweetener for about 4 minutes, until lightened in color, then stir in the vanilla. In a separate bowl, beat the whites until stiff peaks form. Fold the flour and baking powder into the yolk mixture. Gently fold in the whites, making sure not to overmix the batter. Place the batter in a pastry bag or a large zip-top bag with a corner cut off. Pipe the batter onto the lined baking sheet in 4-inch by 1-inch strips, spacing them about 2 inches apart. Bake for 6 to 8 minutes, until light golden. Remove from the oven and allow to cool.

3. Make the coffee dip: In a small bowl, mix the espresso, sweetener, and extracts until well combined. Set aside and allow to cool in the pan.

4. Make the filling: In a small bowl, beat the 4 egg yolks until lightened in color and frothy. Stir in the sweetener. Transfer the egg yolk mixture to a double boiler over medium heat. Stirring constantly, heat the yolks until they are thickened and coat the back of a spoon, 3 to 5 minutes. Pour the yolks into another bowl to stop the cooking. Stir in the rum extract. In a small bowl, whip the heavy cream until stiff peaks form and set aside. Add the mascarpone to the egg yolk mixture and mix to combine. Gently fold the whipped cream into the mascarpone mixture until smooth.

5. To assemble: Arrange 6 ladyfingers flat side down (they absorb more coffee dip that way) in an 8-inch square baking dish. Spoon 1 teaspoon of coffee dip onto each ladyfinger. Layer one-third of the filling over the ladyfingers. Dust with cocoa powder. Repeat two more times, ending with a dusting of cocoa powder. Cover and refrigerate for 1 hour or up to 3 days to set.

NUTRITIONAL INFO (per serving)				
calories	fat	protein	carbs	fiber
293	29g	7g	2g	1g

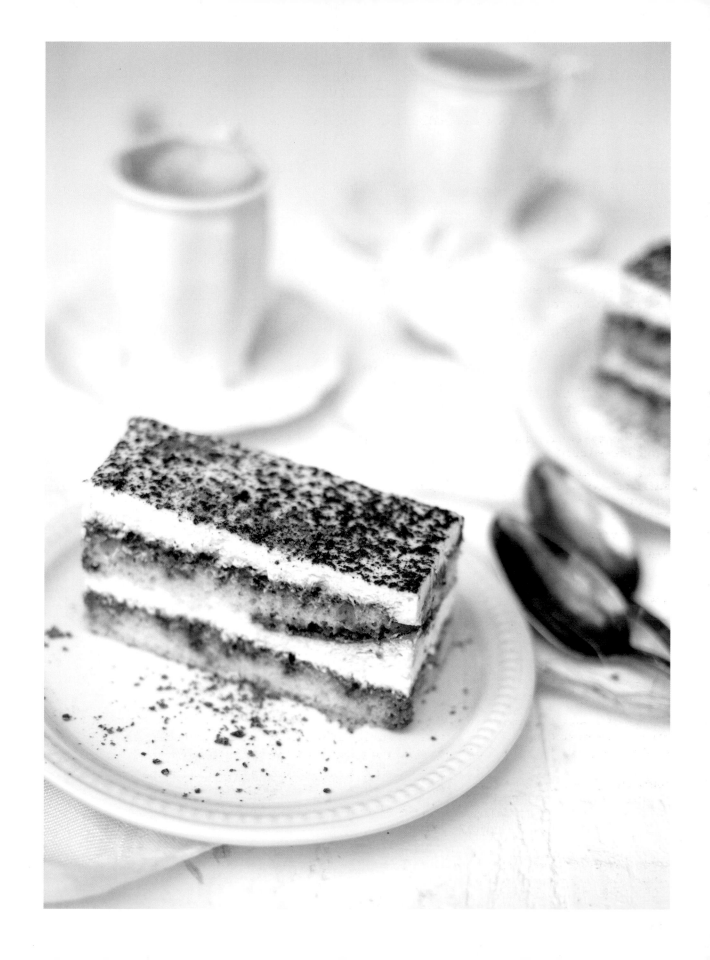

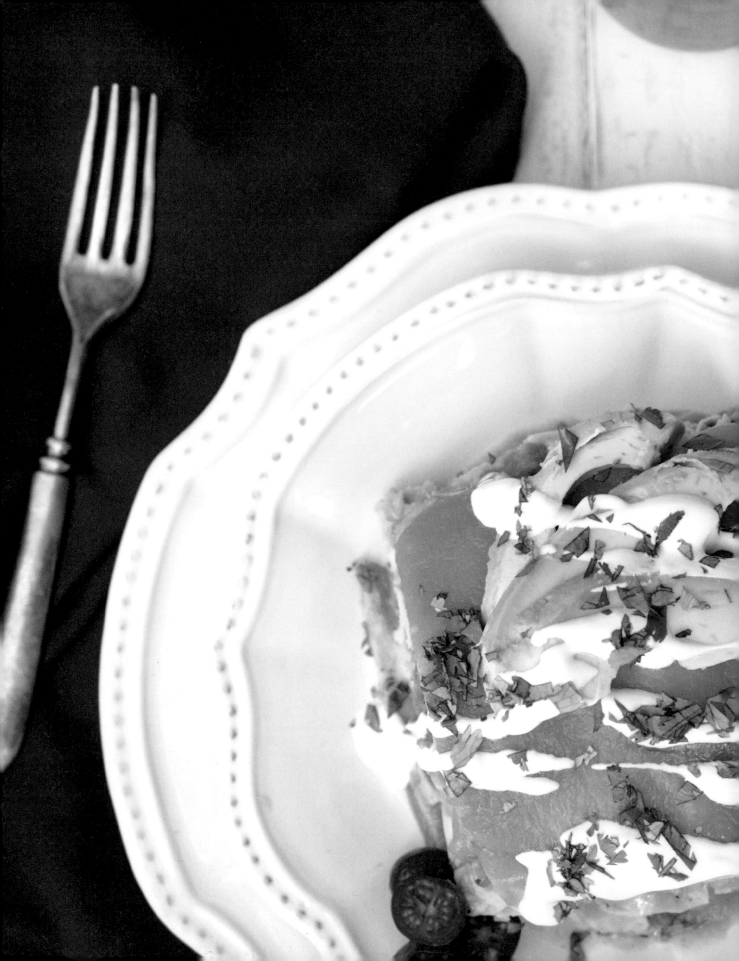

Mexican & Latin American *Fare*

Easy Blender Enchilada Sauce

(L ⌒ H M KETO ▯ ▯ ◗)   prep time: 3 minutes   yield: 2 cups (¼ cup per serving)

If you look at the ingredient lists on jars of store-bought enchilada sauce, you often find gluten and other fillers. This simple enchilada sauce takes just minutes to make but still has an authentic flavor, especially after it gets warm and bubbly in a baked casserole of keto enchiladas. Make sure to use a salsa that does not contain added sugars or vegetable oils.

1 cup store-bought sugar-free salsa

2 tablespoons tomato paste

¾ cup beef or chicken bone broth, homemade (page 356) or store-bought (see note)

¼ cup chili powder

¼ teaspoon ground cumin

¼ teaspoon garlic powder

Place the ingredients in a blender and blend until smooth. Store in an airtight container in the refrigerator for up to 1 week or in the freezer for up to 1 month.

note: *If you are making chicken enchiladas, use chicken broth, and if you are making beef enchiladas, use beef broth.*

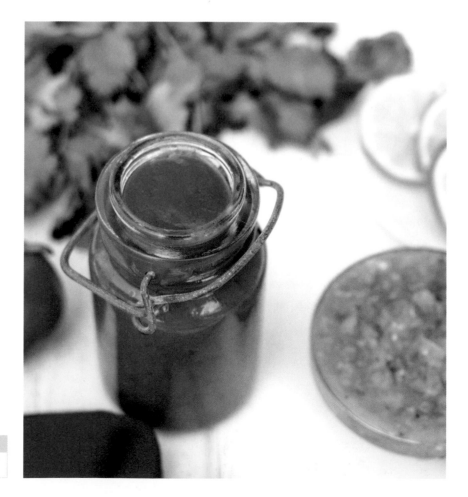

NUTRITIONAL INFO (per serving)				
calories	fat	protein	carbs	fiber
27	1g	1g	4g	2g

Pico de Gallo

prep time: 7 minutes   yield: 2¼ cups (about ½ cup per serving)

Pico de gallo is a great dipping option for keto tortilla chips (page 198). It also can be served with my Chicken Quesadilla (page 206).

1 large tomato, diced (about 1½ cups)

½ cup chopped white onions (about 1 medium)

2 cloves garlic, minced

2 tablespoons fresh lime juice

2 tablespoons chopped fresh cilantro

1 jalapeño pepper, seeded and finely diced

½ teaspoon fine sea salt

Place the ingredients in a small bowl and stir until well combined. Store in an airtight container in the refrigerator for up to 5 days.

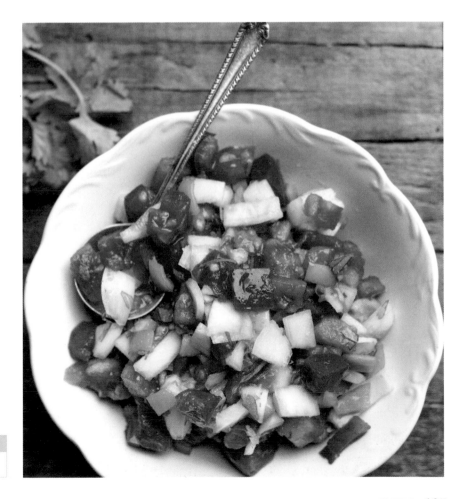

NUTRITIONAL INFO (per serving)				
calories	fat	protein	carbs	fiber
32	0.1g	1g	6g	1g

"Tortilla" Chips with Guacamole

 prep time: 15 minutes, plus at least 1 hour for chips to dry   cook time: at least 2 hours
yield: 64 chips (8 servings) and 3 cups guacamole (½ cup per serving)

It wouldn't be a traditional Mexican restaurant meal without chips and guacamole served when you sit down! To make this guacamole extra-special, I use roasted garlic, which I keep in my freezer at all times for easy flavor bombs to add to dips and salad dressings. If you don't have roasted garlic on hand, raw garlic will work. Happy dipping!

—chips

2 cups grated Parmesan cheese

—guacamole

3 avocados, peeled and pitted

2 plum tomatoes, diced

½ cup diced yellow onions

½ head roasted garlic (page 359), or 2 cloves raw garlic, smashed to a paste

3 tablespoons fresh lime juice, plus more if desired

3 tablespoons chopped fresh cilantro leaves

1 teaspoon fine sea salt

½ teaspoon ground cumin

1. Preheat the oven to 400°F. Line 3 rimmed baking sheets with parchment paper and grease the paper.

2. Make the chips: Place ¼ cup of the cheese on the greased parchment and use your fingers to spread the cheese into a 6-inch circle. Repeat with the remaining cheese, spacing the circles about 2 inches apart. Make 3 circles on two of the baking sheets and 2 circles on the third baking sheet. Bake for 5 minutes or until the cheese is lightly browned and bubbly. Remove from the oven, use a pizza cutter to cut each circle into 8 equal triangles, and allow to cool on the pans for about 1 hour. The chips will crisp up as they cool.

3. When the chips have cooled, make the guacamole: Place the avocados and lime juice in a large bowl and mash until it reaches your desired consistency. Add the rest of the ingredients and stir until well combined. Taste and add more lime juice if desired.

4. Remove the chips from the parchment paper and serve with the guacamole.

5. Store the chips in an airtight container for up to 4 days. The guacamole will keep in the refrigerator for 3 days if tightly covered.

NUTRITIONAL INFO (per serving of chips)				
calories	fat	protein	carbs	fiber
248	16g	15g	2g	0g

NUTRITIONAL INFO (per serving of guac)				
calories	fat	protein	carbs	fiber
174	14g	3g	13g	7g

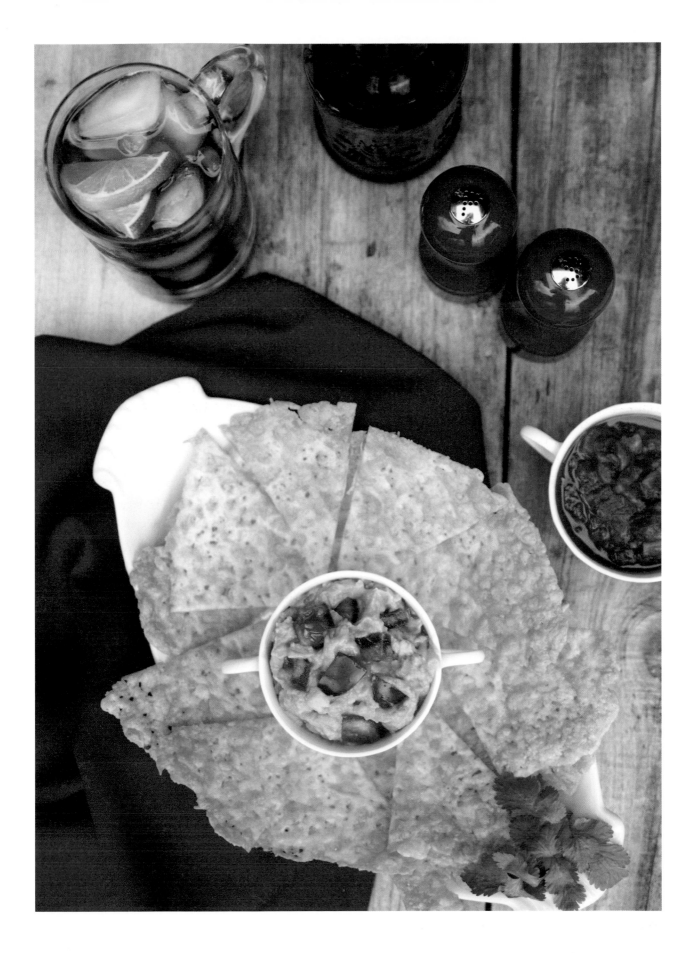

Soft Tortillas

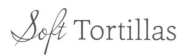

$\left(\begin{smallmatrix} & M & \\ L & \top & H \\ & \text{KETO} & \end{smallmatrix} \quad \boxed{\text{OPTION}} \quad \boxed{\text{OPTION}}\right)$ prep time: 5 minutes   cook time: 50 minutes   yield: 10 tortillas (1 per serving)

These soft tortillas are super-easy to make, and the texture and flavor will remind you of traditional tortillas. They are a little higher in carbohydrates, so if you are trying to keep your carbs lower, try my Keto Tortillas (opposite) instead.

1¼ cups blanched almond flour, or ¾ cup coconut flour

3½ tablespoons psyllium husk powder (no substitutes)

1 teaspoon fine sea salt

2 large eggs (4 eggs if using coconut flour)

1 cup boiling water

2 tablespoons ghee or coconut oil, for the skillet

variation: tomato tortillas. *Simply replace the hot water with an equal amount of hot Easy Blender Enchilada Sauce (page 196).*

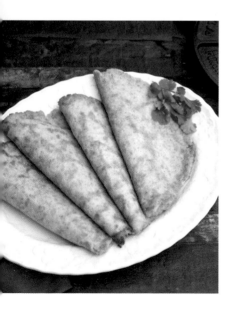

1. In a medium-sized bowl, combine the flour, psyllium husk powder, and salt. Stir in the eggs until a thick dough forms. Add the water and mix until well combined. Let sit for 1 to 2 minutes, until the dough firms up.

2. Lightly grease two 8-inch pieces of parchment paper. Separate the dough into 10 balls (about 2 inches in diameter). Place a ball of dough in the center of one of the greased pieces of parchment. Top it with the other greased piece of parchment. Using a rolling pin, roll out the dough into a circle about ¹⁄₁₆ inch thick. This dough is very forgiving, so if you don't make a circle with the rolling pin, just use your hands to perfect the tortilla. If you have a tortilla press, place the dough, sandwiched between the two pieces of parchment, in the press and press down until the dough flattens to the edge of the press.

3. Heat the ghee in a large skillet over medium-high heat. Remove the tortilla from the parchment paper and place it in the skillet. (If the dough sticks to the parchment, use your fingers to close up any holes.) Cook until lightly browned, about 2 minutes, then flip and cook for another 2 minutes, until cooked through. While the tortilla cooks, roll out and press the second dough ball, regreasing the parchment paper as needed, then cook it as described above, adding more ghee to the skillet if needed. Repeat until all of the tortillas are pressed and cooked.

4. Store in an airtight container in the refrigerator for up to 4 days or in the freezer for up to 1 month.

NUTRITIONAL INFO (per serving)				
calories	fat	protein	carbs	fiber
105	8g	4g	6g	4g

Keto Tortillas

(L $\overset{M}{\underset{KETO}{\curvearrowright}}$ H 🥛 OPTION 🚫)   prep time: 5 minutes   cook time: 32 minutes   yield: 8 tortillas (1 per serving)

If you're looking for a low-carb tortilla, this is the recipe for you. These tortillas have fewer carbs than my Soft Tortillas (opposite) and can be used in any recipe in this book that calls for tortillas.

After making this recipe, you will have leftover egg yolks. You can use them to make recipes such as Green Tea Ice Cream (page 120), Gnocchi (page 146), Traditional Tiramisu (page 192), or Coconut and Thai Basil Ice Cream (page 286).

3 large egg whites

2 tablespoons unflavored egg white protein powder (or whey protein powder if not dairy-sensitive)

2 ounces cream cheese (Kite Hill brand cream cheese style spread if dairy-free), at room temperature

2 tablespoons ghee or coconut oil, for the skillet

1. Whip the egg whites in a clean, dry bowl until very stiff peaks form, about 3 minutes. Fold in the protein powder until just combined. Gently fold in the cream cheese (without deflating the egg whites).

2. Heat the ghee in an 8-inch skillet over medium-high heat until a drop of water sizzles in the pan. Pour ¼ cup of the batter into the skillet and spread with a spatula into a 6-inch circle. Fry until golden brown on both sides, about 2 minutes per side. Repeat with the rest of the batter to make a total of 8 tortillas. Add more ghee to the pan if needed between batches.

3. Store in an airtight container in the refrigerator for up to 4 days or in the freezer for up to 1 month.

NUTRITIONAL INFO (per serving)				
calories	fat	protein	carbs	fiber
78	5g	6g	1g	0g

Breakfast Burritos

(L→H M KETO / OPTION 🚫)   **prep time:** 7 minutes   **cook time:** 28 minutes   **yield:** 4 to 6 servings

14 strips thick-cut bacon

2 teaspoons ghee or unsalted butter (or bacon fat or coconut oil if dairy-free)

¼ cup chopped onions (about 1 small)

2 tablespoons diced bell peppers, any color

4 ounces ground pork

¼ teaspoon fine sea salt

¼ teaspoon ground black pepper

4 large eggs, lightly beaten

½ cup shredded sharp cheddar cheese (omit for dairy-free)

1. Preheat the oven to 400°F. Line a rimmed baking sheet with parchment paper.

2. Weave the bacon strips together to make a 9-inch square on the parchment. Bake for 10 minutes, or until the bacon is starting to cook but is still foldable. Reserve the bacon drippings to make the bacon mayonnaise, or save it for frying eggs.

3. Meanwhile, heat the ghee in a large cast-iron skillet over medium heat. Add the onions and bell peppers and sauté until softened, about 2 minutes. Add the ground pork and season with the salt and pepper. Sauté, breaking up the pork with a spatula, for another 2 minutes, or until the pork is browned and cooked through. Stir in the eggs and scramble until the eggs are cooked through, about 3 minutes. Set aside.

4. Remove the bacon from the oven and place the egg mixture in the center. Top with the cheese, if using, and fold the bacon like a burrito, slightly folding in the edges as you roll. Secure the ends with toothpicks, wrap the burrito in parchment, and place it back in the oven for 15 minutes, or until the bacon is cooked to your liking. These are best served fresh. Store in an airtight container in the refrigerator for up to 5 days. To reheat, place in a lightly greased skillet over medium heat for about 3 minutes.

NUTRITIONAL INFO (per serving, based on 4 servings)				
calories	fat	protein	carbs	fiber
474	39g	29g	2g	0.2g

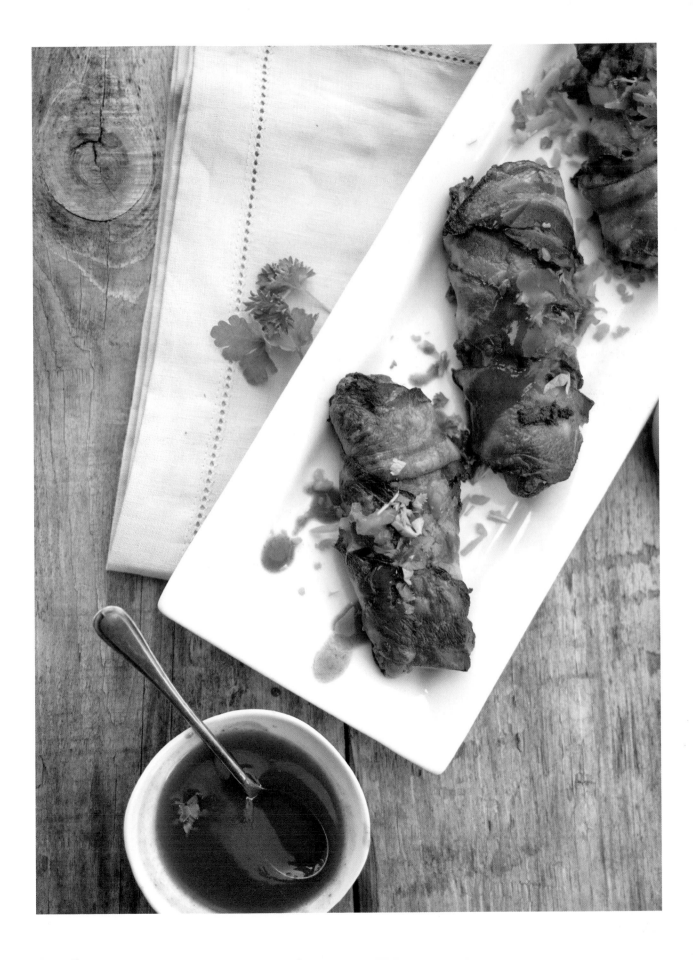

Empanadas

$\left(\begin{smallmatrix} & M & \\ L & \searrow & H \\ & KETO & \end{smallmatrix} \; \diagdown\!\!\!\diagup \; \blacktriangle \right)$ prep time: 12 minutes   cook time: 20 minutes   yield: 16 empanadas (4 per serving)

From the Spanish word *empanar*, meaning "to bake in pastry," empanadas are popular in many Latin American countries. I've replaced the pastry with prosciutto wrappers to convert these handheld beauties into the perfect low-carb snack or appetizer.

1 cup coconut oil, divided

1 pound Mexican-style fresh (raw) chorizo, removed from casings

¼ teaspoon fine sea salt

Pinch of chili powder

Pinch of ground cumin

1 cup diced onions (about 1 large)

16 large slices prosciutto

1 cup shredded Monterey Jack cheese (about 4 ounces)

1 cup store-bought sugar-free salsa, for serving

Sour cream, for serving

Fresh cilantro leaves, for garnish

1. Heat 1½ teaspoons of the oil in a large cast-iron skillet over medium heat. Add the chorizo and season with the salt, chili powder, and cumin. Cook the chorizo for about 5 minutes, breaking it up with a spatula, until browned and cooked through. Set aside on a plate to cool.

2. Place the onions in the same skillet and cook, stirring, for 4 to 5 minutes, until the onions begin to turn golden brown. Remove the onions from the skillet and set aside.

3. Heat the remaining oil in a 4-inch-deep (or deeper) cast-iron skillet over medium heat to 350°F. The oil should be 3 inches deep; add more oil if needed. Line a plate with paper towels.

4. To assemble the empanadas, lay a slice of prosciutto on a flat work surface. Spread 1 tablespoon of the cheese in the middle of the prosciutto, followed by 1 tablespoon of the cooked chorizo and 1 tablespoon of the cooked onions. Wrap the prosciutto tightly around the filling and place it seam side down on a plate. Repeat with the rest of the prosciutto slices and fillings.

5. Place the empanadas, 3 at a time, in the hot oil. Fry for 1 to 2 minutes on each side, until golden brown. Remove from the skillet with a slotted spoon and set on the paper towel–lined plate to drain.

6. Transfer the empanadas to a platter and serve with salsa and sour cream. Garnish with cilantro leaves. Store in an airtight container in the refrigerator for up to 5 days. To reheat, place in a lightly greased skillet over medium heat for about 3 minutes.

NUTRITIONAL INFO (per serving)				
calories	fat	protein	carbs	fiber
575	45g	34g	8g	1g

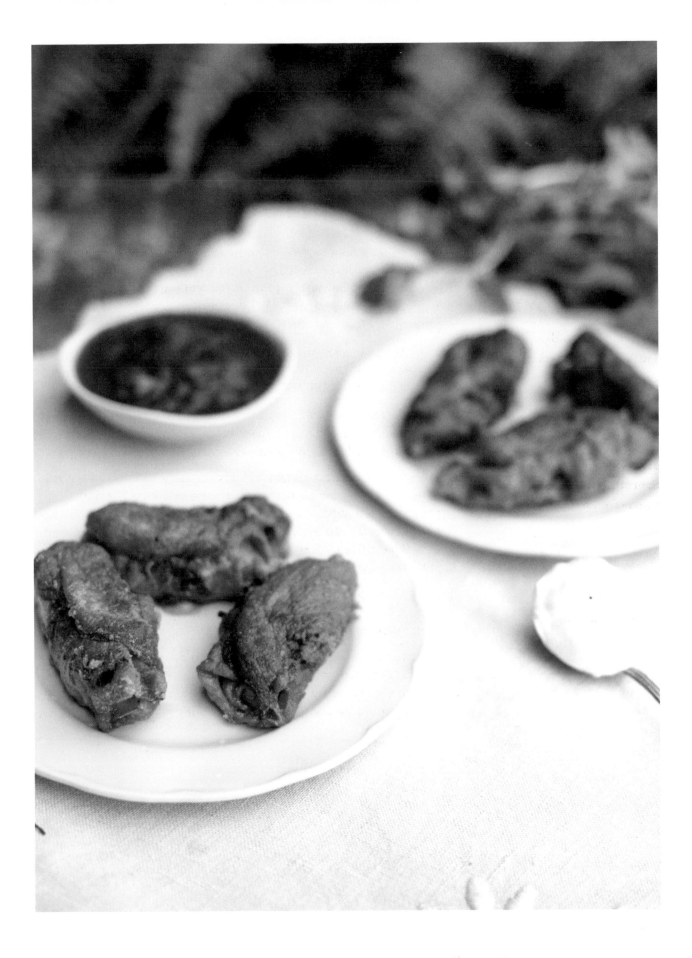

Chicken Quesadilla

(L→H M / KETO OPTION) **prep time:** 5 minutes (not including time to make tortillas) **cook time:** 4 minutes
yield: 2 servings

I store extra tortillas in my freezer for easy meals like this. Another time-saving tip is to buy organic rotisserie chicken from the grocery store and have it on hand for quick meals.

1 tablespoon ghee, coconut oil, or bacon fat

2 Soft Tortillas (page 200) or Keto Tortillas (page 201)

½ cup shredded sharp cheddar or Monterey Jack cheese (about 2 ounces)

½ cup shredded leftover chicken

—for serving

1 cup store-bought sugar-free salsa, or ¼ batch Pico de Gallo (page 197)

1 cup sour cream

Diced avocado or ½ batch Guacamole (page 198)

Lime wedges

1. Heat the ghee in a large skillet over medium-high heat. Place a tortilla in the skillet. Top with half of the cheese, the chicken, and then the rest of the cheese. Place the other tortilla on top of the fillings. Fry the quesadilla until golden and crisp, about 3 minutes. Flip and cook for another 2 minutes, or until the quesadilla is golden and crisp on both sides and the cheese is completely melted.

2. Transfer to a plate, slice into wedges, and serve with salsa, sour cream, diced avocado, and lime wedges. Store in an airtight container in the refrigerator for up to 5 days. To reheat, place in a lightly greased skillet over medium heat for about 3 minutes.

NUTRITIONAL INFO (per serving)				
calories	fat	protein	carbs	fiber
360	27g	24g	6g	4g

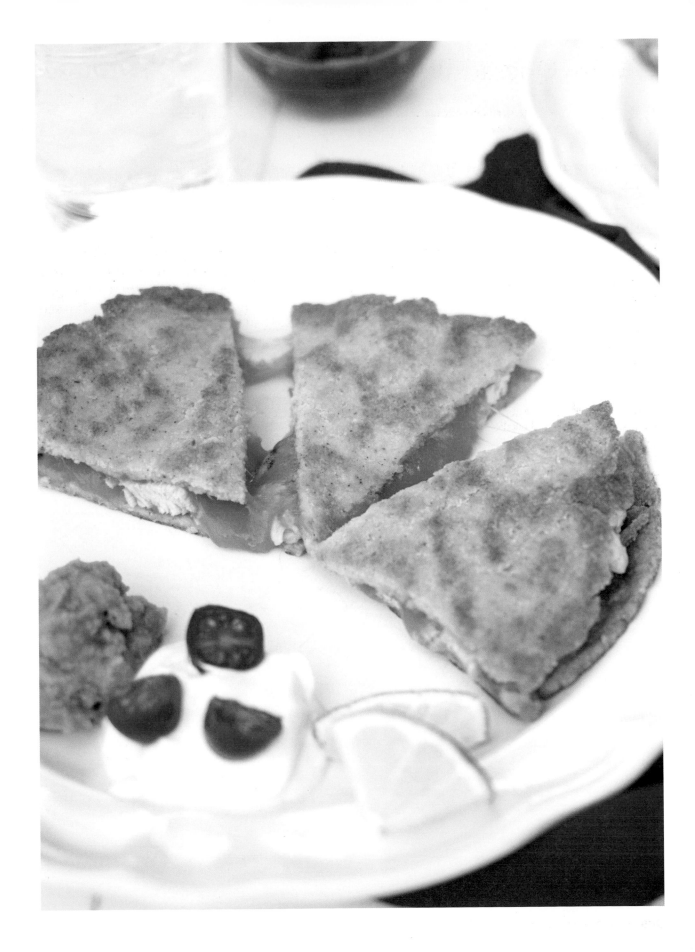

Tortilla Soup

prep time: 10 minutes (not including time to make tortillas)
cook time: 28 minutes   yield: 6 servings

1 tablespoon coconut oil

1 cup chopped white onions

4 cloves garlic, minced

1 tablespoon paprika

2 teaspoons ground cumin

1 teaspoon chili powder

¼ teaspoon cayenne pepper

1 pound boneless, skinless chicken thighs, cut into ½-inch pieces

5 cups chicken bone broth, homemade (page 356) or store-bought

2 cups crushed tomatoes, canned or fresh

¼ cup tomato paste

¼ cup chopped fresh cilantro leaves, plus extra for garnish

2½ teaspoons fine sea salt

2 bay leaves

1 avocado, peeled, pitted, and sliced

Lime wedges, for garnish

1 cup crumbled Cotija cheese (omit for dairy-free)

Soft Tortillas (page 200), Keto Tortillas (page 201), or pork rinds, for serving

1. Heat the oil in a large pot over medium heat. Add the onions, garlic, paprika, cumin, chili powder, and cayenne and sauté for 3 minutes, or until the onions are translucent. Add the chicken and cook for 5 minutes, stirring occasionally, or until the chicken is browned and cooked through.

2. Meanwhile, place the broth, crushed tomatoes, tomato paste, cilantro, and salt in a blender and blend until smooth. Add the mixture to the pot, along with the bay leaves. Increase the heat and simmer for 20 minutes. Remove the bay leaves.

3. Divide the soup among 6 serving bowls. Garnish with additional cilantro, sliced avocado, lime wedges, and cheese, if using. Serve with tortillas. Store in an airtight container in the refrigerator for up to 5 days. To reheat, place in a saucepan over medium heat for about 3 minutes.

NUTRITIONAL INFO (per serving)				
calories	fat	protein	carbs	fiber
295	19g	21g	11g	3g

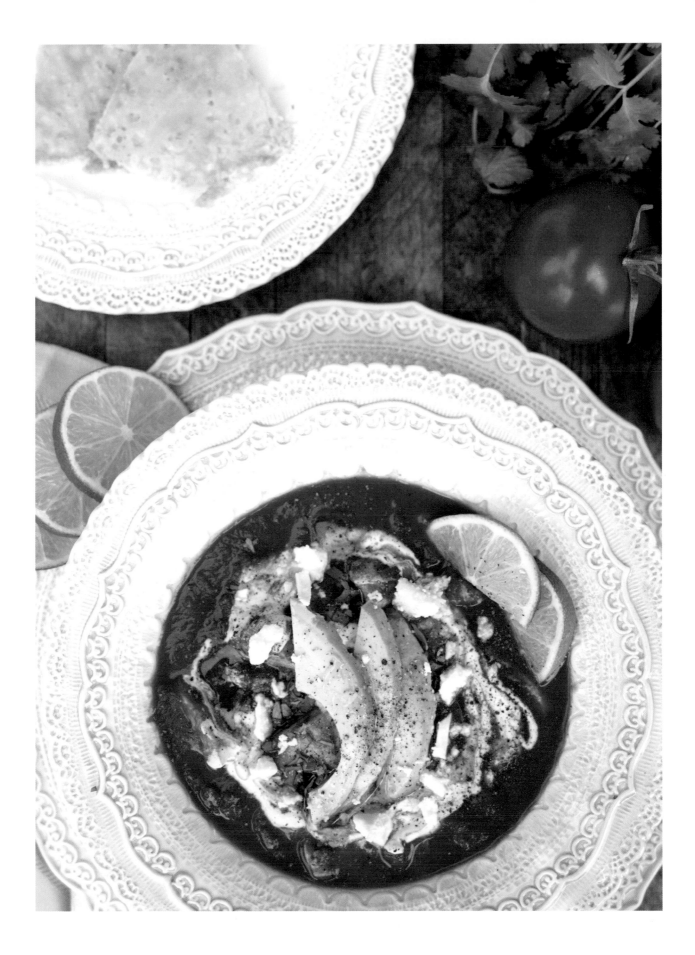

Carne en su Jugo

(L M H KETO   OPTION   OPTION)   prep time: 10 minutes (not including time to make tortillas)
cook time: 4 to 8 hours in a slow cooker   yield: 8 servings

Carne en su jugo means "meat in its juices." It is a simple dish that is packed with flavor!

2 pounds boneless beef roast

1 teaspoon fine sea salt

1 teaspoon ground black pepper

8 medium tomatillos, husks removed

1 medium white onion, chopped

1 cup chopped fresh cilantro, plus extra for garnish

3 cloves garlic, minced

1 to 2 jalapeño peppers, seeded and chopped (optional; see note)

10 strips bacon, finely chopped

1 avocado, peeled, pitted, and diced, for garnish

2 radishes, very thinly sliced, for garnish

2 tablespoons chopped fresh chives, for garnish

8 Soft Tortillas (page 200) or Keto Tortillas (page 201), for serving

1. Season the roast on all sides with the salt and pepper. Place the roast in a 6-quart slow cooker. Cover with 4 cups of water.

2. Place the tomatillos, onion, cilantro, garlic, jalapeño(s), if using, and 1 cup of water in a blender and puree until smooth. Pour the puree into the slow cooker. Cook on low for 8 hours or on high for 4 to 5 hours, until the beef is fork-tender. Using 2 forks, shred the beef in the liquid. Taste the liquid and add more salt, if needed.

3. Place the bacon in a medium-sized cast-iron skillet and fry for 5 minutes, or until crisp.

4. Divide the soup among 8 serving bowls. Garnish each bowl with bacon, avocado, radishes, chives, and cilantro. Serve with tortillas. Store the soup without garnishes in an airtight container in the refrigerator for up to 5 days or in the freezer for up to 1 month. To reheat, place in a saucepan over medium heat for about 3 minutes.

note: *If you prefer a spicy soup, add two seeded and chopped jalapeños. If you like lots of heat, include some of the seeds.*

NUTRITIONAL INFO (per serving)				
calories	fat	protein	carbs	fiber
571	44g	30g	12g	7g

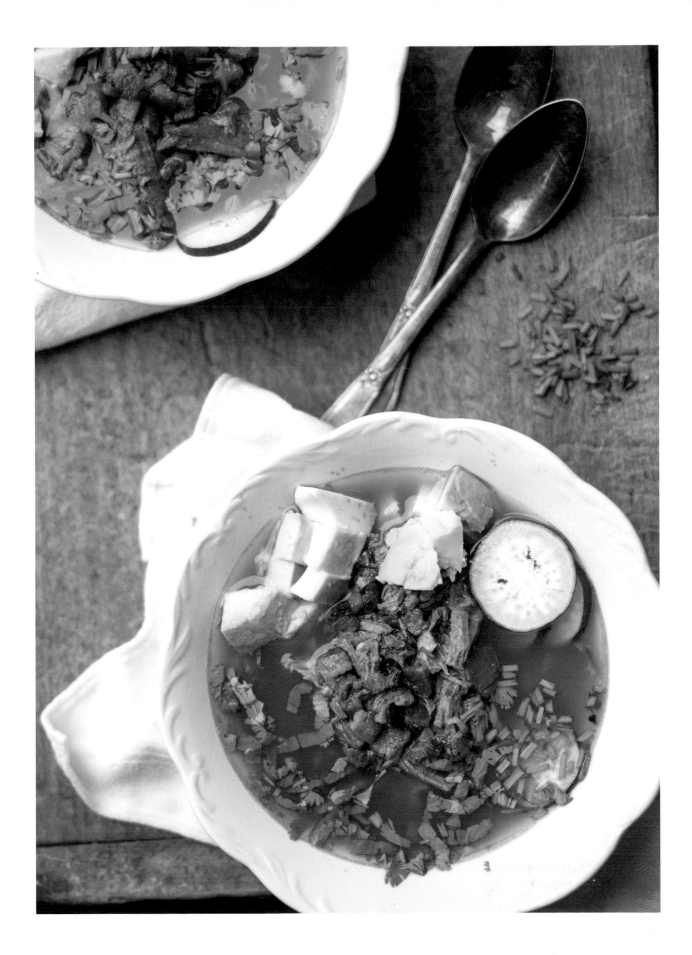

Slow Cooker Posole Soup

(L → M H KETO / OPTION / OPTION) prep time: 12 minutes (not including time to make tortillas)
cook time: 6 hours   yield: 8 servings

San Pedro Cafe is an amazing restaurant in our small town along the St. Croix River. One of the most popular dishes on the menu is posole. Traditionally this soup contains hominy, which is a starchy carbohydrate. I made it keto by replacing the hominy with mushrooms, which give the soup a similar texture.

¼ cup ghee or coconut oil

2 pounds boneless pork butt or pork shoulder, cut into 1-inch cubes

1 pound button or cremini mushrooms, sliced (about 2½ cups)

½ cup diced white onions (about 1 medium)

4 cloves garlic, minced

4 cups chicken bone broth, homemade (page 356) or store-bought

4 cups tomato sauce

2 tablespoons fresh lime juice

½ cup seeded and chopped green chiles

2 teaspoons ground cumin

2 teaspoons dried oregano leaves

½ teaspoon cayenne pepper (or more to desired heat)

¼ cup chopped fresh cilantro, plus extra leaves for garnish (garnish optional)

½ teaspoon fine sea salt

½ batch guacamole, homemade (page 198) or store-bought, for serving (optional)

8 Soft Tortillas (page 200) or Keto Tortillas (page 201), for serving (optional)

1. Heat the ghee in a large skillet over high heat. Add the pork, mushrooms, onions, and garlic and cook, stirring, until the pork is browned on all sides, about 5 minutes.

2. Transfer the pork mixture to a 6-quart slow cooker. Add the broth, tomato sauce, lime juice, chiles, cumin, oregano, cayenne, cilantro, and salt. Cover and cook on low for 6 hours.

3. Serve in bowls with a scoop of guacamole, garnished with cilantro leaves, if desired. Serve with tortillas, if desired. Store in an airtight container in the refrigerator for up to 5 days. To reheat, place in a saucepan over medium heat for about 3 minutes.

NUTRITIONAL INFO (per serving, without tortillas or guacamole)				
calories	fat	protein	carbs	fiber
350	25g	25g	8g	2g

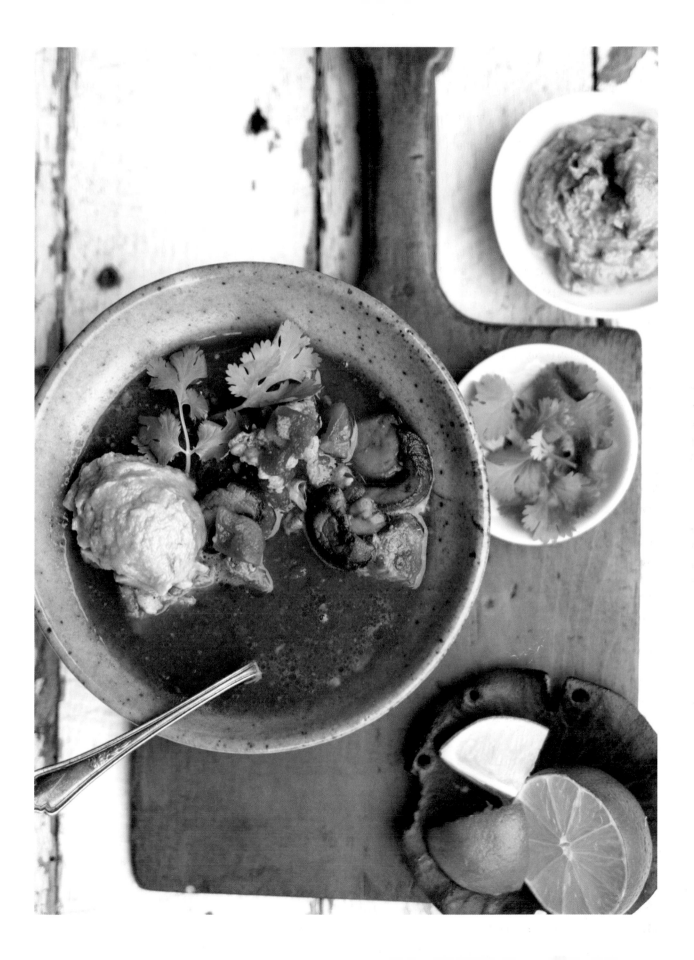

Chicken Enchilada Soup

(L M H KETO / OPTION / OPTION)   **prep time:** 7 minutes (not including time to make tortillas)
cook time: 10 minutes   **yield:** 4 servings

This soup is a flavorful way to use up leftover chicken (or turkey). If you don't have left-over chicken on hand, you can always pick up a roasted chicken from your local grocery store. You can make this soup with raw chicken, but it will increase the cooking time. You can also use leftover turkey.

1 tablespoon ghee or coconut oil

1 green bell pepper, seeded and chopped

½ cup chopped onions (about 1 medium)

1 (15-ounce) can diced tomatoes, or 2 cups diced fresh tomatoes, divided

2 tablespoons tomato paste

1¾ cups chicken bone broth, homemade (page 356) or store-bought

¼ cup chili powder

¼ teaspoon ground cumin

1 clove garlic, minced

1 (8-ounce) package cream cheese (Kite Hill brand cream cheese style spread if dairy-free)

2 cups chopped leftover chicken from 1 roast chicken, or cubed raw boneless, skinless chicken thighs or breasts

Fine sea salt

Fresh cilantro leaves, for garnish

Avocado oil, for drizzling

2 Soft Tortillas (page 200) or Keto Tortillas (page 201), for serving

1. Heat the ghee in a large pot over medium-high heat. Add the bell pepper and onions and cook until the onions are translucent, about 4 minutes. (If using raw chicken, add it to the pot now. Sauté the chicken for 6 minutes, stirring often, until the chicken is browned and cooked through.)

2. Place 1 cup of the diced tomatoes, the tomato paste, broth, chili powder, cumin, garlic, and cream cheese in a blender and blend until very smooth. Add the pureed tomato mixture and remaining 1 cup of diced tomatoes to the pot. If using leftover cooked chicken, add it to the pot now. Give everything a stir and simmer for 5 minutes, or until the soup is nice and hot.

3. Add salt to taste, if desired. Remove from the heat, divide the soup among 4 serving bowls, and garnish with cilantro and a drizzle of avocado oil. Serve with tortillas. Store in an airtight container in the refrigerator for up to 5 days. To reheat, place in a saucepan over medium heat for about 3 minutes.

NUTRITIONAL INFO (per serving)				
calories	fat	protein	carbs	fiber
456	30g	28g	13g	3g

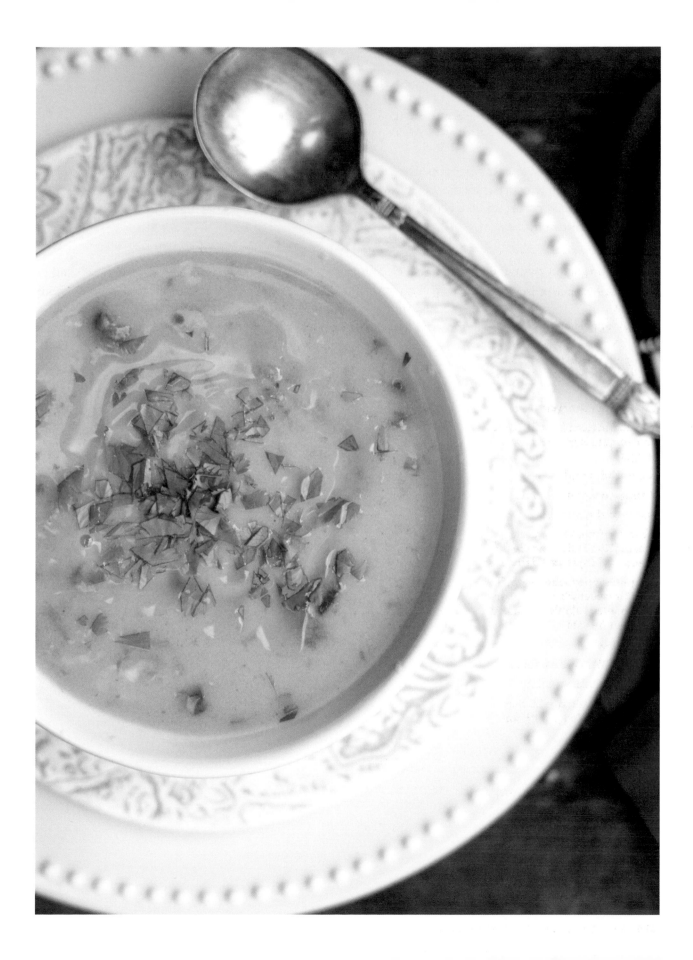

Easy Burrito Bowls

(L ⟶ H · KETO · OPTION 🚫 🚫)   prep time: 5 minutes   cook time: 7 minutes   yield: 4 servings

Last summer, on our way home from the beach, Craig and I started talking about the main complaints we get about eating keto—that it's more expensive and time-consuming than eating out. He suggested that we do a "challenge" to see who could do it faster and for less money, me or Chipotle. While Craig set off to pick up a Chipotle burrito bowl, I made my keto equivalent at home. We made a video of the race to show that eating keto doesn't have to be costly or be a drain on your time. (To see the video, visit my site, MariaMindBodyHealth.com, and type "Easy Chipotle at Home" in the search field.) In a nutshell, not only did the at-home meal take less time to make, but I even had time to clean up before Craig got home with the takeout. (Another bonus: I had leftovers for future meals.)

My homemade version cost $3.90; the equivalent from Chipotle cost $9.97. This pricing is based on using store-bought grass-fed beef. If you want to save even more, you could get a whole, half, or quarter cow each year and store it in the freezer. Beef purchased this way ends up being about half the price of store-bought grass-fed beef, with the savings being greatest for a whole-cow purchase. If you don't have an alternate freezer to store meat purchased in bulk, check out ButcherBox (www.butcher-box.com) to order smaller quantities. They deliver, and they have amazing prices!

It took me 14 minutes to get dinner on the table; it took Craig 22 minutes to get the Chipotle. My winning time was based on having the salsa or guacamole premade (or store-bought, if keto-friendly) and on making use of the time while the ground meat was browning to chop the radicchio, shred the cheese, and chop the cilantro. To save even more time, you could replace the hamburger, which requires sautéing time, with slow-cooked bone-in chicken thighs or pork shoulder. In the morning, throw the meat in a slow cooker with some seasonings and bone broth (page 356) and set it to low. When you get home, all you have to do is shred the meat, throw it over some chopped lettuce, and top it with cheese, salsa, guacamole, and sour cream!

1 pound ground beef

½ cup tomato sauce

2½ teaspoons chili powder

2½ teaspoons ground cumin

¾ teaspoon paprika

¾ teaspoon fine sea salt

4 cups chopped lettuce or radicchio

—toppings

½ cup shredded cheddar cheese (omit for dairy-free)

1 cup store-bought sugar-free salsa

½ cup sour cream (omit for dairy-free)

½ batch guacamole, homemade (page 198) or store-bought

1. Place the ground beef, tomato sauce, spices, and salt in a large skillet over medium heat. Sauté, stirring often, until the beef is cooked through, about 5 minutes. Remove from the heat.

2. Divide the lettuce among 4 bowls. Top with the ground beef, cheese (if using), salsa, sour cream (if using), and guacamole. Store in an airtight container in the refrigerator for up to 5 days. To reheat, place the ground beef in a lightly greased skillet over medium heat for about 3 minutes.

NUTRITIONAL INFO (per serving)				
calories	fat	protein	carbs	fiber
483	37g	28g	7g	2g

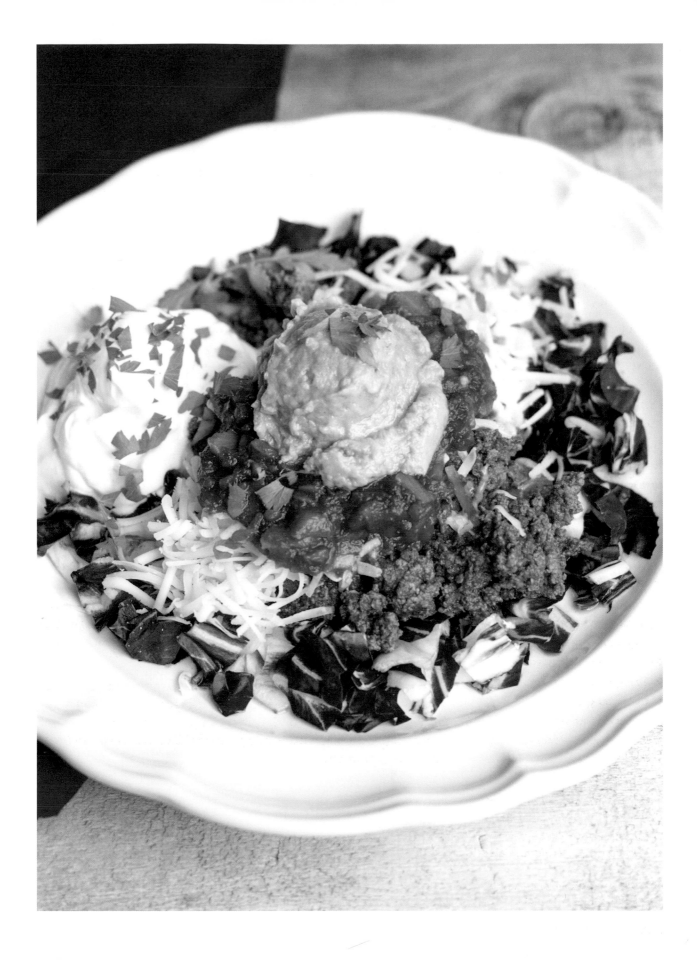

Burritos

(L M H KETO · OPTION · OPTION) **prep time:** 6 minutes (not including time to make tortillas) **cook time:** 5 minutes **yield:** 4 servings

—fillings

2 cups shredded lettuce

2 cups shredded leftover chicken, beef, or pork (see tip)

1 cup diced tomatoes (about 1 medium)

1 avocado, diced

Fresh cilantro leaves, for garnish

4 Soft Tortillas (page 200) or Keto Tortillas (page 201)

1. Divide the fillings equally among the 4 tortillas, placing the fillings in the center of the tortilla. Tuck the sides of the tortilla over the filling, then roll the long edge up and over the filling. Serve immediately.

2. Store the fillings and tortillas in separate airtight containers in the refrigerator for up to 5 days. To reheat the tortillas, place in a lightly greased skillet over medium heat for about 3 minutes.

busy family tip: *If you don't have leftover meat on hand, place bone-in chicken thighs, beef roast, or pork butt (aka pork shoulder) in a slow cooker. Add a jar of sugar-free, preferably organic, salsa to the slow cooker and cook on low for 6 to 8 hours, until you can pull the meat apart with a fork. You now have awesome shredded meat for filling the burritos!*

NUTRITIONAL INFO (per serving)				
calories	fat	protein	carbs	fiber
398	21g	40g	12g	7g

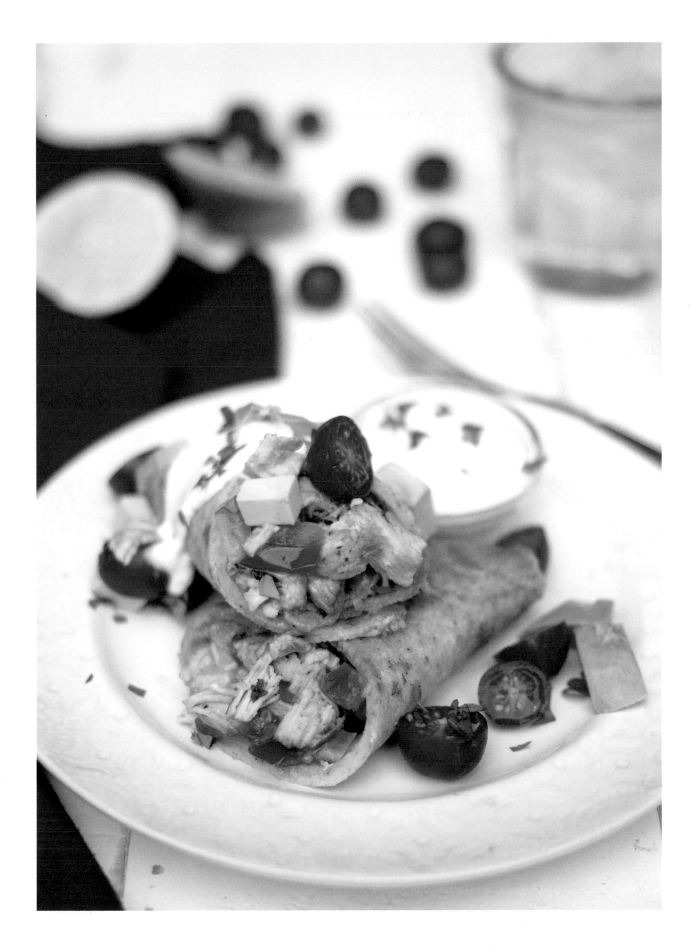

Enchiladas

(LᴹH KETO · OPTION · OPTION) **prep time:** 5 minutes (not including time to make sauce) **cook time:** 20 minutes
yield: 6 servings

1 batch Easy Blender Enchilada Sauce (page 196)

8 large cabbage leaves, Soft Tortillas (page 200), or Keto Tortillas (page 201)

4 cups shredded leftover beef or chicken

1 cup shredded cheddar cheese (about 4 ounces)

½ cup sliced black olives

1 (4-ounce) can green chiles

Fresh cilantro leaves, for garnish

Crumbled Cotija or shredded cheddar cheese, for garnish

1. Preheat the oven to 350°F. Spread the enchilada sauce in the bottom of a 13 by 9-inch baking dish.

2. If using cabbage leaves, bring a large pot of water to a boil. Add the cabbage leaves and cook for 5 minutes, or until the leaves are soft. Remove the leaves from the water and drain well.

3. Lay a cabbage leaf or tortilla on a flat work surface. Fill it with ½ cup of the shredded beef, 2 tablespoons of the cheddar, 1 tablespoon of the black olives, and 1 tablespoon of the chiles. Fold the sides of the cabbage leaf or tortilla over the filling to enclose it. Place the cabbage or tortilla roll on top of the enchilada sauce, with the folded sides facing up. Repeat with the remaining wrappers and filling ingredients.

4. Bake for 15 minutes, or until the cheddar is melted. Garnish with cilantro and Cotija. Store in an airtight container in the refrigerator for up to 5 days. To reheat, place in a lightly greased skillet over medium heat for about 3 minutes.

busy family tip: *If you don't have leftover chicken from another meal ready to use, pick up a roasted organic chicken from your grocery store and shred the meat. That's my cheater trick to make this dish even easier! You can also prepare this dish up to 3 days ahead and store it, unbaked and covered, in the refrigerator. Bake it when you are in need of a quick and easy weeknight dinner.*

NUTRITIONAL INFO (per serving)				
calories	fat	protein	carbs	fiber
598	40g	48g	10g	4g

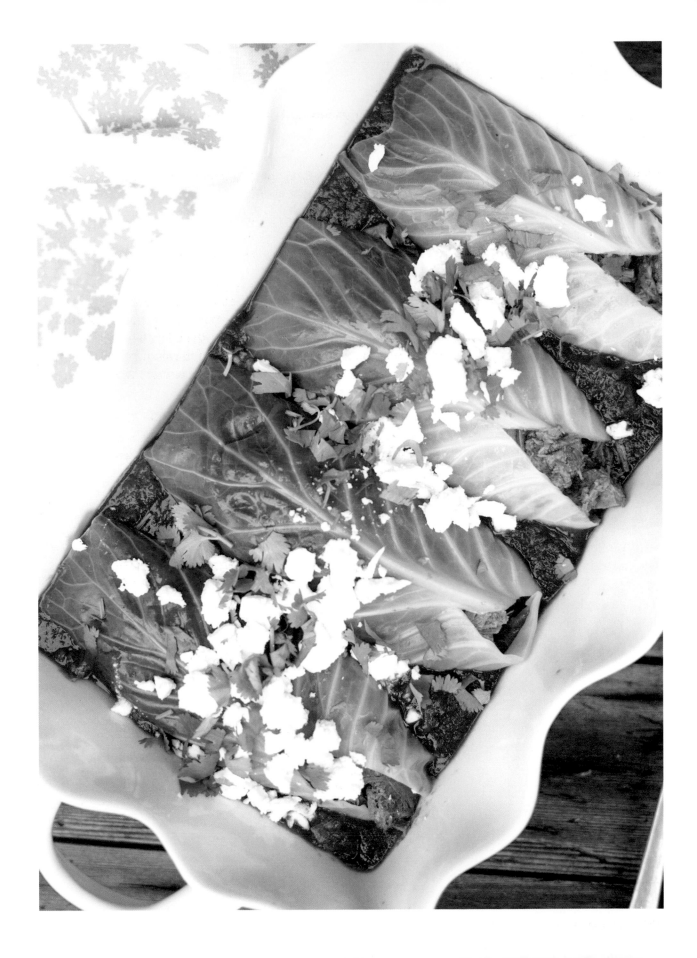

Steak Fajitas

(M / L↷H / KETO / OPTION / OPTION) prep time: 10 minutes, plus 1 hour to marinate (not including time to make tortillas)
cook time: 10 minutes   yield: 6 servings

⅓ cup avocado oil

⅓ cup fresh lime juice (about 3 limes)

¼ cup chopped fresh cilantro leaves

1 tablespoon chili powder

2 teaspoons ground cumin

½ teaspoon crushed red pepper

4 cloves garlic, minced

1 pound flank steak

1 small onion, thinly sliced

1 green bell pepper, thinly sliced

1 red bell pepper, thinly sliced

1 yellow bell pepper, thinly sliced

2 teaspoons fine sea salt

2 tablespoons ghee, coconut oil, or avocado oil, for frying

2 tablespoons chopped fresh cilantro leaves, for garnish

—for serving

6 Soft Tortillas (page 200) or Keto Tortillas (page 201)

6 cups shredded lettuce

1 cup shredded Monterey Jack cheese (about 4 ounces) (omit for dairy-free)

6 tablespoons sour cream (omit for dairy-free)

6 tablespoons store-bought sugar-free salsa

1 lime, cut into 6 slices

Diced avocado, for garnish (optional)

1. Place the avocado oil, lime juice, cilantro, chili powder, cumin, crushed red pepper, and garlic in a 13 by 9-inch baking dish. Stir to combine, then add the steak, onion, and bell peppers. Turn the steak and toss the vegetables to coat them well in the marinade. Cover the baking dish, place in the refrigerator, and marinate for 1 hour or overnight.

2. Remove the steak from the marinade and pat dry. Season the steak with salt on both sides.

3. Heat the ghee in a large cast-iron skillet over medium-high heat. Sear the steak on both sides for 3 to 5 minutes, until done to your liking (see the chart on page 232 for doneness temperatures). The exact cooking time will depend on the thickness of the steak. Remove the steak from the skillet and allow to rest for 8 minutes before slicing.

4. Meanwhile, remove the vegetables from the marinade and add them to the skillet (discard the marinade). Sauté the vegetables over medium-high heat, stirring often, until crisp-tender, about 5 minutes.

5. Place the vegetables on a platter. Slice the steak against the grain into ⅛-inch-thick slices and place the slices on the platter with the veggies. Garnish the meat and veggies with chopped cilantro.

6. Serve with the tortillas, lettuce, cheese, sour cream, salsa, lime slices, and avocado. Store in an airtight container in the refrigerator for up to 5 days. To reheat, place in a lightly greased skillet over medium heat for about 3 minutes.

tip: *I prepare the toppings and marinate the steak and veggies the night before for an easy dinner the next day. All I have to do is sauté the meat and veggies and set out all the toppings. Easy as pie!*

NUTRITIONAL INFO (per serving)				
calories	fat	protein	carbs	fiber
525	40g	27g	17g	7g

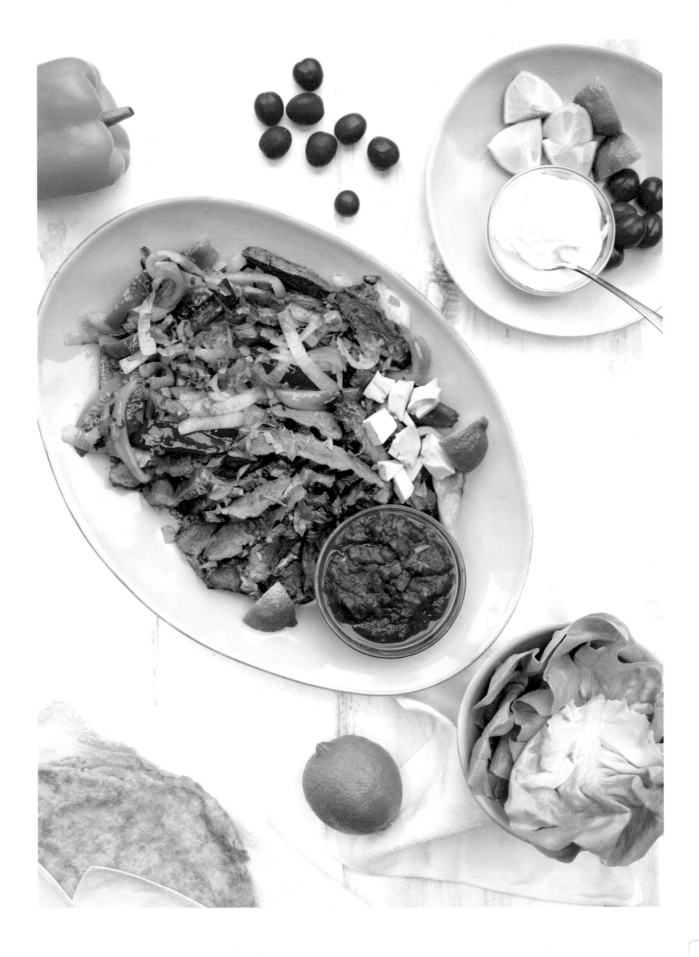

Cheesy Chile Rellenos

(L $\underset{\text{KETO}}{\overset{\text{M}}{\rightarrow}}$ H 🍽️)   prep time: 10 minutes   cook time: 10 minutes   yield: 2 servings

2 medium poblano chiles

Fine sea salt and ground black pepper

—filling

1½ cups shredded Monterey Jack cheese (about 6 ounces)

2 ounces cream cheese, at room temperature

—coating

2 large eggs, separated, at room temperature

½ teaspoon fine sea salt

¼ cup ghee or coconut oil, for frying

½ cup Easy Blender Enchilada Sauce (page 196), warmed, for serving

1. Lay a chile on a cutting board so that it sits flat naturally without rolling. Using a knife, make two cuts, forming a "T" by first slicing down the middle of the chile lengthwise from stem to tip, then making a second cut perpendicular to the first about ½ inch from the stem, slicing only halfway through the chile (be careful not to cut off the stem end completely). Carefully open the flaps to expose the interior of the chile and, using the paring knife, carefully cut out and remove the core.

2. Scrape the inside with a small spoon to remove the seeds, ribs, and any remaining core. Repeat with the other chile. Coring and removing the seeds from the chiles is easier before roasting.

3. Roast the chiles: If you have a gas stove, turn a burner to medium-high heat. Place 1 chile directly on the burner and roast, turning occasionally with tongs, until blackened and blistered on all sides, 5 to 7 minutes. If you don't have a gas stove, use the broiler to roast them: Preheat the broiler to high and place a rack in the upper third of the oven. Place the chiles directly on the rack. Broil, turning occasionally with tongs, until the chiles blacken and blister on all sides, 8 to 10 minutes. (The chiles will be softer if you use the broiler rather than a direct flame, so be careful not to tear them while stuffing.)

4. Transfer the roasted chiles to a large heatproof dish. Cover the dish tightly with plastic wrap or a baking sheet and let the chiles steam until cool enough to handle, about 15 minutes. Using a butter knife, scrape away and discard the skins, being careful not to tear the chiles; set the chiles aside.

5. Season the inside and outside of the chiles with salt and pepper. Stuff each chile with the cheeses. Set aside.

6. Using a hand mixer, whip the egg whites in a small bowl until soft peaks form. In another small bowl, whisk the egg yolks. Gently fold the yolks into the whites. Dip each chile into the egg mixture to coat the entire chile; if the coating doesn't stick, use the alternative coating method described in Step 7.

7. Heat the ghee in a medium-sized skillet over medium heat. Place the coated chiles in the skillet and fry on all sides until golden brown, 2 to 3 minutes per side. If the egg coating didn't stick to the chiles when completing Step 6, dollop about 3 tablespoons of the coating into the hot oil in the shape of a chile, lay a chile on top

NUTRITIONAL INFO (per serving)				
calories	fat	protein	carbs	fiber
799	71g	31g	7g	1g

of the coating mixture, and then dollop another 3 tablespoons of the egg mixture over the top of the chile and smooth it out with a spoon to cover the entire chile. Repeat to coat the second chile.

8. To serve, divide the warmed enchilada sauce between 2 shallow bowls and place a chile in each bowl. Store in an airtight container in the refrigerator for up to 5 days. To reheat, place in a lightly greased skillet over medium heat for about 3 minutes.

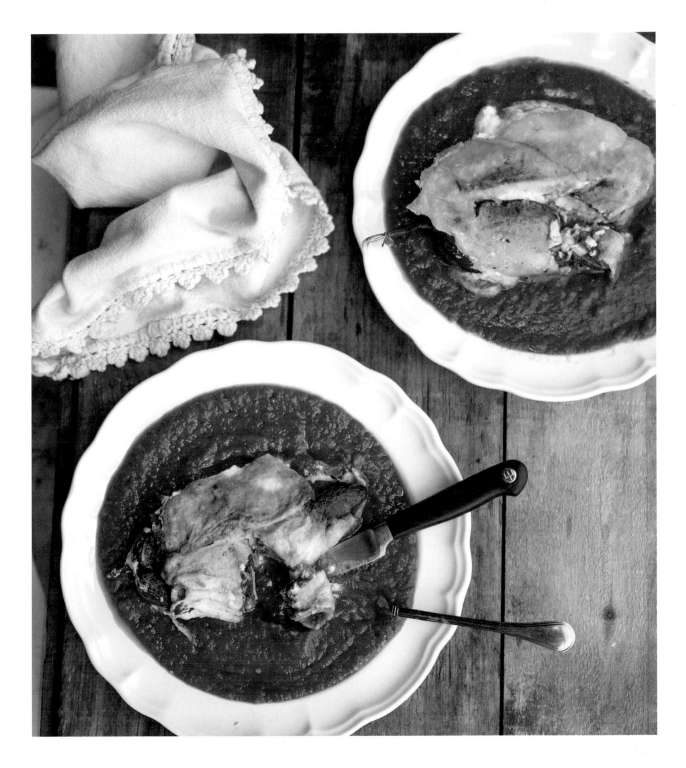

Enchiladas Verdes Lasagna

(L M H KETO · OPTION · OPTION · OPTION)   prep time: 10 minutes   cook time: 25 minutes   yield: 6 servings

This Mexican dish is made by creating alternating layers of tortillas and filling—sort of like Italian lasagna!

I'm a traditional German girl who is not a fan of spicy food. If you are like me, you may want to add only half a serrano chile; however, if you are like my Ethiopian boys, who love spicy food, you may want to increase it to two chiles!

—salsa verde

1 pound green tomatillos, husks removed

½ cup chicken bone broth, home-made (page 356) or store-bought

½ cup chopped fresh cilantro leaves

¼ cup diced onions (about 1 small)

1 clove garlic, minced

1 serrano chile (or more to desired heat), seeded

½ teaspoon fine sea salt

1 tablespoon ghee or coconut oil, for frying

—filling

2 cups shredded cooked chicken

—tortillas

6 thin slices deli chicken (about the size of an 8-inch tortilla), or 6 Soft Tortillas (page 200) or Keto Tortillas (page 201)

—for serving

1 avocado, sliced

½ cup sour cream (omit for dairy-free)

½ cup crumbled Cotija cheese or other Mexican cheese (optional; omit for dairy-free)

Chopped fresh cilantro, for garnish (optional)

1. Preheat the oven to 375°F.

2. Make the salsa verde: Place the tomatillos, broth, cilantro, onions, garlic, chile, and salt in a blender and puree until smooth. Heat the ghee in a small saucepan over medium-high heat. Pour the toma-tillo mixture into the pan and simmer for about 15 minutes, until it thickens a bit. Taste and adjust the seasoning to your liking.

3. Assemble the lasagna: Place one-third of the shredded chicken in an 8-inch square baking dish. Place 2 slices of chicken on top of the shredded chicken. Pour one-third of the sauce over the chicken slices. Repeat the layers two more times: shredded chicken, chicken slices, sauce. Bake for 10 minutes, or until hot and bubbly.

4. Serve with sliced avocado, sour cream, and Cotija cheese, if using. Garnish with cilantro, if desired. Store in an airtight container in the refrigerator for up to 5 days. To reheat, place in a baking dish in a preheated 375°F oven for about 3 minutes.

NUTRITIONAL INFO (per serving)				
calories	fat	protein	carbs	fiber
368	21g	34g	8g	3g

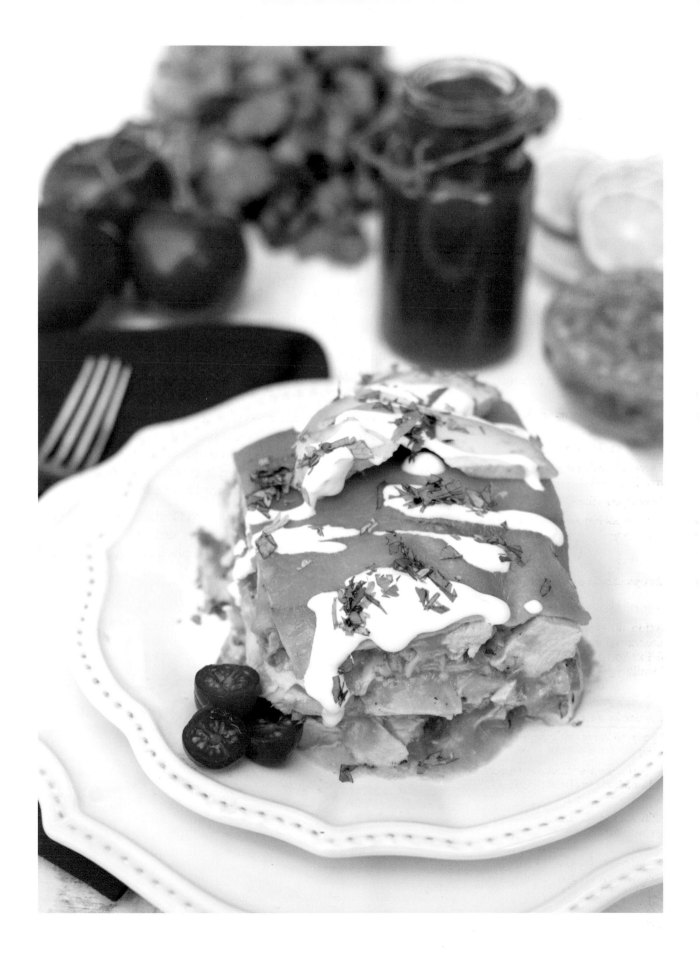

Chicken Thigh Chili Verdes

(L →H M KETO OPTION) prep time: 7 minutes   cook time: 35 minutes   yield: 8 servings

3 tablespoons coconut oil or avocado oil

8 bone-in, skin-on chicken thighs

Fine sea salt and ground black pepper

1 batch Salsa Verde (page 226)

Fresh cilantro leaves, for garnish

1 avocado, sliced, for serving

½ cup sour cream, for serving (omit for dairy-free)

2 limes, quartered, for serving

1. Heat the oil in a large cast-iron skillet over medium-high heat. Pat the chicken thighs dry and season them liberally with salt and pepper. Place the chicken, skin side down, in the skillet and cook for 10 minutes per side, or until the skin is golden brown.

2. Pour the salsa into the skillet with the chicken, reduce the heat, and simmer for about 15 minutes, until the chicken is cooked through.

3. Garnish with cilantro and serve with avocado, sour cream (if using), and lime wedges. Store in an airtight container in the refrigerator for up to 5 days. To reheat, place in a lightly greased skillet over medium heat for about 3 minutes.

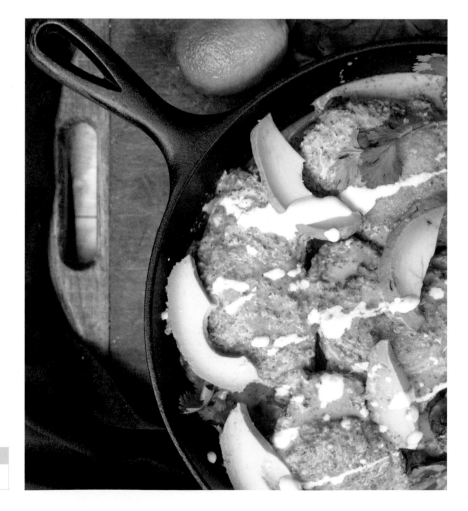

NUTRITIONAL INFO (per serving)				
calories	fat	protein	carbs	fiber
304	23g	17g	7g	2g

Simple Pollo Asado

prep time: 4 servings   cook time: 6 minutes   yield: 3 or 6 hours in a slow cooker

—sauce

1 cup chicken bone broth, homemade (page 356) or store-bought

½ cup chopped onions (about 1 medium)

4 scallions, chopped

3 cloves garlic, chopped

2 tablespoons fresh lime juice

¼ cup chopped fresh cilantro, plus extra for garnish

1 tablespoon chopped fresh thyme leaves

2 tablespoons smoked paprika

1 tablespoon ground cumin

1 teaspoon fine sea salt

½ teaspoon ground black pepper

8 bone-in, skin-on chicken thighs

1. In a food processor or blender, puree the broth, onions, scallions, garlic, lime juice, cilantro, thyme, paprika, cumin, salt, and pepper until smooth. Pour the sauce into a 4-quart slow cooker and add the chicken. Cover and cook on low for 6 hours or on high for 3 hours.

2. When the chicken is fork-tender, place the thighs, skin side up, on a rimmed baking sheet. Preheat the broiler to high. Broil the chicken for 6 minutes, or until the chicken skin is browned and crisp.

3. Transfer the chicken to a serving plate and serve with the sauce from the slow cooker. Garnish with cilantro. Store in an airtight container in the refrigerator for up to 5 days. To reheat, place in a baking dish in a preheated 375°F oven for about 5 minutes.

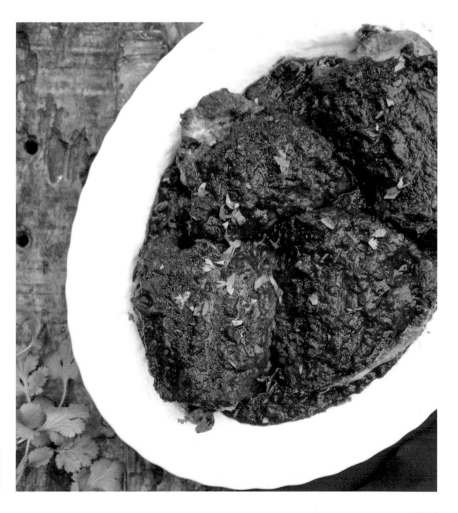

NUTRITIONAL INFO (per serving)				
calories	fat	protein	carbs	fiber
345	21g	33g	6g	1g

Mouthwatering Carnitas

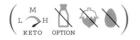

prep time: 5 minutes   cook time: 3 to 4 hours or 8 hours in a slow cooker
yield: 6 servings

I went to a super-cute restaurant in Maui called Fred's Mexican Café. I know what you're thinking: "What are you doing eating Mexican food when you can eat fresh seafood?!" But after weeks of fish, which I'm not a huge fan of, I needed something different. The waitress, who was from Wisconsin, was such a peach!

I told her I wanted the carnitas, but instead of tortillas, I asked if she could throw it on a bed of lettuce so that I could make a salad. She smiled. When she came back, I had the most beautiful and tasty dish covered in guacamole, sour cream, salsa, and fresh cilantro. It was just what I needed!

Carnitas are basically "confit pork," and confit is a French cooking method. My best tip for a great confit is to control the temperature and keep the meat there long enough for the collagen to break down without losing moisture. This is why I use fat rather than water in my recipe. Using fat instead of water helps in three ways:

1. It helps retain moisture. I recommend cooking the pork in the smallest cooking vessel you can find and fitting the pork as tightly as possible so that it cooks in its own fat as it renders. The fat that coats the meat will help retain moisture because it doesn't allow the moisture to evaporate.

2. It helps control the temperature better, distributing heat more evenly.

3. It delivers fat-soluble flavor molecules. The spices and oils from the lime are fat-soluble and are infused with fats!

2 teaspoons chili powder

2 teaspoons ground cumin

2 teaspoons fine sea salt

3 pounds boneless pork butt (aka pork shoulder), cut into 6 pieces

½ cup sliced red onions (about 1 medium)

4 cloves garlic, minced

½ cup melted lard or coconut oil

About 4 cups pork, beef, or chicken bone broth (enough to cover the pork), homemade (page 356) or store-bought

Juice of 2 limes

Coconut oil, ghee, or lard, for frying

Lettuce wraps, for serving

1 batch Pico de Gallo (page 197), for serving

¼ cup diced red onions, for serving

baking option: *After slow-cooking the pork, preheat the oven to 450°F. Cut the pork into 1-inch chunks. Place the carnitas on a rimmed baking sheet in a single layer. Bake for 15 to 20 minutes, until the pork is browned.*

NUTRITIONAL INFO (per serving)				
calories	fat	protein	carbs	fiber
592	51g	30g	4g	1g

1. Combine the chili powder, cumin, and salt in a small bowl. Using your hands, rub the mixture all over the pieces of pork.

2. Place the onions and garlic in a 4-quart slow cooker. Set the pork on top of the onions and garlic. Cover the pork with the melted lard. Add enough broth to cover the pork, then add the lime juice. Cover and cook on low for 8 hours or on high for 3 to 4 hours, until the pork is fork-tender and starting to fall apart. Low and slow will create more tender carnitas.

3. Place the pork on a cutting board and slice it into 1-inch chunks. Discard the liquid from the slow cooker.

4. Heat the oil in a large cast-iron skillet over medium-high heat. Place the pork in the skillet and fry until crisp on all sides, about 1 minute per side. Remove from the heat and serve in lettuce wraps. Store in an airtight container in the refrigerator for up to 3 days. To reheat, place the pork mixture in a skillet over medium heat and sauté for about 3 minutes.

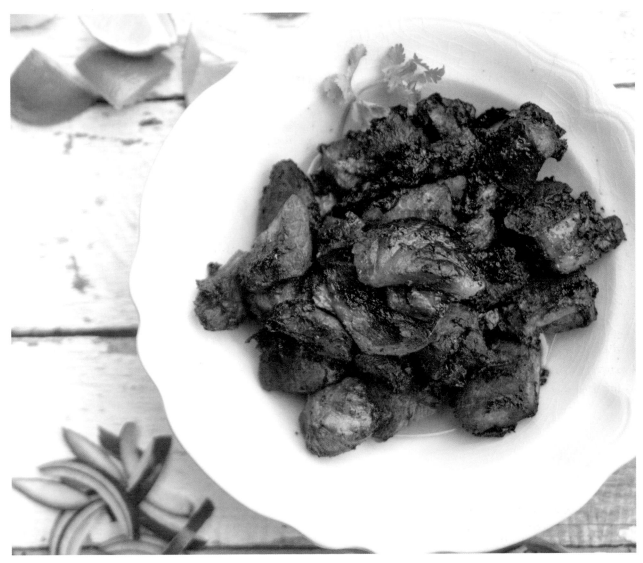

Carne Asada Tacos

(LM TH KETO · OPTION · OPTION · OPTION) **prep time:** 10 minutes, plus time to marinate steak (not including time to make tortillas or pico de gallo) **cook time:** 8 to 12 minutes **yield:** 8 servings

—marinade

½ cup chopped fresh cilantro

⅓ cup avocado oil

2 tablespoons coconut vinegar or apple cider vinegar

2 tablespoons fresh lime juice

2 tablespoons Swerve confectioners'-style sweetener or equivalent amount of liquid or powdered sweetener (see page 31)

1 tablespoon wheat-free tamari, or ¼ cup coconut aminos

2 teaspoons fine sea salt, if using coconut aminos (less salty)

1 teaspoon ground black pepper

1 teaspoon ground cumin

4 cloves garlic, smashed to a paste or minced

1 jalapeño pepper, seeded and minced

2 pounds flank or skirt steak

8 Soft Tortillas (page 200), Keto Tortillas (page 201), or large lettuce leaves

—suggested fillings

Shredded lettuce

Diced avocado

Lime wedges

1 batch Pico de Gallo (page 197)

¼ cup fresh cilantro leaves

1 radish, thinly sliced

1. Make the marinade: Place the cilantro, oil, vinegar, lime juice, sweetener, tamari, salt, black pepper, cumin, garlic, and jalapeño in a large baking dish and stir to combine.

2. Slice the steak in half. Place the steaks in the dish and turn to coat in the marinade. Cover the baking dish, place in the refrigerator, and marinate for 3 hours or overnight.

3. Preheat a grill to medium-high heat or heat up a large cast-iron skillet over medium-high heat. Remove the steaks from the marinade, scraping off any pieces of herbs or garlic from the steaks (discard the marinade). Place the steaks on the grill or in the skillet and sear for about 3 minutes per side, or until cooked to your liking (see the chart below). Remove the steaks from the grill and place on a cutting board to rest for 10 minutes before slicing.

4. Meanwhile, set out the tortillas and taco fillings.

5. Using a sharp knife, slice the steaks across the grain. Assemble the tacos with the carne asada and other fillings of your choice. These are best served fresh, but extra carne asada and fillings can be stored in separate airtight containers in the refrigerator for up to 3 days. To reheat the carne asada, place in a baking dish in a preheated 350°F oven for about 3 minutes.

busy family tip: *I store tortillas in the freezer to make it easier to pull together meals like this!*

Temperature	Doneness
140°F–145°F	Medium
130°F–135°F	Medium-rare
120°F–125°F	Rare

NUTRITIONAL INFO (per serving, without fillings)				
calories	fat	protein	carbs	fiber
386	27g	28g	7g	4g

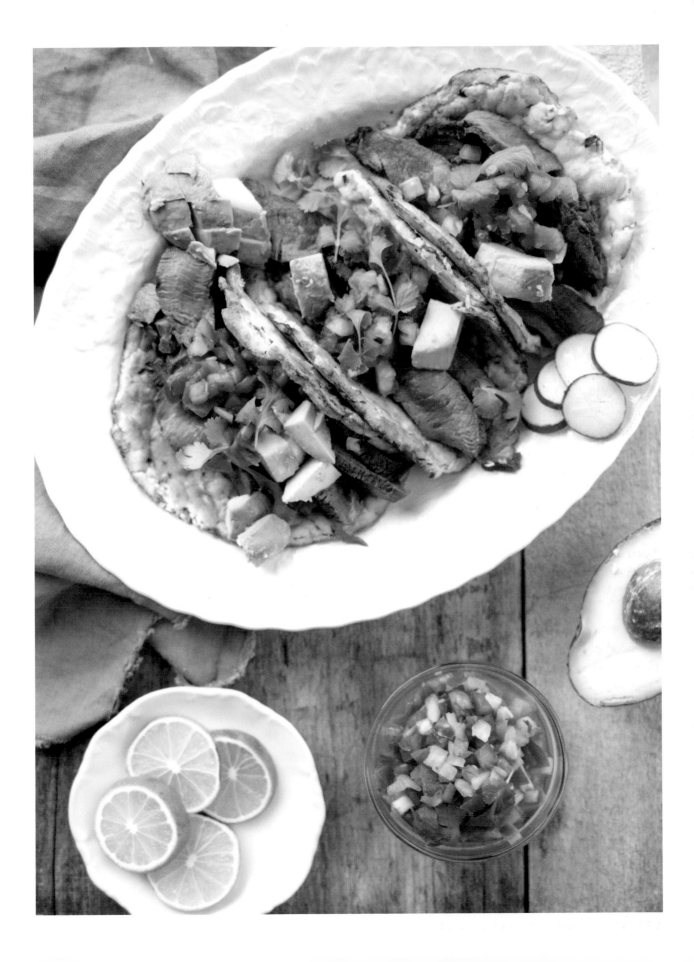

Smoky Refried "Beans"

(LMH KETO · OPTION) prep time: 5 minutes · cook time: 20 minutes · yield: 8 servings

Most of you know that refried beans are traditionally made with pinto beans. Sure, they seem harmless: no corn syrup, no trans fats, no "plastic package" surrounding this food item . . . so what's wrong with eating beans?

Well, beans are very high in carbs. Sure, they have protein, too, but the ratio of carbohydrate to protein is 4:1. Beans also contain lectins, which are indigestible proteins found in plants. Lectins attach to the lower intestine, which can create unpleasant inflammatory responses and lead to awful bowel issues, such as irritable bowel syndrome, colitis, and Crohn's disease. Lectins also increase your risk of developing leptin resistance. Leptin is the hormone that signals to your brain that you are full, and when it malfunctions, overeating is often the result. This is why I suggest a bean-free diet. My passion is to make the keto diet as tasty as possible so that you can be successful! I think you will totally enjoy this bean-free recipe, which is low in starch and has no lectins.

1 medium eggplant, or 2 large zucchini

4 strips bacon, chopped

1 cup chopped onions (about 1 large)

1 clove garlic, minced

1 tablespoon seeded and minced jalapeño pepper

1 tablespoon chili powder

1 teaspoon ground cumin

½ teaspoon fine sea salt

Pinch of cayenne pepper

½ teaspoon chopped fresh oregano

½ cup crumbled queso fresco or shredded cheddar cheese (optional)

¼ cup minced fresh cilantro, for garnish (optional)

1. Peel and cube the eggplant. Place the eggplant and bacon in a large cast-iron skillet over medium-high heat. Stir-fry until the bacon is crisp and the eggplant is very soft, about 10 minutes. Using a slotted spoon, transfer the eggplant and bacon to a food processor; leave the bacon fat in the pan. Puree the eggplant and bacon until smooth.

2. Cook the onions in the skillet with the bacon fat over medium-high heat, stirring, until soft, about 3 minutes. Add the garlic, jalapeño, chili powder, cumin, salt, and cayenne and cook, stirring, until fragrant, 45 seconds to 1 minute. Stir in the eggplant puree and oregano. Cook, stirring with a heavy wooden spoon, until the mixture forms a thick paste, 5 to 10 minutes, adding water 1 tablespoon at a time to keep it from getting dry.

3. Sprinkle with the cheese and cilantro, if using, and serve. Store in an airtight container in the refrigerator for up to 5 days. To reheat, place in a lightly greased skillet over medium heat for about 3 minutes.

vegetarian option: *Peel and slice the eggplant, wrap it in foil, and smoke it in a wood smoker for 2 hours. This gives the eggplant a smoky flavor without using bacon.*

NUTRITIONAL INFO (per serving)				
calories	fat	protein	carbs	fiber
107	8g	6g	6g	2g

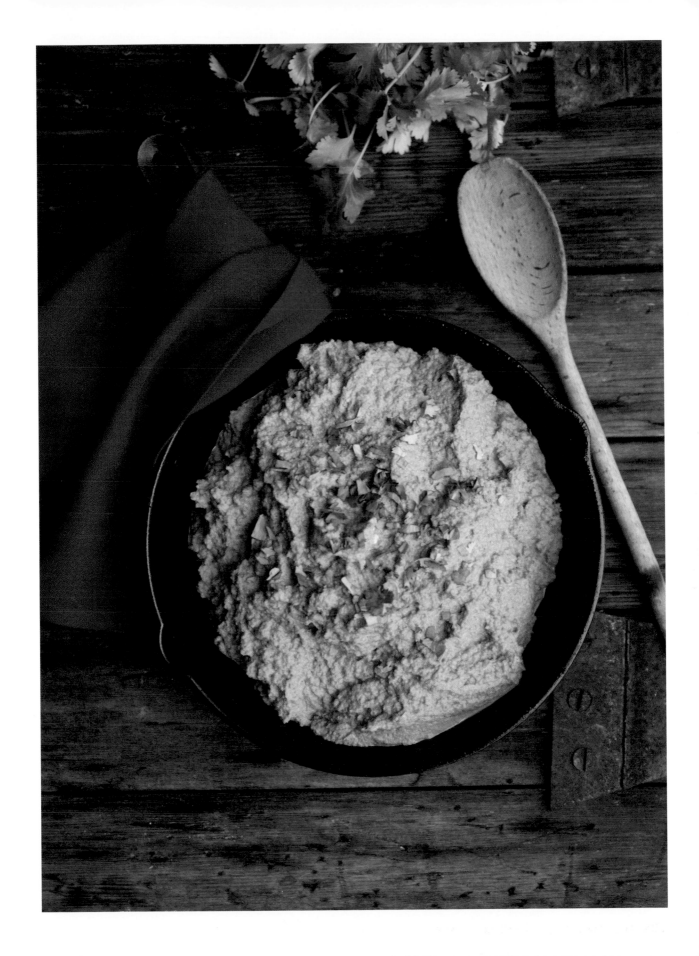

Piña Colada

(L →M H ⬢ 🥛 🚫 🌰) prep time: 3 minutes   yield: 4 servings

If you enjoyed this Puerto Rican classic before going keto and thought you'd never be able to imbibe again, try my version. It has all the flavor without the sugar.

1 cup full-fat coconut milk

¼ cup fresh lime juice (about 2 limes)

¼ cup Swerve confectioners'-style sweetener or equivalent amount of liquid or powdered sweetener (see page 31)

2 teaspoons coconut-pineapple Stur (optional, for color and more flavor)

1 teaspoon pineapple extract

½ teaspoon rum extract

2 cups crushed ice

1. Place the coconut milk, lime juice, sweetener, pineapple Stur (if using), pineapple extract, rum extract, and ice in a blender and puree until smooth. Pour into glasses and enjoy!

2. This drink is best served fresh, but extras can be stored in an airtight container in the freezer for up to 1 month. Thaw for a few minutes before serving.

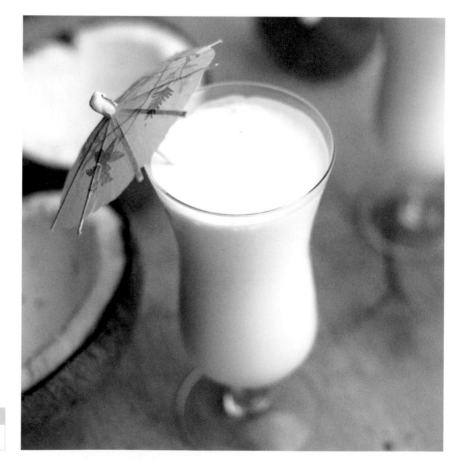

NUTRITIONAL INFO (per serving)				
calories	fat	protein	carbs	fiber
92	9g	1g	2g	0.1g

Fried Ice Cream

(L M H KETO) prep time: 10 minutes, plus 15 minutes to freeze (not including time to make bread or ice cream)
cook time: 8 minutes   yield: 2 servings

6 slices Keto Bread (page 362), crusts removed

1 cup Keto Vanilla Ice Cream (page 342)

2 tablespoons ghee or coconut oil, for frying

2 teaspoons ground cinnamon

2 teaspoons Swerve confectioners'-style sweetener or equivalent amount of liquid or powdered sweetener (see page 31)

1. Arrange the bread slices on a piece of parchment paper so that the slices overlap just a touch in the center. Using a rolling pin or your hands, flatten out the bread. Place ½ scoop of keto ice cream in the center of the bread. Roll up the bread and use your fingers to seal the edges. Place in the freezer for about 15 minutes.

2. Heat the ghee in a small saucepan over medium heat to 350°F.

3. Combine the cinnamon and sweetener in a small serving bowl. Stir well and set next to the stove.

4. Fry the wrapped ice cream in the ghee until golden brown, about 90 seconds per side. Add more ghee to the pan, if needed.

5. Remove from the pan and place in the bowl with the cinnamon mixture. Spoon the mixture all over the fried ice cream. Serve immediately.

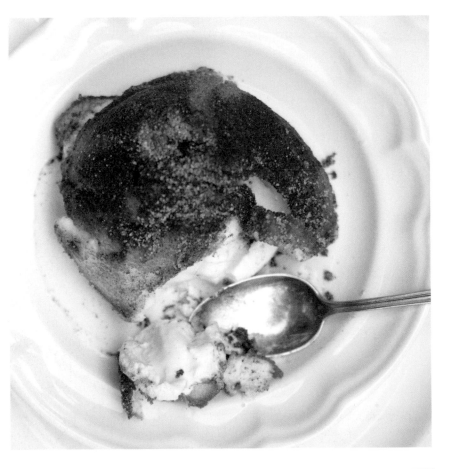

NUTRITIONAL INFO (per serving)				
calories	fat	protein	carbs	fiber
429	36g	23g	5g	3g

Flan

(L →H M KETO | OPTION 🥛 🚫) **prep time:** 15 minutes **cook time:** 10 minutes **yield:** 6 servings

Flan is a baked custard dessert served in a caramel sauce. Traditionally it's made with milk, but to make it a keto dessert, I use heavy cream instead. The Conquistadors brought flan to the New World colonies, and it is now a classic dessert in the majority of Latin American countries. Though it's not traditional, I sometimes like to garnish flan with crumbled bacon to add a salty, smoky accent. It's delicious!

2 cups heavy cream (or canned coconut milk if dairy-sensitive)

1 cup Swerve confectioners'-style sweetener or equivalent amount of liquid or powdered sweetener (see page 31)

5 large eggs

2 teaspoons vanilla extract

1 teaspoon ground cinnamon

—caramel sauce
  (omit if dairy-sensitive)

6 tablespoons unsalted butter

1 cup Swerve confectioners'-style sweetener or equivalent amount of powdered stevia or erythritol

½ cup heavy cream

1 teaspoon ground cinnamon

1. Place an oven rack in the middle of the oven and preheat the oven to 325°F.

2. Make the flan: Place the cream, sweetener, eggs, vanilla, and cinnamon in a blender or food processor and process until smooth. Divide the mixture evenly among six 3-ounce custard cups or ramekins.

3. Place the ramekins in a large roasting pan and add enough hot water to come halfway up the sides of the ramekins. Loosely cover the pan with foil and bake until the flan has barely set (a knife inserted halfway between the edge and the center should come out clean), 35 to 40 minutes. Let cool in the water bath, then place in the refrigerator to chill thoroughly.

4. Make the caramel sauce: Before you begin, make sure you have everything ready to go—have the ingredients next to the pan and ready to put in. Work fast or the sweetener will burn. Heat the butter in a heavy-bottomed 2- or 3-quart saucepan over high heat. As soon as it comes to a boil, watch for brown flecks; this is browned butter. Immediately add the sweetener, cream, and cinnamon and whisk until the caramel is smooth. Let cool in the pan for a couple minutes, then pour into a jar and let cool to room temperature. Stir before using.

5. To serve, run a knife around the edges, then unmold each flan onto a small serving plate. Pour the caramel sauce over each flan, allowing it to cover the top and run down the sides. Store in an airtight container in the refrigerator for up to 3 days.

busy family tip: *The caramel can be made up to 2 weeks ahead and stored in the refrigerator. The flans can be made up to 3 days ahead and stored in the fridge.*

NUTRITIONAL INFO (per serving)				
calories	fat	protein	carbs	fiber
495	55g	5g	1g	0.2g

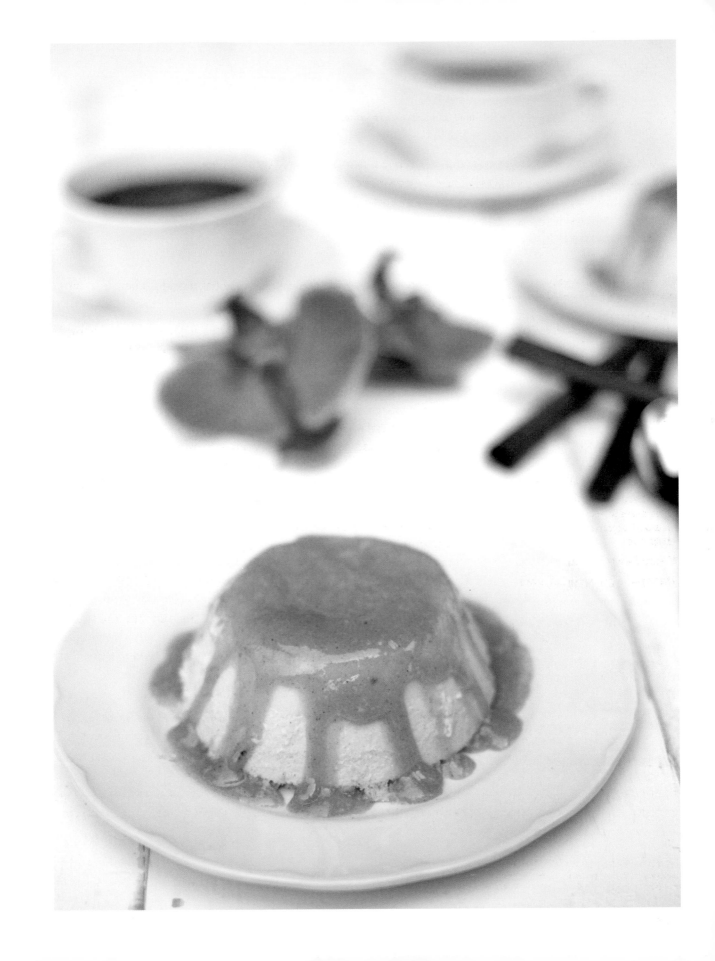

Churros

$\left(\begin{smallmatrix} & M & \\ L & \circlearrowright & H \\ & KETO & \end{smallmatrix}\right)$ **prep time:** 8 minutes   **cook time:** 10 minutes to bake, or 2 minutes to fry   **yield:** 8 servings

Churros are a type of donut, shaped somewhat like a cruller, but much thinner. The Portuguese and Spanish brought their taste for churros to the New World colonies, and they remain very popular today, in various forms, in Mexico and many Latin American countries. They are traditionally deep-fried; here I give you two options, a fried version and an oven-baked version.

1¾ cups shredded mozzarella cheese (about 7 ounces)

1 ounce cream cheese

¾ cup blanched almond flour

3 tablespoons Swerve confectioners'-style sweetener or equivalent amount of powdered sweetener (see page 31), plus extra for dusting

1 large egg

1 teaspoon almond extract

1 teaspoon vanilla extract

⅛ teaspoon fine sea salt

—cinnamon coating

1 tablespoon ground cinnamon

1 tablespoon Swerve confectioners'-style sweetener or equivalent amount of powdered stevia or erythritol

—glaze

¼ cup Swerve confectioners'-style sweetener or equivalent amount of liquid or powdered sweetener

1 to 2 tablespoons unsweetened cashew milk or heavy cream

1 tablespoon coconut oil, for frying

1. If baking the churros, preheat the oven to 400°F and grease a rimmed baking sheet with ghee or butter.

2. Make the dough: Place the mozzarella and cream cheese in a medium-sized microwavable bowl and microwave on high for 1 to 2 minutes, until the cheese is entirely melted. Stir well. To the bowl, add the almond flour, sweetener, egg, extracts, and salt. Using a hand mixer on high speed, mix the ingredients together until well combined. Roll into ½-inch-thick by 3-inch-long logs.

3. Make the cinnamon coating: Combine the cinnamon and sweetener in a shallow dish. Set aside.

4. Make the glaze: In a small bowl, combine the sweetener and just enough cashew milk to make a thin glaze. If it gets too thin, add a tablespoon of sweetener, and if it is too thick, add a splash of milk. Mix until smooth and set aside.

5. To fry the churros, heat 1 tablespoon of coconut oil in a large cast-iron skillet over medium heat. Fry the logs in batches for 1 minute on each side, adding more oil to the pan if needed, until golden brown on all sides.

   To bake the churros, place the logs on the greased baking sheet and bake for 9 minutes, or until the logs are golden brown and the dough is fully cooked and springy in the center.

6. As soon you remove the churros from the skillet or oven, roll them in the cinnamon coating. Once cool, drizzle the glaze over each churro. Store in an airtight container in the refrigerator for up to 5 days. To reheat, place in a lightly greased skillet over medium heat for about 3 minutes.

NUTRITIONAL INFO (per serving)				
calories	fat	protein	carbs	fiber
153	13g	9g	3g	1g

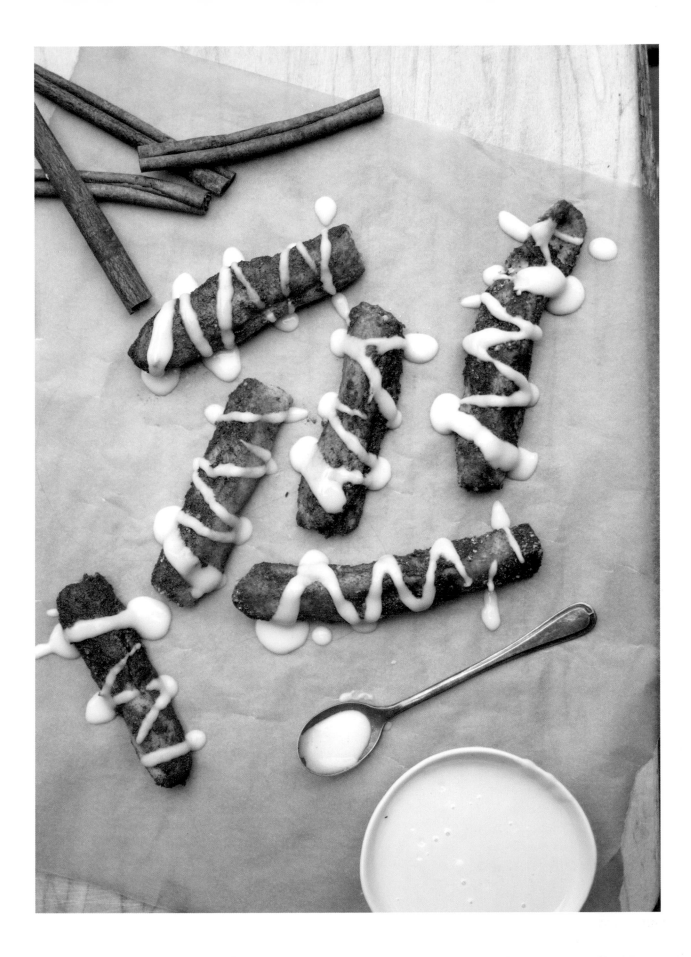

Tres Leches Cake

(L →M H / KETO)   **prep time:** 10 minutes   **cook time:** 50 minutes   **yield:** 8 servings

—cake

5 large eggs, separated

1 cup Swerve confectioners'-style sweetener or equivalent amount of liquid or powdered sweetener (see page 31), divided

1/3 cup unsweetened cashew milk or almond milk

1 teaspoon vanilla extract

1 cup blanched almond flour

1½ teaspoons baking powder

—leches

1 cup full-fat coconut milk

½ cup unsweetened cashew milk or almond milk

2 cups heavy cream, divided

¼ cup Swerve confectioners'-style sweetener or equivalent amount of liquid or powdered sweetener

1. Preheat the oven to 350°F. Coat the bottom of a 9-inch springform pan with coconut oil spray.

2. Make the cake: In a medium-sized bowl, use a hand mixer to beat the egg yolks with ¾ cup of the sweetener until lightened in color and doubled in volume. Stir in the milk, vanilla, almond flour, and baking powder.

3. In a small bowl, beat the egg whites until soft peaks form. Gradually add the remaining ¼ cup of sweetener and continue to beat until firm but not dry. Gently fold the whites into the egg yolk mixture, then pour the batter into the prepared pan. Bake for 45 to 50 minutes, until a cake tester inserted into the center of the cake comes out clean. Allow to cool in the pan for 10 minutes.

4. Loosen the edge of the cake with a knife before removing the ring of the pan. Let the cake cool completely, then transfer to a deep serving plate. Use a two-prong meat fork or cake tester to pierce the surface of the cake in several places.

5. Make the leches: Mix together the coconut milk, cashew milk, ¼ cup of the heavy cream, and the sweetener. Discard 1 cup of this milk mixture or cover and refrigerate it for later use. Slowly pour the remaining milk mixture over the cake until absorbed. Whip the remaining 1¾ cups of heavy cream until soft peaks form.

6. To serve as a traditional cake, frost the cake with the whipped cream and cut into slices. To serve as a layered dessert in individual glasses, as pictured, cut the cake into cubes and divide them among 8 glasses. Top the cake with about one-third of the whipped cream, then add the rest of the cake to the glasses. Top with the rest of the whipped cream, reserving some for piping on the very top for a pretty presentation.

7. Store the cake in an airtight container in the refrigerator for up to 4 days.

NUTRITIONAL INFO (per serving)				
calories	fat	protein	carbs	fiber
329	34g	7g	3g	2g

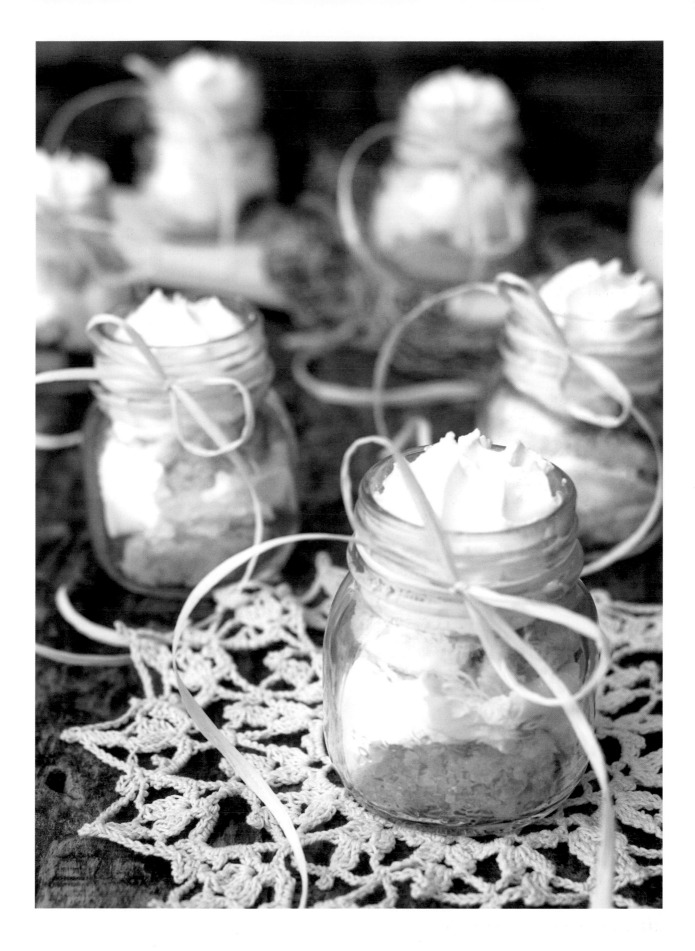

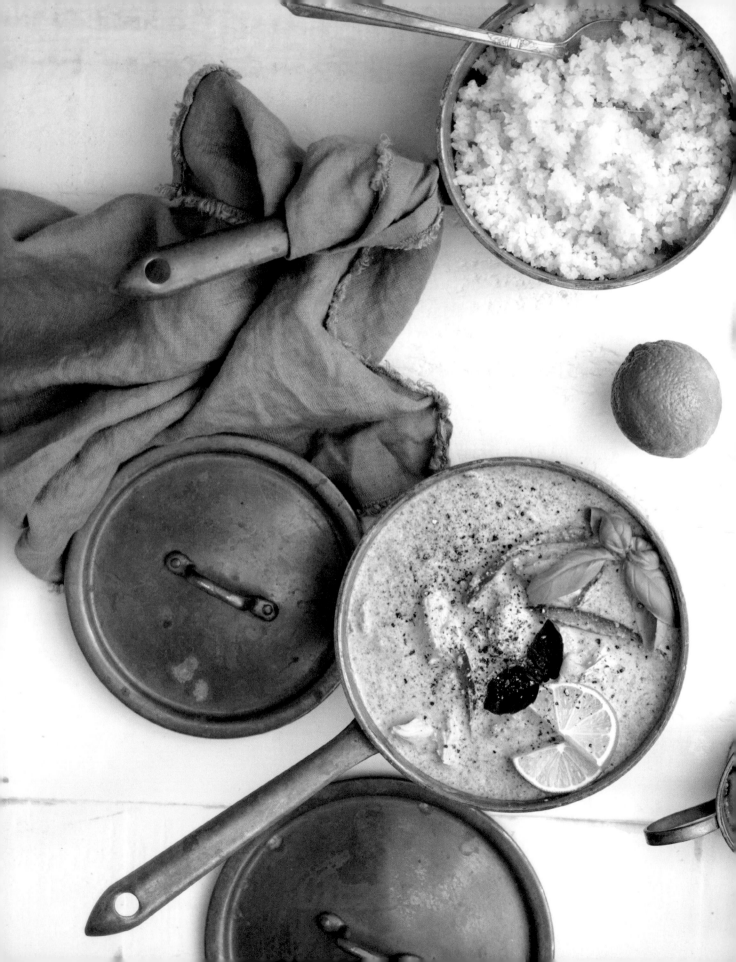

Indian, Thai, & Other Southeast Asian *Cuisine*

WARNING! Thai restaurants usually add sugar or honey to their dishes. If you prefer this sweeter taste, feel free to add a touch of natural sweetener, such as Swerve or stevia glycerite, to my Thai recipes. If you have been eating keto for a while and your sweet tooth is gone, you likely will not miss the sweetness.

Sinangag

(L—M—H KETO   OPTION)   **prep time:** 5 minutes   **cook time:** 7 minutes   **yield:** 8 servings

Sinangag—rice fried with a lot of garlic—is a common Filipino side dish. My keto version of Sinangag, made with cauliflower rice, goes well with several of my recipes, such as Malai Curry Shrimp (page 278), pictured below, and Fish Palak (page 280).

4 cups riced cauliflower (see page 363)

1½ teaspoons fine sea salt

3 tablespoons ghee, coconut oil, or avocado oil

3 cloves garlic, minced

1. Place the riced cauliflower and salt in a large bowl and mix well. Heat the ghee in a wok or large cast-iron skillet over medium-high heat. Add the garlic and stir-fry until golden brown and crisp, about 2 minutes. Stir in the riced cauliflower and cook until the rice is tender, about 4 minutes. Remove from the wok and place in a serving bowl.

2. Store in an airtight container in the refrigerator for up to 4 days. To reheat, place in a sauté pan over medium heat for about 3 minutes, stirring often.

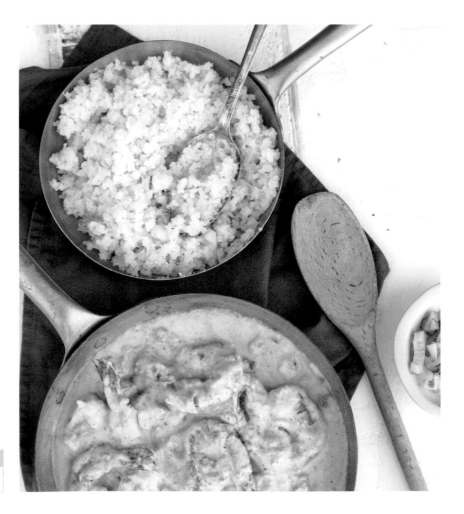

NUTRITIONAL INFO (per serving)				
calories	fat	protein	carbs	fiber
65	6g	1g	3g	1g

Thai Basil Fried "Rice"

(L M H KETO · OPTION)   prep time: 5 minutes   cook time: 7 minutes   yield: 4 servings

2 tablespoons ghee, coconut oil, or avocado oil

2 cloves garlic, minced

1 tablespoon grated fresh ginger

2 cups riced cauliflower (see page 363)

2 tablespoons fish sauce

1 large egg, lightly beaten

Fine sea salt

Fresh Thai basil leaves, for garnish

1. Heat the ghee in a large cast-iron skillet or wok over medium-high heat. Add the garlic and ginger and sauté for 1 minute, until fragrant. Add the riced cauliflower and fish sauce and stir-fry for 5 minutes, until the cauliflower is soft.

2. Add the egg and stir-fry until the egg is cooked through, about 1 minute. Season to taste with salt and garnish with Thai basil. Serve immediately. Store in the refrigerator for up to 4 days. To reheat, place in a sauté pan over medium heat for about 3 minutes, stirring often.

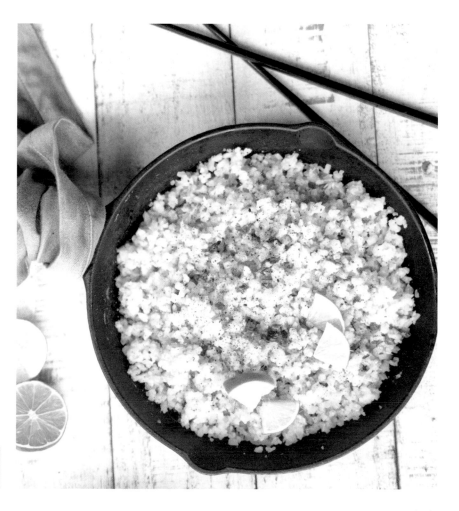

NUTRITIONAL INFO (per serving)				
calories	fat	protein	carbs	fiber
111	9g	5g	4g	1g

Vietnamese Imperial Rolls

(L ⟶ᴹ H · KETO ▯ ⊘ ◗)   prep time: 12 minutes   cook time: 15 minutes   yield: 20 rolls (2 rolls per serving)

—filling

1 pound ground chicken or ground pork

2 cups chopped button mushrooms (about 1 pound)

1 cup thinly shredded cabbage

¼ cup diced red onions (about 1 small)

2 cloves garlic, minced

2 teaspoons grated fresh ginger

1 teaspoon fish sauce

1 teaspoon wheat-free tamari, or 1 tablespoon plus 1 teaspoon coconut aminos

20 strips bacon

—dipping sauce

¼ cup chicken or beef bone broth, homemade (page 356) or store-bought

2 tablespoons Swerve confectioners'-style sweetener or equivalent amount of liquid or powdered sweetener (see page 31)

2 tablespoons fresh lime juice

1 tablespoon fish sauce

Sliced scallions, for garnish

1. Preheat the oven to 400°F.

2. Make the filling: Place the ground chicken, mushrooms, cabbage, onions, garlic, ginger, fish sauce, and tamari in a large bowl. Mix well with your hands.

3. Lay 1 bacon strip vertically on a sushi mat or sheet of parchment paper. Spoon 2 to 3 tablespoons of the filling onto the end of the bacon. Pick up the bottom left corner of the bacon strip and fold it tightly over the filling, at an angle. Then roll the bacon forward, straight out in front of you. Now repeat the first fold, except from the opposite direction, rolling the bacon from right to left at an angle, then rolling the bacon forward, straight out in front of you. Repeat this left-forward-right folding motion to the end of strip (the ends may be exposed, and that's okay). Place the roll on a rimmed baking sheet to catch the drippings. Repeat until all the bacon strips are filled.

4. Bake the rolls for 15 minutes, or until the bacon is crisp. Remove from the oven and set aside.

5. Make the dipping sauce: Place the broth, sweetener, lime juice, and fish sauce in a small bowl and stir to combine well.

6. To serve, drizzle some of the sauce over the rolls and garnish with scallions. Serve with extra sauce on the side for dipping. Store in an airtight container in the refrigerator for up to 4 days. To reheat, place in a preheated 400°F oven for 5 minutes, or until the bacon is crispy again.

NUTRITIONAL INFO (per serving)				
calories	fat	protein	carbs	fiber
271	18g	23g	3g	1g

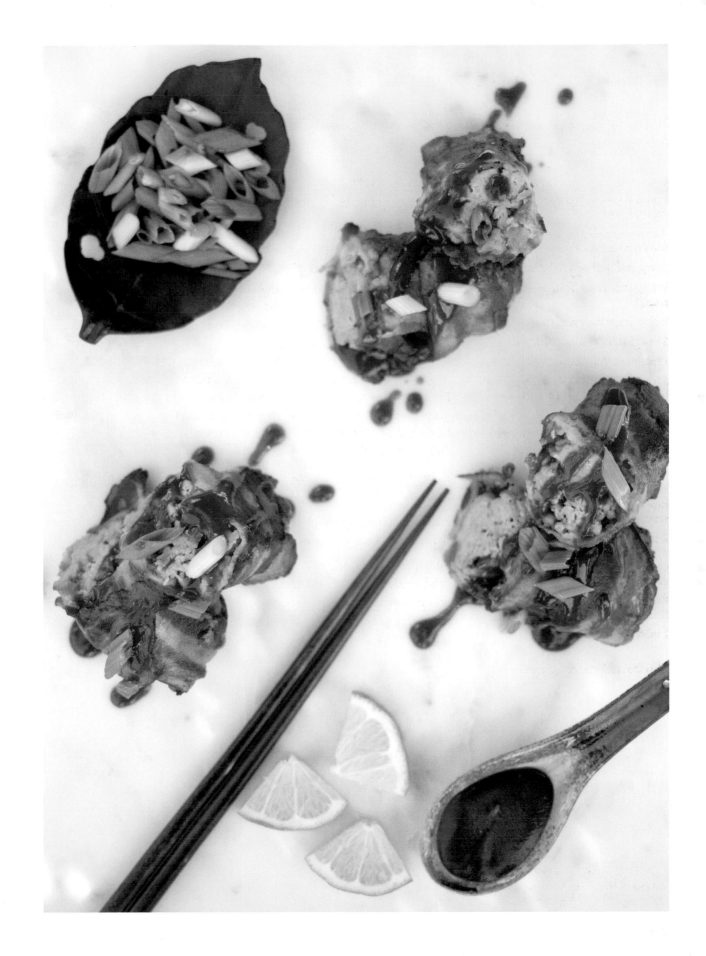

Tom Ka Gai (Coconut Chicken Soup)

(L M↑H KETO 🥛 🚫 🥑)   prep time: 5 minutes   cook time: 30 minutes   yield: 4 servings

In 2009, I ran the Hawaii marathon with some friends. The night before the race, we went out to dinner to "carb load." Well, I didn't, but my friends asked how I was going to perform well the next day if I didn't eat any carbs. My running friends were shocked when the man we were staying with chimed in and said, "I heard people can run marathons with 'fat-loading' instead." I just smiled.

My pre-race meal was Tom Ka Gai, and it was divine! It was my first taste of this dish, and I will never forget it. Our hosts were local Hawaiians, and they knew the best places to eat. We ate at a tiny restaurant hidden away on a side street. Our hosts warned us that the food would take a long time to get to the table because the owner made everything to order, but assured us that it would be the best Thai food we had ever eaten, and worth the wait. They weren't lying. It did take a long time, but the taste was incredible. The cook didn't even take issue with my request for my soup to be prepared without sugar.

1 tablespoon coconut oil

3 shallots, chopped

1½ cups chicken bone broth, homemade (page 356) or store-bought

1 (13½-ounce) can full-fat coconut milk

2 tablespoons red curry paste

1 tablespoon grated fresh ginger

3 stalks fresh lemongrass, tough outer layers removed, cut into thirds

1 teaspoon fine sea salt

1 pound boneless, skinless chicken thighs, cut into 2-inch pieces

¼ cup chopped fresh cilantro leaves

2 scallions, cut into ½-inch pieces

Juice of 1 lime

2 cups Zoodles (page 360), for serving (optional)

2 tablespoons finely diced red onions or sliced scallions, for garnish

Fresh cilantro or Thai basil leaves, for garnish

Avocado oil or extra-virgin olive oil, for drizzling

1. Heat the coconut oil in a large cast-iron skillet or wok over medium heat. Add the shallots and stir-fry until tender, about 2 minutes. Whisk in the broth, coconut milk, curry paste, and ginger, then add the lemongrass. Simmer, uncovered, for 20 minutes, or until the soup has thickened a bit.

2. Sprinkle the salt all over the chicken, then add the chicken to the soup. Cover the pan and poach the chicken until cooked through, about 10 minutes. Stir in the cilantro, scallions, and lime juice. Remove the stalks of lemongrass.

3. If using zoodles, divide them among 4 bowls, then ladle the soup over the top. Garnish with diced red onions, cilantro or Thai basil leaves, and a drizzle of oil. Store in an airtight container in the refrigerator for up to 3 days. To reheat, place in a saucepan over medium heat for about 3 minutes.

NUTRITIONAL INFO (per serving)				
calories	fat	protein	carbs	fiber
390	28g	25g	9g	2g

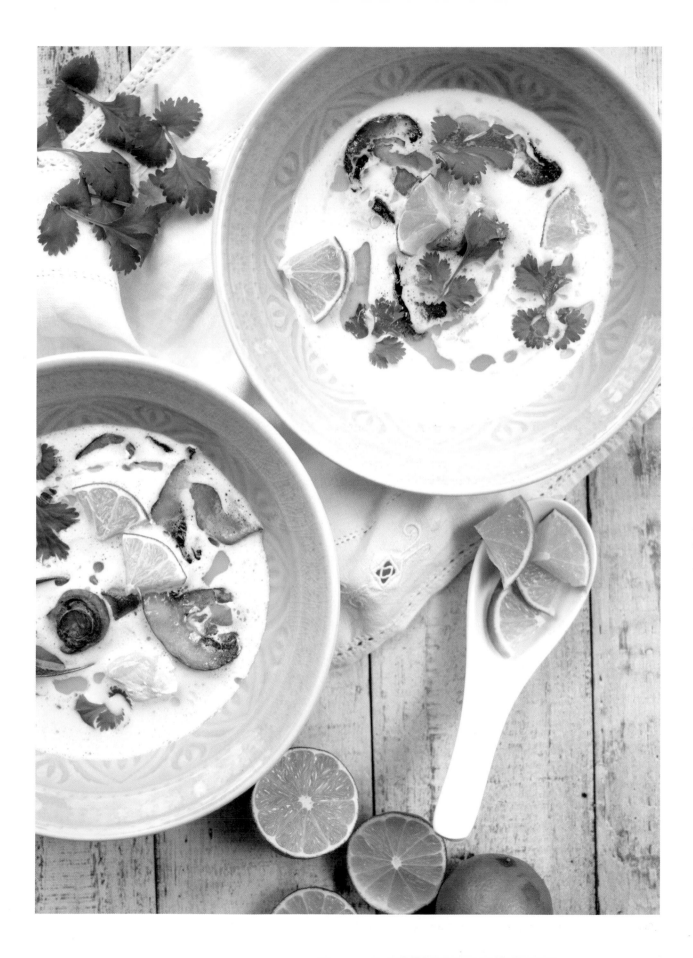

Tom Yum Gai (Hot-and-Sour Chicken Soup)

(L M H KETO) prep time: 7 minutes   cook time: 12 minutes   yield: 6 servings

6 cups chicken bone broth, homemade (page 356) or store-bought

1/3 cup fish sauce

3 tablespoons Swerve confectioners'-style sweetener or equivalent amount of liquid or powdered sweetener (see page 31) (optional)

8 kaffir lime leaves (or increase the amount of lime juice by 2 tablespoons)

2 stalks fresh lemongrass, tough outer layers removed, cut into 2-inch pieces

8 very thin slices fresh ginger

1 pound boneless, skinless chicken thighs, cut into bite-sized pieces (see tip)

1½ cups sliced button mushrooms (about 8 ounces)

½ to 1 green Thai chile, sliced

¼ cup plus 1 tablespoon fresh lime juice (2 to 3 limes)

Ground black pepper

Fresh cilantro leaves, for garnish

Lime or lemon wedges, for garnish (optional)

1. Place the broth, fish sauce, sweetener (if using), lime leaves, lemongrass, and ginger in a large pot over medium-high heat. Bring to a boil and cook for 5 minutes. Add the chicken, mushrooms, and Thai chile and simmer for 5 minutes, or until the chicken is cooked through.

2. Stir in the lime juice. Remove and discard the lime leaves, lemongrass, and ginger. Season to taste with black pepper and serve garnished with cilantro leaves and lime wedges, if desired. Store in an airtight container in the refrigerator for up to 4 days or in the freezer for up to 1 month. To reheat, place in a saucepan over medium heat for about 3 minutes, stirring often.

busy family tip: *Using leftover chicken will speed up this recipe. Simply replace the raw chicken thighs with 4 cups diced cooked chicken and add it at the end of cooking just to heat through.*

NUTRITIONAL INFO (per serving)				
calories	fat	protein	carbs	fiber
198	12g	21g	3g	1g

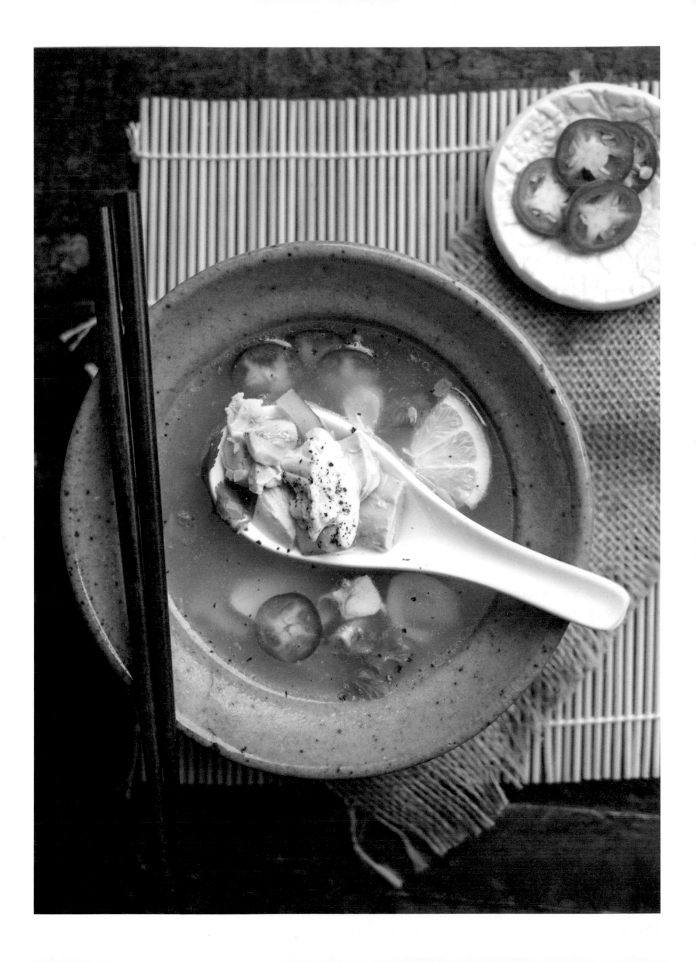

Pho

(L M T H KETO) 　 prep time: 12 minutes　cook time: 7 hours　yield: 8 servings

Pho is an intensely flavorful soup that you do not want to rush. The roasting of the bones and long cooking of the broth really bring the taste to another level.

3 pounds beef soup bones

1 cup chopped onions (about 1 large)

6 thin slices fresh ginger

2 tablespoons coconut aminos

2 tablespoons fish sauce

2 teaspoons fine sea salt

2 star anise

2 large zucchini, 10 to 12 inches long, spiral-sliced into noodles (about 4 cups)

1½ pounds beef top sirloin, thinly sliced

¼ cup chopped fresh cilantro

1 tablespoon chopped scallions

Fresh Thai basil or cilantro leaves, for garnish

2 limes, quartered, for serving

1. Preheat the oven to 425°F. Place the beef bones on a rimmed baking sheet and roast until browned, about 40 minutes.

2. Place the bones, onions, ginger, coconut aminos, fish sauce, salt, and star anise in a large pot. Cover with 3 quarts of water. Bring to a boil, then reduce the heat to low and simmer for 6 hours.

3. Strain the broth through a colander; discard the bones, onions, ginger, and star anise. Taste the broth and adjust the seasoning to your liking.

4. Divide the zucchini noodles among 4 serving bowls and top with the sliced beef, cilantro, and scallions. Divide the hot broth among the bowls. Stir and let sit until the beef is cooked to medium-rare, 1 to 2 minutes.

5. Serve fresh, garnished with Thai basil leaves and accompanied by lime wedges. The broth can be made up to 4 days ahead and stored in an airtight container in the refrigerator; or it can be frozen for up to 1 month. Store the zucchini noodles in a separate airtight container in the refrigerator for up to 5 days. To reheat the broth, place in a saucepan over medium heat for about 3 minutes, stirring often.

NUTRITIONAL INFO (per serving)				
calories	fat	protein	carbs	fiber
163	9g	15g	6g	2g

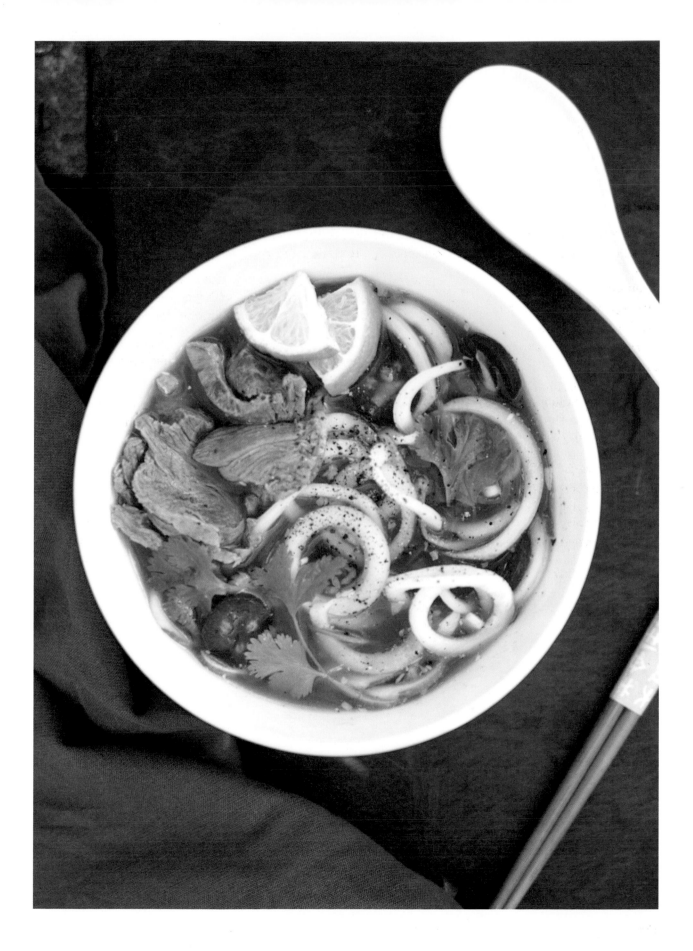

Pho Gà (Vietnamese Chicken Noodle Soup)

prep time: 5 minutes   cook time: 4 or 8 hours in a slow cooker   yield: 12 servings

1 whole chicken (about 3 pounds)

1 tablespoon fine sea salt

2½ teaspoons ground black pepper

4 cups thinly shredded cabbage (about 1 pound)

1 cup chopped fresh cilantro, plus extra for garnish

½ small onion, sliced

6 cloves garlic, smashed to a paste or minced

¼ cup unseasoned rice vinegar or apple cider vinegar

2 tablespoons fish sauce

2 teaspoons grated fresh ginger

4 serrano chiles or jalapeño peppers, thinly sliced

1 star anise

1 cinnamon stick

1 to 2 tablespoons fresh lime juice

Scallions, sliced on the diagonal, for garnish (optional)

1. Season the outside of the chicken with the salt and pepper. Place the chicken in a 4-quart slow cooker. Add the cabbage, cilantro, onion, garlic, vinegar, fish sauce, ginger, chiles, star anise, and cinnamon stick. Add enough water to cover the chicken. Cover the slow cooker and cook on low for 8 hours or on high for 4 hours, until the chicken is tender and falling off the bone. Remove the star anise and cinnamon stick.

2. Transfer the chicken to a cutting board. Slice the meat into cubes and discard the bones. Return the chicken to the slow cooker, then stir in the lime juice. Taste and adjust the seasoning to your liking. Add more chiles for heat, if desired. Serve garnished with cilantro leaves and sliced scallions, if desired. Store in an airtight container in the refrigerator for up to 5 days or in the freezer for up to 1 month. To reheat, place in a saucepan over medium heat for about 2 minutes, stirring often.

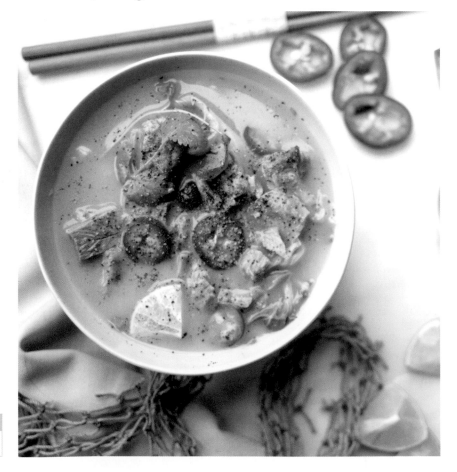

NUTRITIONAL INFO (per serving)				
calories	fat	protein	carbs	fiber
258	17g	22g	3g	1g

Vietnamese Salad

(L M H KETO · OPTION)   prep time: 7 minutes   cook time: 90 minutes   yield: 4 servings

1 medium zucchini

1 medium yellow squash

1 red or green jalapeño pepper, seeded and thinly sliced

¼ small onion, thinly sliced

¼ cup fresh cilantro leaves

¼ cup fresh Thai basil leaves

2 tablespoons fresh mint leaves

1 tablespoon MCT oil, avocado oil, or extra-virgin olive oil

1 tablespoon fish sauce

1 tablespoon fresh lime juice

1 tablespoon Swerve confectioners'-style sweetener or equivalent amount of liquid or powdered sweetener (see page 31)

¼ cup chopped pili nuts or macadamia nuts, for garnish (omit for nut-free)

1. Using a spiral slicer, swirl the zucchini and yellow squash into thin noodles. Place the noodles in a large bowl and add the jalapeño, onion, cilantro, Thai basil, and mint; toss gently to combine.

2. Make the dressing: In a small bowl, whisk together the oil, fish sauce, lime juice, and sweetener until well combined. Adjust the seasoning to your liking.

3. Pour the dressing over the vegetables and stir well to combine. Garnish with pili nuts, if desired. Store in an airtight container in the refrigerator for up to 4 days.

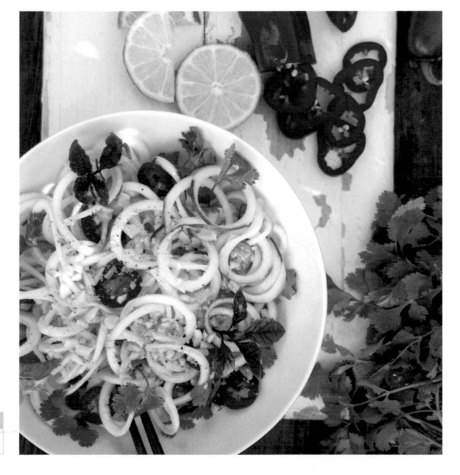

NUTRITIONAL INFO (per serving)				
calories 106	fat 9g	protein 3g	carbs 6g	fiber 2g

Thai Curry Stew

(L M H KETO) **prep time:** 5 minutes **cook time:** 3 or 7 hours plus 20 minutes in a slow cooker
yield: 8 servings

3 (13½-ounce) cans full-fat coconut milk

3 tablespoons fish sauce

3 tablespoons Swerve confectioners'-style sweetener or equivalent amount of liquid or powdered sweetener (see page 31)

3 tablespoons yellow curry paste

3 tablespoons grated fresh ginger

1 tablespoon fresh lime juice

6 shallots, thinly sliced

4 cloves garlic, minced

1½ pounds boneless beef roast, such as chuck roast or beef bottom round, cut into 1-inch cubes

2 red bell peppers, cut into 1-inch pieces

Fine sea salt and ground black pepper

Fresh cilantro leaves, for garnish

1 lime, quartered, for serving

1. In a 4-quart slow cooker, whisk together the coconut milk, fish sauce, sweetener, curry paste, ginger, lime juice, shallots, and garlic until well combined. Add the beef, cover, and cook on low for 7 hours or on high for 3 hours, until the beef is fork-tender.

2. Add the bell peppers to the slow cooker. Cover and cook for another 20 minutes to soften the peppers. Season to taste with salt and black pepper. Garnish with cilantro leaves and serve with lime wedges. Store in the refrigerator for up to 4 days. To reheat, place in a saucepan over medium heat for about 3 minutes, stirring often.

NUTRITIONAL INFO (per serving)				
calories	fat	protein	carbs	fiber
490	40g	19g	10g	2g

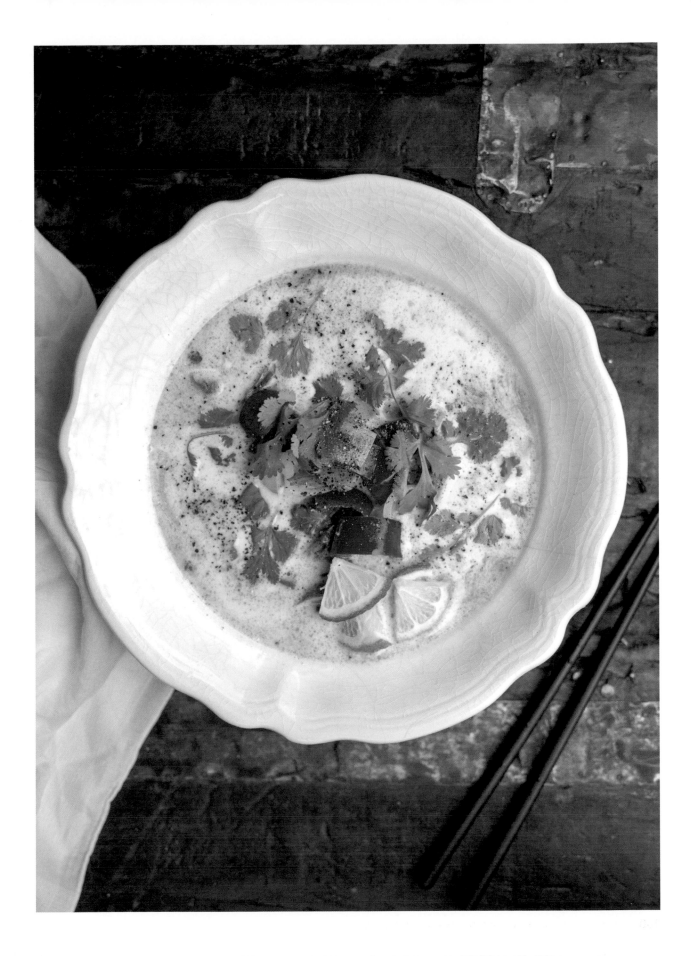

Crab Curry "Rice"

(L M H KETO OPTION)   prep time: 5 minutes   cook time: 8 minutes   yield: 4 servings

I grew up in Medford, Wisconsin, which wasn't very diverse when it came to the food scene. So when I met Craig, who lived in Minneapolis, he wanted to expose me to new and exotic flavors. I was a little apprehensive, but I was hooked after my first experience at an authentic Thai restaurant! I ordered a crab and egg curry and told them to skip the side of rice. The eggs were scrambled into such small curds that they reminded me of rice!

2 pounds snow crab or king crab clusters, thawed if frozen

8 large eggs

1⅓ cups full-fat coconut milk

2 teaspoons curry powder

1 teaspoon fine sea salt

¼ teaspoon grated fresh ginger

¼ cup (½ stick) unsalted butter (or coconut oil if dairy-sensitive)

Roughly chopped fresh cilantro, for garnish

Sliced scallions, for garnish

1 lime, quartered, for serving (optional)

1. Cut each crab shell lengthwise. Heat a large pot of salted water over medium heat. Add the crab legs to the pot and simmer until completely heated, about 5 minutes.

2. Meanwhile, make the "rice": Place the eggs, coconut milk, curry powder, salt, and ginger in a medium-sized bowl and stir until well combined.

3. In a large saucepan, melt the butter over medium heat. Add the egg mixture and cook, whisking constantly, until the mixture thickens and small curds form, about 7 minutes.

4. Place the curry "rice" on a platter and top with the crab claw pieces. Garnish with cilantro and scallions and serve with lime wedges, if desired. Store in the refrigerator for up to 4 days. To reheat, place in a sauté pan over medium heat for about 3 minutes, stirring often.

NUTRITIONAL INFO (per serving)				
calories	fat	protein	carbs	fiber
615	38g	67g	2g	0.1g

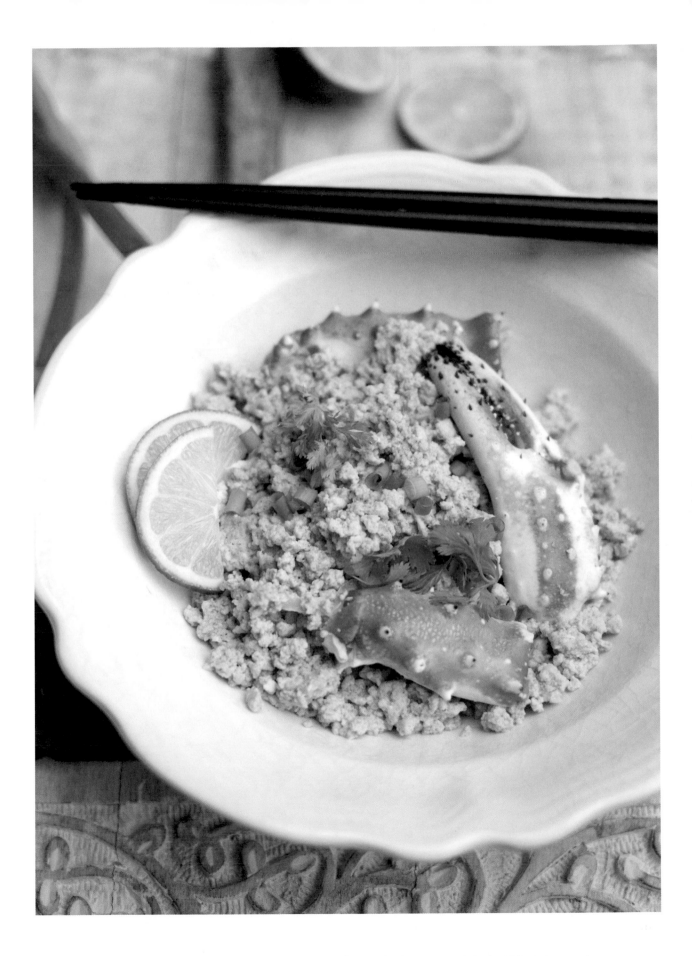

Pad Thai

(L—M—H KETO [icon] OPTION [icon]) prep time: 12 minutes cook time: 16 minutes yield: 4 servings

2 large zucchini, 10 to 12 inches long, spiral-sliced into noodles (about 4 cups)

Fine sea salt

1 cup chicken bone broth, homemade (page 356) or store-bought

¾ cup Swerve confectioners'-style sweetener or equivalent amount of liquid or powdered sweetener (see page 31)

3 tablespoons coconut vinegar or apple cider vinegar

1 tablespoon sunflower seed butter or almond butter

1 teaspoon fish sauce

½ teaspoon cayenne pepper

1 tablespoon coconut oil

1 pound boneless, skinless chicken thighs, cut into ¾-inch pieces

Ground black pepper

2 cloves garlic, minced

1 teaspoon grated fresh ginger

4 large eggs, lightly beaten

¼ cup chopped fresh chives or scallions, for garnish

Handful of sunflower seeds or chopped macadamia nuts, for garnish

Fresh cilantro leaves, for garnish

1. Place the zucchini noodles in a colander in the sink. Sprinkle with salt and allow the moisture to drain from the noodles for 5 minutes. Squeeze the zucchini noodles gently to release the remaining excess moisture.

2. Meanwhile, whisk together the broth, sweetener, vinegar, sunflower seed butter, fish sauce, and cayenne in a small bowl. Set aside.

3. Heat the oil in a large skillet or wok over medium-high heat. Season the chicken on all sides with a few pinches each of salt and pepper. Add the chicken to the pan and stir-fry until the chicken is cooked through, about 4 minutes. Remove the chicken from the pan and set aside, reserving the drippings.

4. Add the garlic and ginger to the pan and stir-fry for 2 minutes, until fragrant. Stir in the eggs and sauté until the eggs are set, about 2 minutes. Add the sauce to the eggs and stir to combine. Reduce the heat and simmer, stirring frequently, about 3 minutes. Add the cooked chicken and stir to combine.

5. To serve, divide the zucchini noodles among 4 bowls. Top each bowl with one-quarter of the chicken mixture. Garnish with chives, sunflower seeds, and cilantro leaves. Pad Thai is best served fresh, but leftover noodles and chicken mixture can be stored in separate airtight containers in the refrigerator for up to 4 days. To reheat, place the chicken mixture in a saucepan over medium heat for about 4 minutes, stirring occasionally, then add the noodles and heat for about 30 more seconds.

NUTRITIONAL INFO (per serving)				
calories	fat	protein	carbs	fiber
329	20g	30g	9g	2g

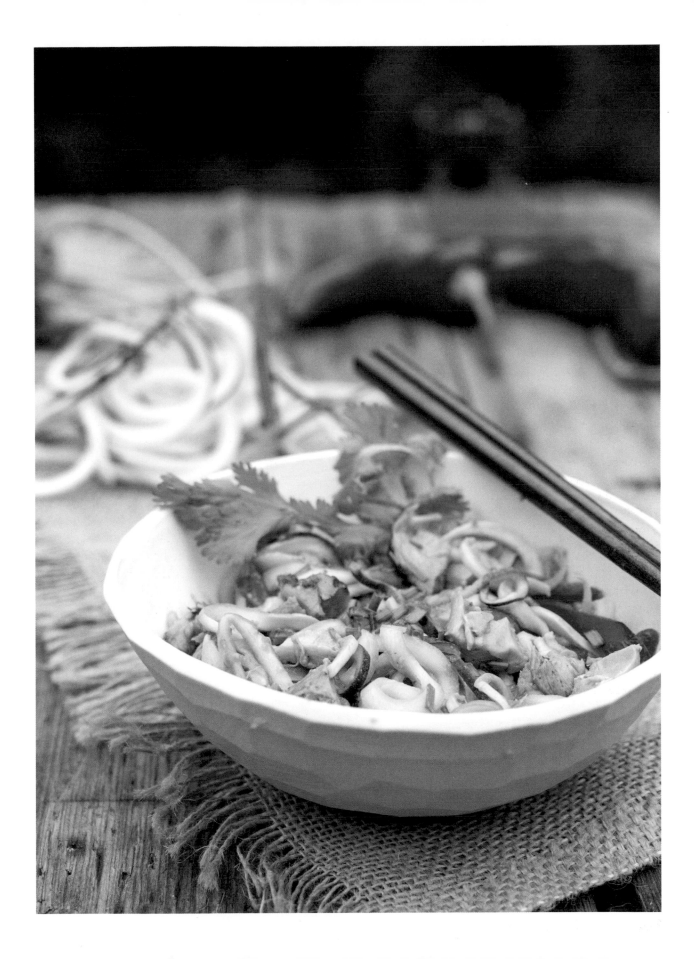

Larb

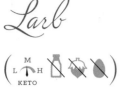

prep time: 8 minutes   cook time: 7 minutes   yield: 4 servings

—sauce

½ cup fresh lime juice (about 4 limes)

¼ cup fish sauce

1 tablespoon Swerve confectioners'-style sweetener or equivalent amount of liquid or powdered sweetener (see page 31)

—filling

1 tablespoon coconut oil

¼ cup diced onions (about 1 small)

2 cloves garlic, minced

2 tablespoons minced fresh lemongrass

2 teaspoons grated fresh ginger

1 pound ground chicken

½ teaspoon fine sea salt

—for serving

1 head Boston lettuce, leaves separated, for the wrappers

1 bunch scallions, chopped

½ bunch fresh basil, chopped

½ bunch fresh cilantro, chopped

½ bunch fresh mint, chopped

1. Make the sauce: Place the lime juice, fish sauce, and sweetener in a small bowl. Stir well and set aside.

2. Make the filling: Heat the oil in a large cast-iron skillet over medium-high heat. Add the onions, garlic, lemongrass, and ginger and sauté for 3 minutes, or until the onions are soft. Add the ground chicken, season with the salt, and cook, stirring often, breaking up the chicken with a spatula, until the chicken is browned and cooked through, about 4 minutes. Add the sauce and stir well to combine.

3. Serve with the lettuce leaves, scallions, and herbs. Store in separate airtight containers in the refrigerator for up to 4 days. To reheat the chicken filling, place in a sauté pan over medium heat for about 3 minutes, stirring often.

NUTRITIONAL INFO (per serving)				
calories	fat	protein	carbs	fiber
333	16g	36g	11g	3g

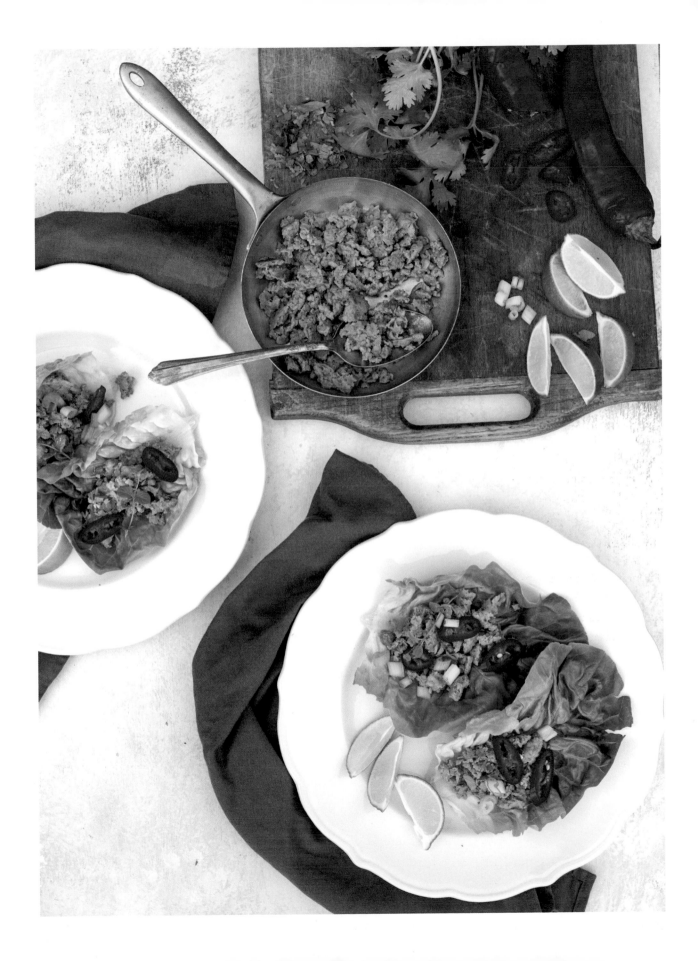

Yellow Chicken Thighs Adobo

(L ⟶ H M KETO 🥛 🥜 🥚) prep time: 7 minutes   cook time: 90 minutes   yield: 4 servings

If you're looking to bulk up this dish, try serving it over Zero-Carb Fried "Rice" (page 44) or Cauliflower Fried Rice (page 46).

2 tablespoons turmeric powder

2 tablespoons coconut oil, divided

¼ cup chopped white onions (about 1 small)

3 cloves garlic, chopped

1 tablespoon grated fresh ginger

½ teaspoon crushed red pepper

1 (13½-ounce) can full-fat coconut milk

¼ cup coconut vinegar or apple cider vinegar

2 tablespoons Swerve confectioners'-style sweetener or equivalent amount of liquid or powdered sweetener (see page 31)

2 tablespoons black peppercorns

4 bay leaves

4 bone-in, skin-on chicken thighs

Fine sea salt and ground black pepper

1. Toast the turmeric in a medium-sized cast-iron skillet over medium heat, stirring constantly, until aromatic, about 30 seconds. Add 1 tablespoon of the oil, the onions, garlic, ginger, and crushed red pepper. Stir and cook for 6 minutes. Stir in the coconut milk, vinegar, sweetener, peppercorns, and bay leaves. Bring to a boil, then reduce the heat to low and simmer for 20 minutes, or until the sauce has thickened a bit.

2. Meanwhile, season the chicken well on all sides with salt and pepper. Heat the remaining 1 tablespoon of oil in a large cast-iron skillet over medium-high heat. Place the chicken thighs, skin side down, in the skillet. Cook for 8 minutes per side, or until golden brown.

3. Pour the sauce over the chicken. Cover and cook over medium heat for 1 hour, or until the chicken is fork-tender and cooked through. Remove the bay leaves and peppercorns before serving. Store in an airtight container in the refrigerator for up to 4 days. To reheat, place in a skillet over medium heat for about 3 minutes.

NUTRITIONAL INFO (per serving)				
calories	fat	protein	carbs	fiber
371	31g	17g	6g	1g

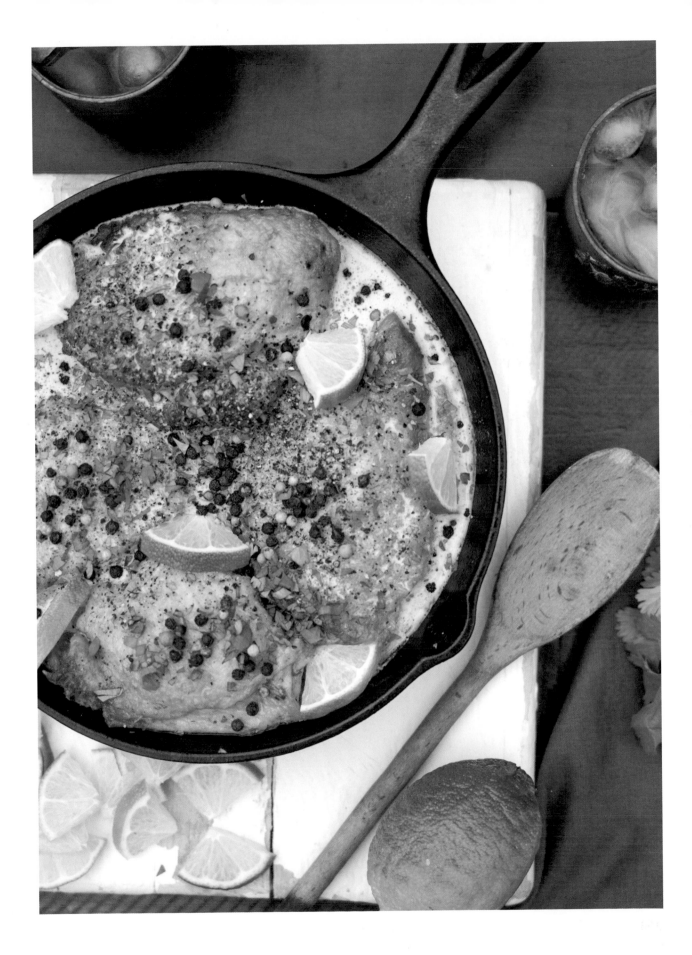

Chicken Korma

(L M H KETO OPTION) prep time: 6 minutes cook time: 30 minutes yield: 4 servings

¼ cup ghee or unsalted butter

1 cup chopped onions (about 1 large)

½ cup sour cream

2 tablespoons Swerve confectioners'-style sweetener or equivalent amount of liquid or powdered sweetener (see page 31)

4 cloves garlic, minced

2 teaspoons garam masala

2 teaspoons turmeric powder

2 teaspoons fine sea salt

1 pound boneless, skinless chicken breasts or thighs, chopped into ¾-inch pieces

⅓ cup sliced almonds, for garnish (omit for nut-free)

Fresh cilantro leaves, for garnish

1. Preheat the oven to 350°F. Lightly grease a 2-quart baking dish.

2. Heat the ghee in a large skillet over medium heat. Add the onions and cook for 3 minutes, or until soft.

3. Place the cooked onions, sour cream, sweetener, garlic, garam masala, and turmeric in a blender or food processor and puree until smooth. Place the chicken in the greased baking dish and pour the onion puree over the chicken.

4. Bake for 20 minutes, or until the chicken is cooked through. Garnish with sliced almonds, if using, and cilantro leaves. Store in an airtight container in the refrigerator for up to 4 days. To reheat, place on a rimmed baking sheet in a preheated 350°F oven or toaster oven for about 5 minutes.

NUTRITIONAL INFO (per serving)				
calories	fat	protein	carbs	fiber
339	27g	14g	9g	2g

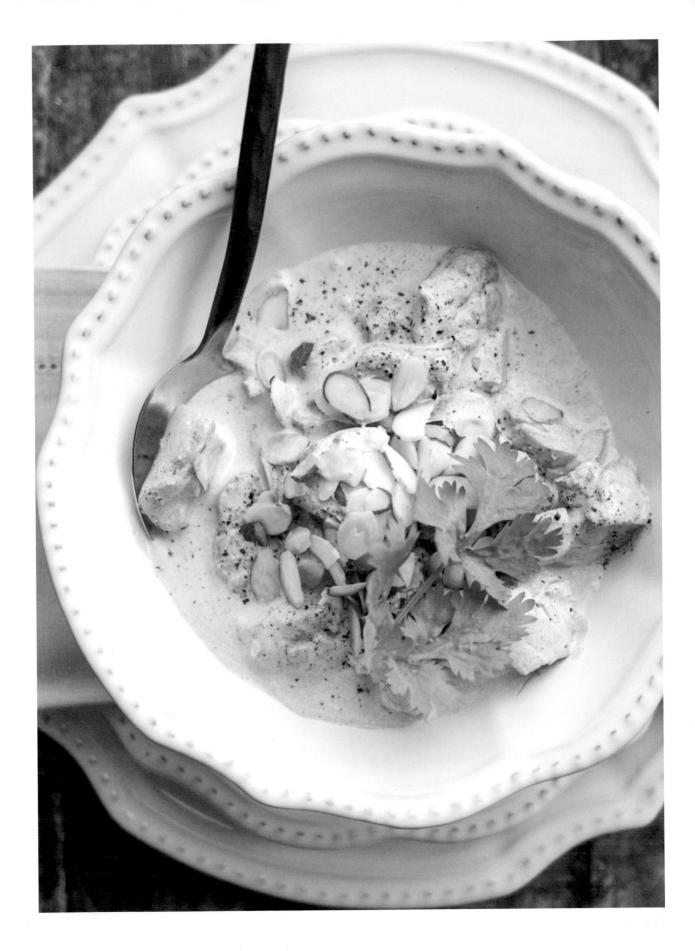

Green Curry Chicken

(L M H KETO · OPTION)
prep time: 5 minutes (not including time to make sinangag)
cook time: 15 minutes   yield: 2 servings

1½ tablespoons coconut oil

2 tablespoons green curry paste

½ pound boneless, skinless chicken thighs, cut into bite-sized pieces

½ cup full-fat coconut milk

¼ cup chicken bone broth, homemade (page 356) or store-bought

¼ cup fresh lime juice (about 2 limes)

¼ cup Thai basil leaves, plus extra for garnish

1 tablespoon fish sauce

1 tablespoon Swerve confectioners'-style sweetener or equivalent amount of liquid or powdered sweetener (see page 31)

1 red chile, seeded and cut into thick strips

¼ batch Sinangag (page 246), for serving (optional)

1. Heat the oil in a medium-sized saucepan over medium heat. Add the curry paste and cook for 1 minute to open up the flavors. Add the chicken and stir until well coated. Stir in the coconut milk, broth, lime juice, Thai basil, fish sauce, sweetener, and chile. Bring to a boil, then reduce the heat and simmer, uncovered, for 10 minutes, or until the chicken is cooked through and the sauce has thickened a bit.

2. Remove from the heat, garnish with Thai basil, and serve with sinangag, if desired. Store in an airtight container in the refrigerator for up to 4 days. To reheat, place in a saucepan over medium heat for about 5 minutes, stirring occasionally.

NUTRITIONAL INFO (per serving)				
calories	fat	protein	carbs	fiber
489	37g	27g	15g	5g

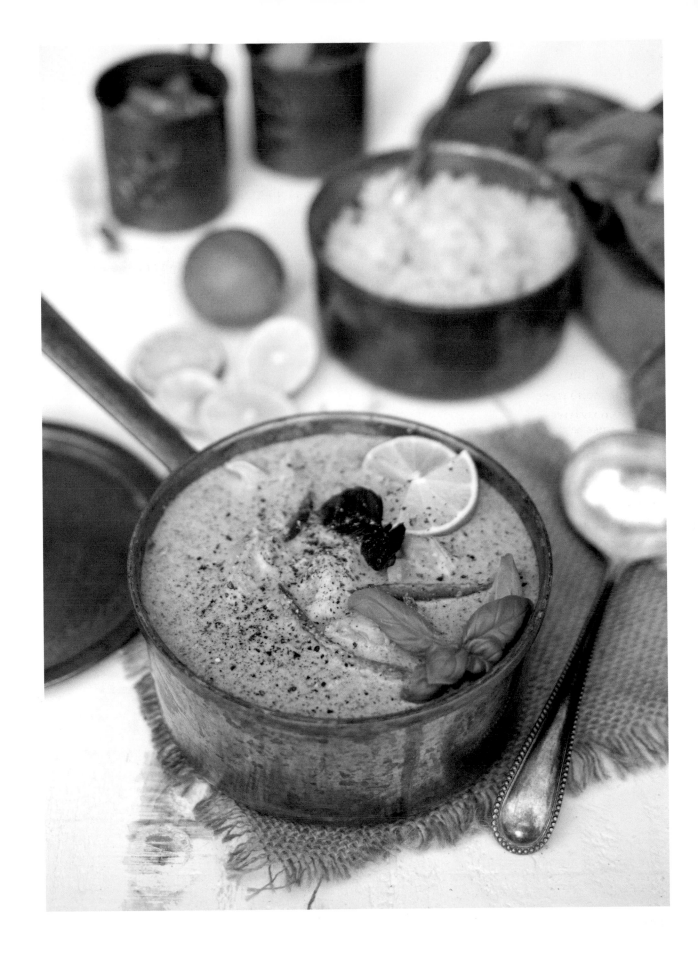

Red Curry Shrimp

prep time: 5 minutes   cook time: 14 minutes

yield: 4 servings (3 large shrimp per serving)

1 tablespoon ghee (or avocado oil if dairy-free), plus 1 teaspoon if pan-frying the shrimp

½ cup diced shallots (about 4 large)

1½ cups chicken bone broth, homemade (page 356) or store-bought

1 (13½-ounce) can full-fat coconut milk

1½ tablespoons red curry paste

¼ cup chopped fresh cilantro, plus extra for garnish (optional)

¼ cup thinly sliced scallions, plus extra for garnish (optional)

¼ teaspoon fine sea salt

12 jumbo shell-on shrimp, butterflied and deveined

Fine sea salt and ground black pepper

1 tablespoon fresh lime juice

1. Heat the ghee in a large cast-iron skillet or wok over medium heat. Add the shallots and sauté until tender, about 2 minutes. Whisk in the broth, coconut milk, and curry paste. Reduce the heat and simmer, uncovered, for 10 minutes, or until the mixture has reduced a bit. The longer you simmer it, the thicker the sauce will be. Add the cilantro, scallions, and salt and continue to simmer.

2. Pat the shrimp dry and season with a couple pinches each of salt and pepper. Preheat a grill to high, or heat the 1 teaspoon of oil in a large cast-iron skillet over high heat. Add the shrimp, shell side up. Cook until the shrimp turns pink, about 3 minutes. Transfer the shrimp to the skillet with the curry.

3. Stir in the lime juice. Serve garnished with cilantro and scallions, if desired. Store in an airtight container in the refrigerator for up to 3 days. To reheat, place in a saucepan over medium heat for a few minutes.

NUTRITIONAL INFO (per serving)				
calories	fat	protein	carbs	fiber
270	21g	14g	6g	1g

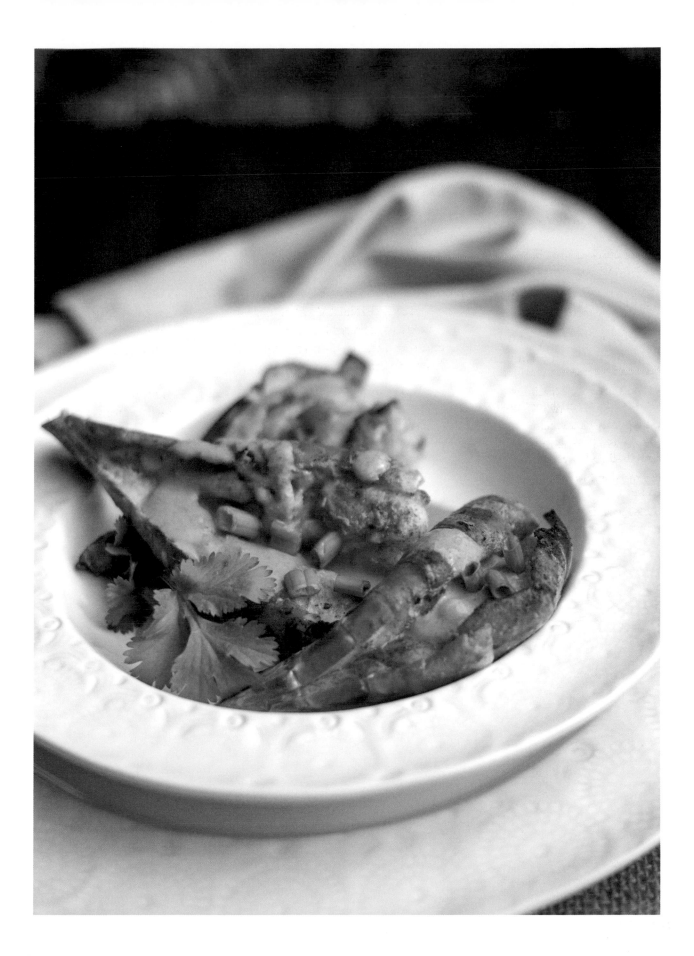

Coconut Curry Chicken and Pancakes

(L M H KETO   OPTION)   prep time: 5 minutes   cook time: 15 minutes   yield: 2 servings

1 tablespoon ghee or unsalted butter (or avocado oil if dairy-free)

¼ cup diced onions (about 1 small)

2 cloves garlic, minced

½ pound boneless, skinless chicken thighs, cut into ¾-inch pieces

Fine sea salt

½ cup full-fat coconut milk (or sour cream if not dairy-sensitive, for a thicker sauce)

1 teaspoon ground cumin

1 teaspoon smoked paprika

1 teaspoon turmeric powder

1 teaspoon ground black pepper

¼ teaspoon cayenne pepper

—pancakes

2 raw large eggs

2 hard-boiled eggs

4 ounces cream cheese (Kite Hill brand cream cheese style spread for dairy-free)

¼ teaspoon fine sea salt

1 tablespoon coconut oil, for the pan

Sliced scallions, for garnish

Lime quarters, for serving

1. Heat the ghee in a large cast-iron skillet over medium heat. Add the onions and garlic and sauté until tender, about 2 minutes.

2. Season the chicken well on all sides with salt and add to the skillet. Sauté, stirring occasionally, until the chicken is cooked through, about 4 minutes.

3. Add the coconut milk, cumin, paprika, turmeric, black pepper, and cayenne. Reduce the heat and simmer, uncovered, for 10 minutes, or until the liquid has reduced a bit. The longer the sauce simmers, the thicker it will be. Taste and adjust the seasoning and spices to your liking.

4. Meanwhile, make the pancakes: Place the raw eggs, hard-boiled eggs, cream cheese, sweetener, and salt in a blender and puree until very smooth. Heat the coconut oil in a large skillet over medium-high heat until a drop of water sizzles in the skillet. Pour three 3-inch circles of batter into the skillet. Cook for 3 to 5 minutes per side, until golden brown. Repeat with the remaining batter to make a total of 8 pancakes, adding more oil to the skillet if needed.

5. Garnish the curry chicken mixture with scallions and lime quarters and serve with the pancakes. Store the curry and pancakes in separate airtight containers in the refrigerator for up to 4 days. To reheat the pancakes, place in a lightly greased skillet over medium heat for a few minutes. To reheat the curry, place in a saucepan over medium-low heat, stirring often, until warmed through.

NUTRITIONAL INFO (per serving)				
calories	fat	protein	carbs	fiber
347	28g	17g	4g	1g

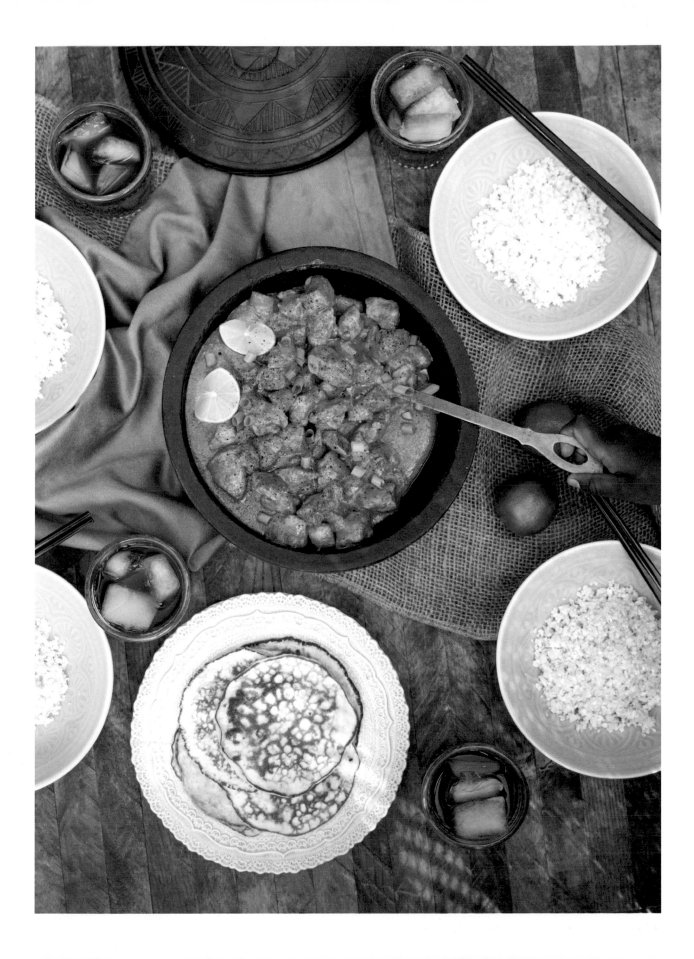

Kofta with Cilantro Sauce

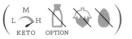

prep time: 5 minutes, plus 15 minutes to soak skewers   **cook time:** 15 minutes
yield: 4 servings

—kofta

1 pound ground lamb or ground beef

¼ cup diced red onions (about 1 small)

3 tablespoons chopped fresh parsley

1 tablespoon ground coriander

3 cloves garlic, smashed to a paste

1½ teaspoons ground cinnamon

1 teaspoon ground cumin

1 teaspoon fine sea salt

¼ teaspoon ground black pepper

¼ teaspoon cayenne pepper

¼ teaspoon ginger powder

—cilantro sauce

2 teaspoons ghee or coconut oil

¼ cup minced shallots (about 4 medium)

1 clove garlic, minced

½ cup chopped fresh cilantro

½ cup chopped fresh parsley

2 teaspoons grated fresh ginger

½ teaspoon ground cumin

¼ teaspoon crushed red pepper

¼ cup beef or chicken bone broth, homemade (page 356) or store-bought

2 tablespoons fresh lime juice or lemon juice

Fine sea salt and ground black pepper

—for garnish (optional)

Diced red onions

Lime or lemon wedges

Chopped fresh cilantro

1. Preheat a grill to medium heat. Place 12 bamboo skewers, about 8 inches in length, in water to soak for 15 minutes.

2. Make the kofta: In a large bowl, mix together the ingredients for the kofta until well combined. Form the mixture into 12 balls. Place each ball around a skewer and use your hands to flatten it, making it about 6 inches long and 1¼ inches thick.

3. Make the sauce: Heat the ghee in a medium-sized cast-iron skillet over medium-high heat. Add the shallots and sauté for 1 minute. Add the garlic and sauté for another minute. Add the cilantro, parsley, fresh ginger, cumin, and crushed red pepper. Reduce the heat and simmer for 2 minutes. Transfer the herb mixture to a small food processor or blender and add the broth. Puree until very smooth. Stir in the lime juice just before serving. Taste and season with salt and pepper.

4. Grease the hot grill grates with avocado oil or melted coconut oil. Place the skewers on the grill and cook on all sides for about 4 minutes total for medium-rare kofta (or longer if you prefer the meat more well-done). Serve 3 skewers per person with sauce on the side. Garnish the kofta with diced red onions, lime or lemon wedges, and cilantro, if desired. Store the kofta and sauce in separate airtight containers in the refrigerator for up to 4 days. To reheat the kofta, place in a lightly greased skillet over medium heat for a few minutes.

busy family tip: *The kofta mixture can be made and formed onto the skewers up to 2 days ahead. Store the skewers in an airtight container in the refrigerator until ready to grill. The sauce can be made up to 2 days ahead and stored in an airtight container in the refrigerator until ready to serve.*

NUTRITIONAL INFO (per serving)				
calories	fat	protein	carbs	fiber
332	25g	21g	6g	1g

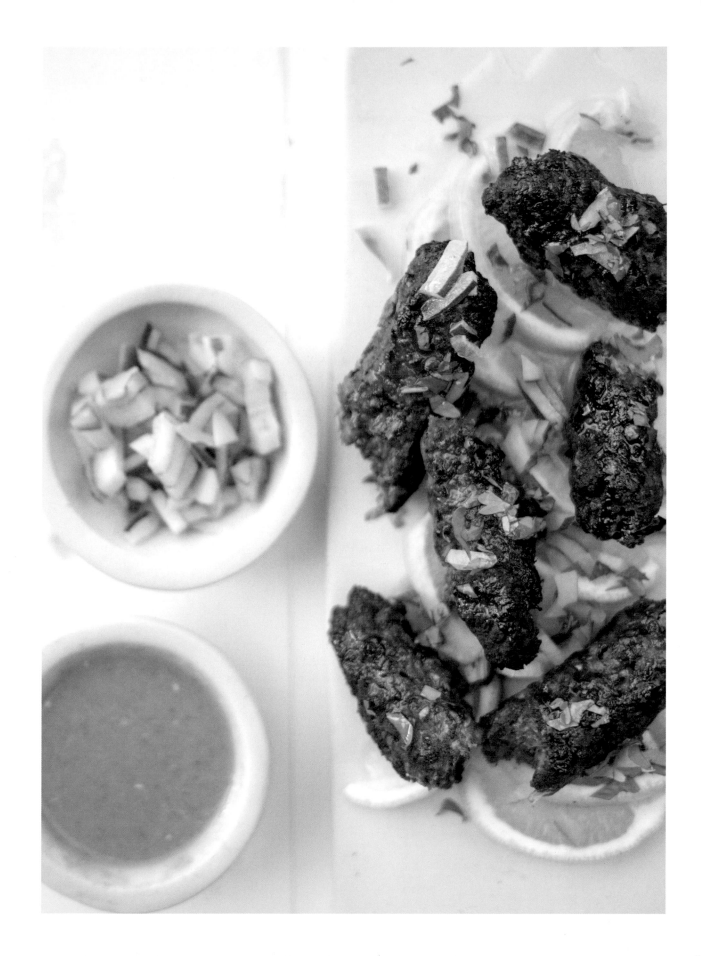

Malai Curry Shrimp

(L—H KETO / OPTION) prep time: 7 minutes (not including time to make sinangag)
cook time: 17 minutes   yield: 4 servings

2 tablespoons coconut oil, divided, for the pan

½ cup diced onions (about 1 medium)

5 cloves garlic, minced

1 tablespoon grated fresh ginger

1 teaspoon ground cardamom

½ teaspoon turmeric powder

¼ teaspoon chili powder

¾ cup full-fat coconut milk

¼ cup chicken bone broth, homemade (page 356) or store-bought

4 bay leaves

1 cinnamon stick

1 pound large shrimp, peeled and deveined, with tails on

2 tablespoons fresh lemon juice

Fine sea salt and fresh ground pepper

½ batch Sinangag (page 246), for serving (optional)

1. Heat 1 tablespoon of the oil in a large cast-iron skillet over medium-high heat. Add the onions and sauté for 1 minute. Add the garlic and sauté for another minute. Add the ginger, cardamom, turmeric, and chili powder and cook for 2 minutes. Transfer the mixture to a blender or food processor, add the coconut milk and broth, and puree until smooth. Set aside.

2. Heat the remaining 1 tablespoon of oil in the skillet over medium-high heat. Add the bay leaves and cinnamon stick and cook for 1 minute, until fragrant.

3. Add the shrimp and sauté for 2 minutes, or until the shrimp are just starting to turn pink. Pour the coconut milk mixture into the skillet, reduce the heat, and simmer, uncovered, for 10 minutes, or until the sauce has thickened a bit. Stir in the lemon juice and season with salt and pepper to taste. Serve over sinangag, if desired. Store in separate airtight containers in the refrigerator for up to 4 days. To reheat the shrimp, place in a lightly greased skillet over medium heat for a few minutes.

NUTRITIONAL INFO (per serving)				
calories	fat	protein	carbs	fiber
358	20g	31g	14g	3g

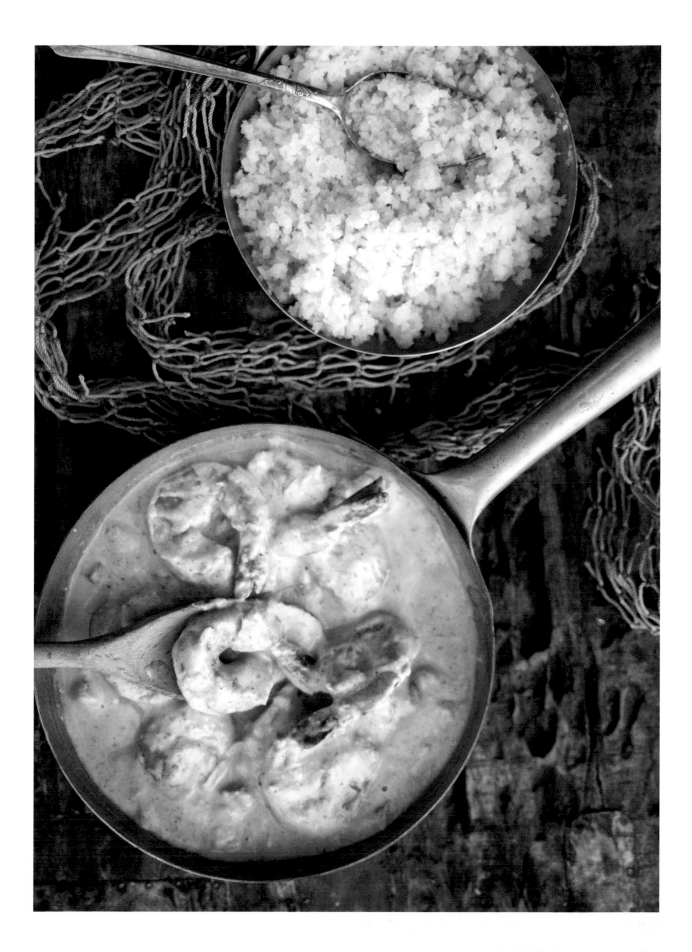

Fish Palak

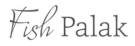 prep time: 5 minutes (not including time to make sinangag)
cook time: 15 minutes   yield: 4 servings

This classic Indian takeout dish is filled with delicious spices. You can also make it with chicken if you prefer: simply replace the halibut with the same amount of boneless, skinless chicken thighs cut into bite-sized pieces.

2 tablespoons coconut oil, divided, for the pan

¼ teaspoon ground cloves

2 cinnamon sticks

2 bay leaves

½ cup diced onions (about 1 medium)

6 cloves garlic, minced

1 (7-ounce) can diced green chiles

1 teaspoon ground coriander

¼ teaspoon cayenne pepper (optional)

4 cups fresh spinach, chopped

1 pound halibut steaks, cut into bite-sized cubes

Fine sea salt and ground black pepper

¾ cup sour cream (or coconut cream if dairy-free)

½ batch Sinangag (page 246), for serving (optional)

1. Heat 1 tablespoon of the oil in a wok or large cast-iron skillet over medium heat. Add the cloves, cinnamon sticks, and bay leaves and stir-fry for 1 minute. Add the onions and stir-fry for another minute, until the onions are soft. Stir in the garlic, chiles, and coriander, and, if you desire a spicier palak, add the cayenne as well. Stir-fry for another minute. Add the spinach and stir-fry for 5 minutes, or until the spinach is wilted. Remove and discard the cinnamon sticks and bay leaves.

2. Transfer the spinach mixture to a blender or food processor (or use an immersion blender) and puree until smooth and thick. Set aside.

3. Make the fish: Wipe out the pan you used to make the palak. Heat the remaining 1 tablespoon of oil in the pan over medium heat. Generously season the fish on all sides with salt and pepper. Place the fish in the pan and stir-fry on all sides until cooked through, about 5 minutes. Remove from the heat and set aside.

4. Pour the spinach puree into the pan with the fish. Turn the heat to medium and gently stir in the sour cream until well combined. Heat for a minute or two, just long enough to warm the sour cream. Serve over sinangag, if desired. Store in an airtight container in the refrigerator for up to 4 days. To reheat, place in a lightly greased skillet over medium heat for a few minutes.

NUTRITIONAL INFO (per serving)				
calories	fat	protein	carbs	fiber
384	20g	28g	16g	3g

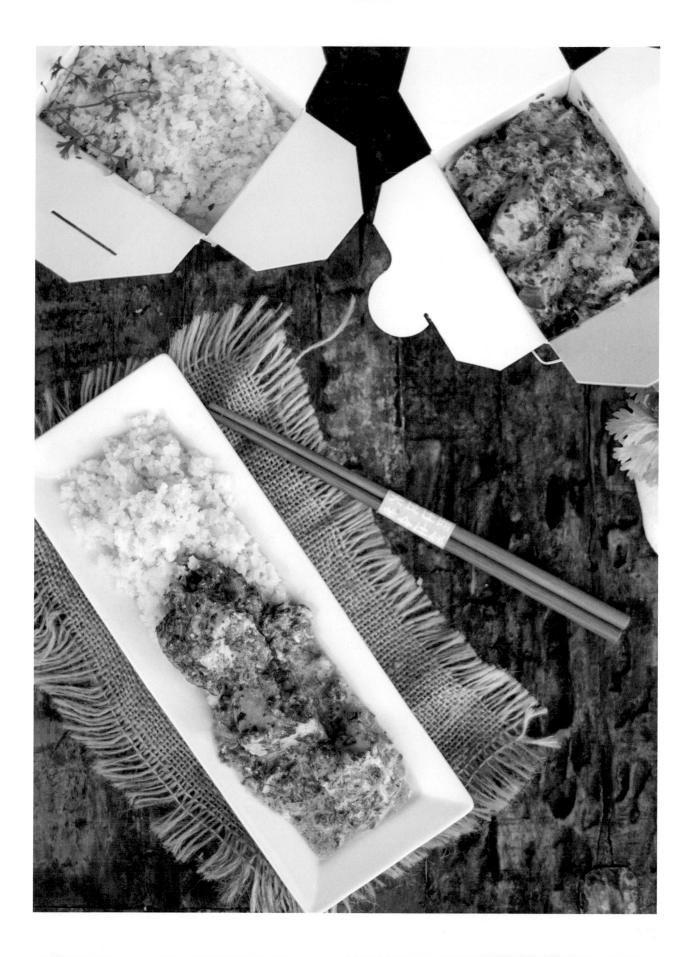

Thai Red Beef Curry

(L M H KETO) prep time: 5 minutes cook time: 9 minutes yield: 4 servings

1 (13½-ounce) can full-fat coconut milk

2 teaspoons Swerve confectioners'-style sweetener or equivalent amount of liquid or powdered sweetener (see page 31)

2 teaspoons fish sauce

1 tablespoon red curry paste

1 red bell pepper, sliced

1 small onion, sliced

12 ounces beef tenderloin, thinly sliced

2 tablespoons fresh lime juice

½ teaspoon fine sea salt

Fresh mint or basil leaves, for garnish

1 lime, quartered, for serving

1. Place the coconut milk, sweetener, and fish sauce in a large cast-iron skillet or pot over medium-high heat. Whisk in the curry paste until well combined. Bring to a boil and boil for 1 minute, then add the bell pepper and onion. Reduce the heat and simmer, uncovered, for 5 minutes, or until the onion is soft. Add the beef and cook for 3 to 5 minutes for medium-rare to medium-done beef. (*Note:* Do not cook the beef much longer than this, or it will become tough.)

2. Remove from the heat and stir in the lime juice and salt. Taste and adjust the seasoning to your liking. Garnish with mint and serve with lime wedges. Store in an airtight container in the refrigerator for up to 4 days. To reheat, place in a lightly greased skillet over medium heat for a few minutes.

NUTRITIONAL INFO (per serving)				
calories	fat	protein	carbs	fiber
393	30g	20g	10g	2g

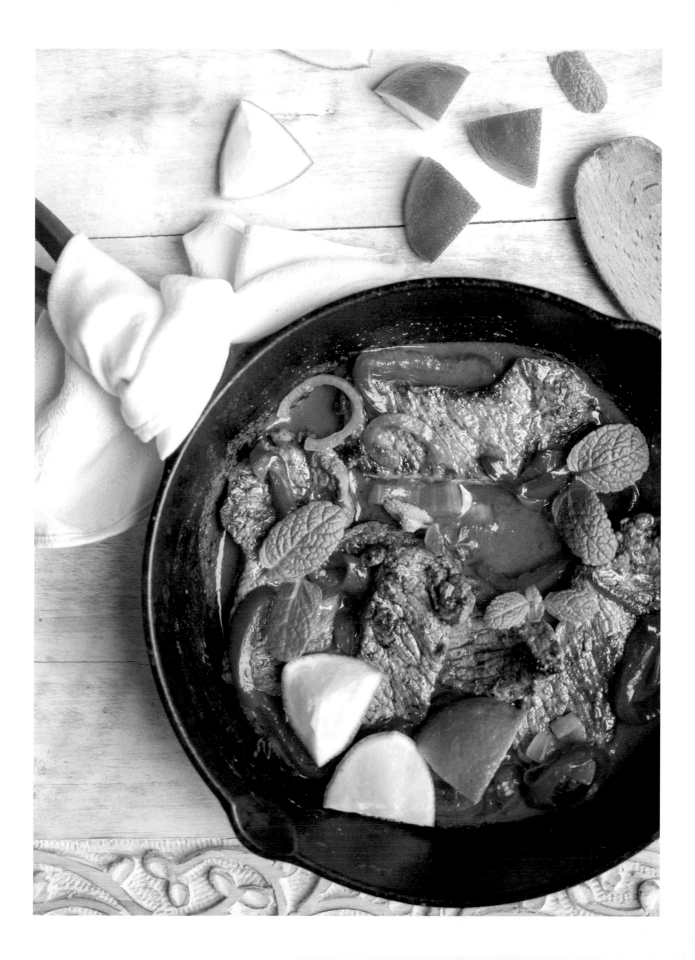

Oven-Baked Curried Turkey Legs

(L M H KETO   OPTION)   **prep time:** 5 minutes   **cook time:** 1 hour 50 minutes   **yield:** 4 servings

1 tablespoon ghee or coconut oil, for the pan

2 turkey legs

1 teaspoon fine sea salt, divided

¼ teaspoon ground black pepper

3 shallots, finely diced

½ cup diced celery (about 4 stalks)

1½ tablespoons red curry paste

1½ cups chicken bone broth, homemade (page 356) or store-bought

1 (13½-ounce) can full-fat coconut milk

¼ cup chopped fresh cilantro, plus extra for garnish

2 scallions, sliced into ½-inch pieces, plus thinly sliced scallions for garnish

1 tablespoon fresh lime juice

1 lime, sliced or quartered, for serving

1. Preheat the oven to 300°F. Heat the ghee in a Dutch oven over medium-high heat.

2. Pat the turkey legs dry with a paper towel and season well on all sides with ½ teaspoon of the salt and the pepper. Sear the turkey legs in the Dutch oven until golden brown, about 3 minutes per side. Remove the turkey from the pot and set aside, keeping the drippings in the pot.

3. Add the shallots and celery to the Dutch oven and sauté until tender, about 2 minutes. Remove the pot from the heat. Whisk in the curry paste, broth, and coconut milk, then add the remaining ½ teaspoon of salt, the cilantro, and scallions.

4. Return the turkey legs to the Dutch oven. Place the pot in the oven and bake, uncovered, for 1 hour 40 minutes, or until the turkey is cooked through and the meat is fork-tender.

5. Just before serving, stir in the lime juice. Serve with lime wedges and garnish with more cilantro and scallions, if desired. Store in an airtight container in the refrigerator for up to 4 days. To reheat, place in a baking dish in a preheated 300°F oven for about 5 minutes.

NUTRITIONAL INFO (per serving)				
calories	fat	protein	carbs	fiber
401	24g	37g	7g	1g

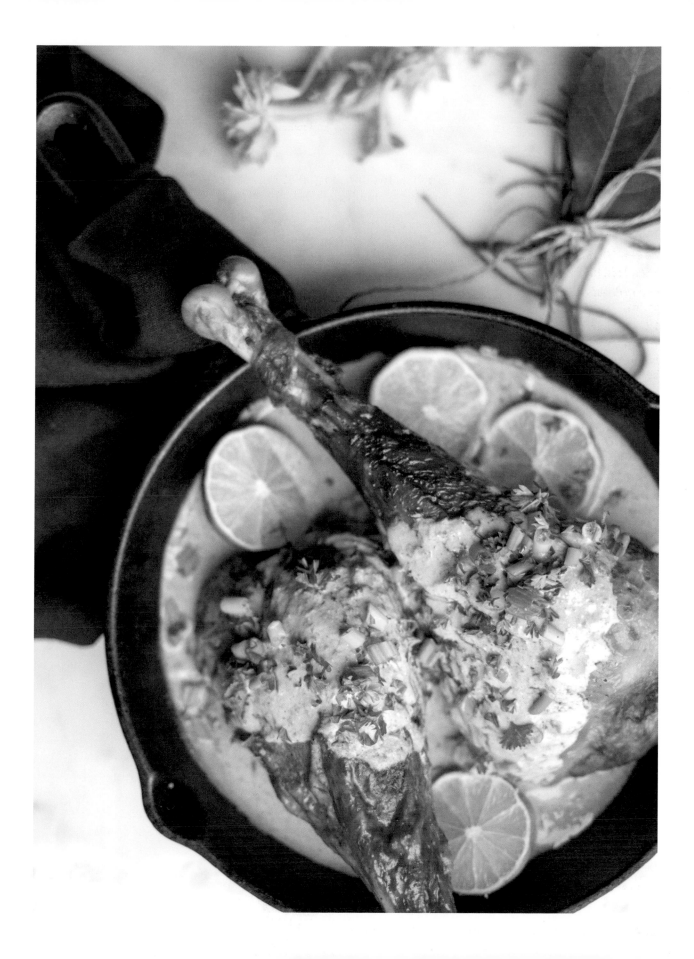

Coconut and Thai Basil Ice Cream

(L → M → H KETO   OPTION   OPTION)   **prep time:** 5 minutes, plus time to churn   **cook time:** a few seconds
yield: 3 cups (½ cup per serving)

⅓ cup fresh Thai basil leaves

1 (13½-ounce) can full-fat coconut milk

1 cup unsweetened cashew milk (or hemp milk if nut-free)

4 ounces mascarpone cheese (omit for dairy-free)

6 large egg yolks

½ cup Swerve confectioners'-style sweetener or equivalent amount of liquid or powdered sweetener (see page 31)

Seeds scraped from 1 vanilla bean (about 8 inches long), or 1 teaspoon vanilla extract

¼ teaspoon fine sea salt

—special equipment

Ice cream maker

1. Bring a medium-sized pot of salted water to a boil. Add the Thai basil leaves and blanch for a few seconds. Quickly drain the leaves and rinse with cold running water to retain the bright green color. Gently squeeze the leaves to release the moisture.

2. Put the blanched Thai basil in a blender and add the coconut milk, cashew milk, mascarpone, egg yolks, sweetener, vanilla bean seeds, and salt. Puree until very smooth. Taste the mixture and adjust the sweetness to your liking, keeping in mind that when frozen, it will taste less sweet.

3. Pour the mixture into an ice cream maker and churn according to the manufacturer's instructions. Store in an airtight container in the freezer for up to 1 month.

variation: coconut and thai basil ice pops. *After completing Step 2, pour the ice cream mixture into three 4-well ice pop molds and freeze until set, about 2 hours. Makes 12 ice pops.*

NUTRITIONAL INFO (per serving)				
calories	fat	protein	carbs	fiber
236	23g	5g	2g	0.1g

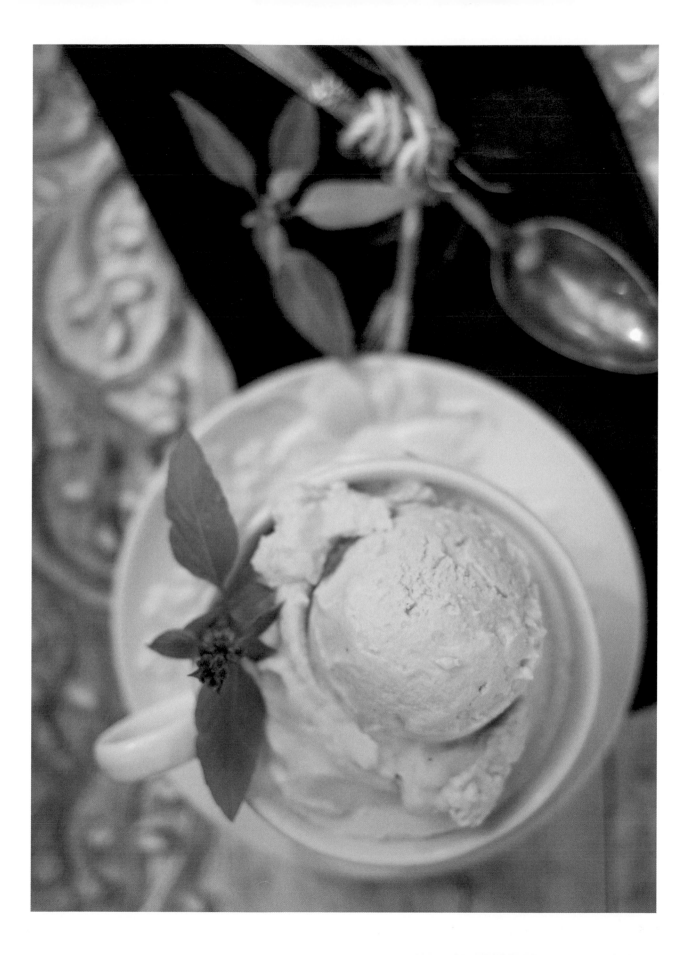

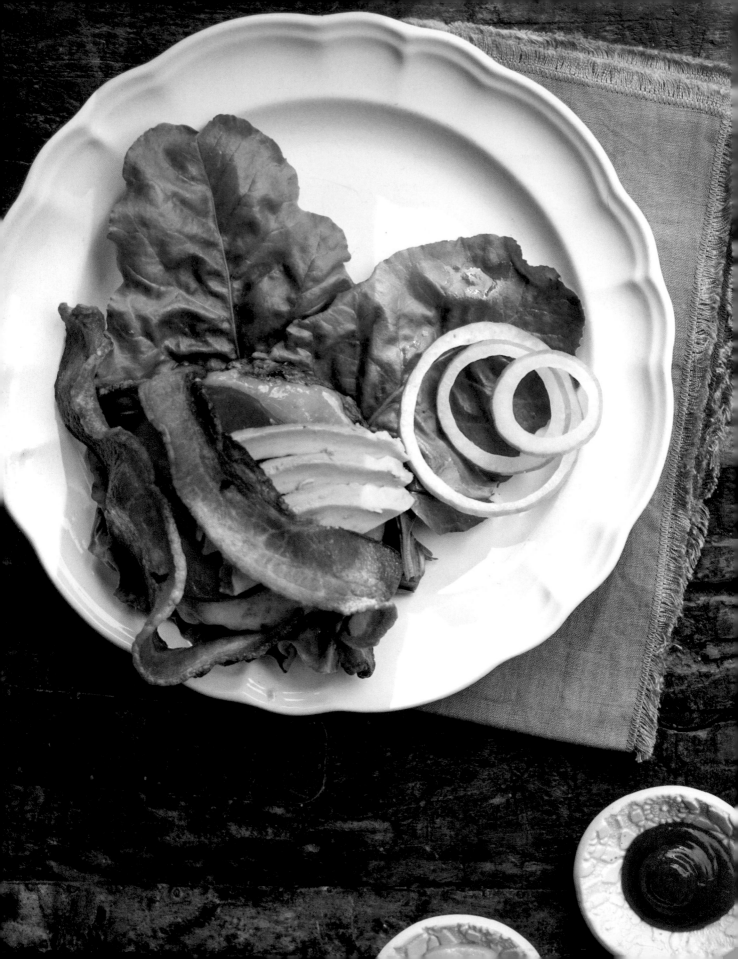

Fast-Casual
Favorites

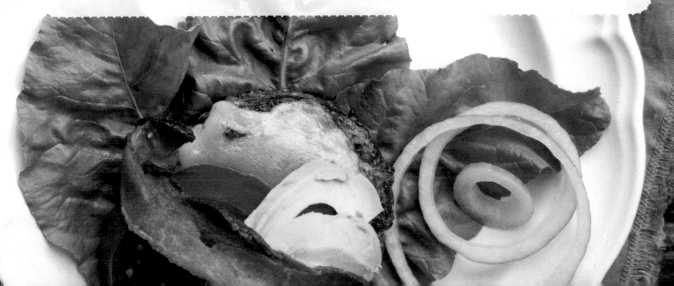

Keto Ketchup

1½ cups beef or chicken bone broth, homemade (page 356) or store-bought

1 (7-ounce) jar tomato paste

2 tablespoons apple cider vinegar or coconut vinegar

1 tablespoon Swerve confectioners'-style sweetener or equivalent amount of liquid or powdered sweetener (see page 31)

1 teaspoon garlic powder

1 teaspoon onion powder

1 teaspoon fine sea salt

Place all the ingredients in a medium-sized bowl and whisk until smooth. Taste and adjust the seasoning to your liking, adding more sweetener or salt, if desired. Store in an airtight container in the refrigerator for up to 12 days.

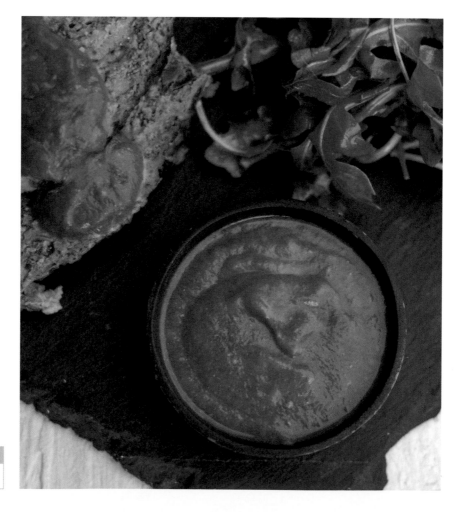

NUTRITIONAL INFO (per serving)				
calories	fat	protein	carbs	fiber
5	0g	0.3g	1g	0.3g

Creamy "Honey" Mustard

(L M H KETO 🔒 🚫 OPTION)   **prep time:** 5 minutes   **yield:** 1 cup (1 tablespoon per serving)

½ cup mayonnaise, homemade (page 357) or store-bought

½ cup prepared yellow mustard

¼ cup Swerve confectioners'-style sweetener or equivalent amount of liquid or powdered sweetener (see page 31)

1 tablespoon coconut vinegar or apple cider vinegar

⅛ teaspoon fine sea salt

Place all the ingredients in a small bowl and whisk to combine. Taste and adjust the seasoning to your liking, adding more sweetener or salt, if desired. Store in an airtight container in the refrigerator for up to 5 days.

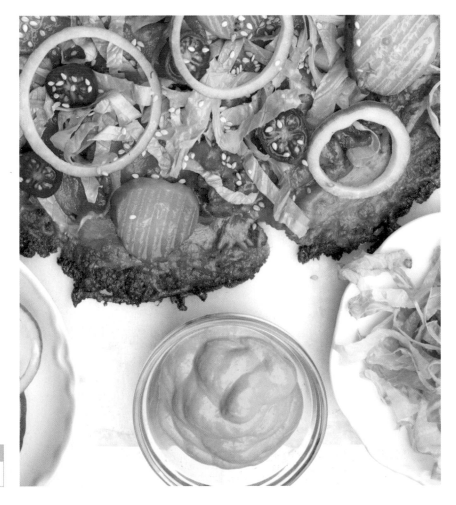

NUTRITIONAL INFO (per serving)				
calories	fat	protein	carbs	fiber
45	5g	0g	0g	0g

Sausage Breakfast Sandwiches
with Zero-Carb English Muffins

(L M→H KETO · OPTION · OPTION)   **prep time:** 7 minutes   **cook time:** 25 minutes   **yield:** 2 sandwiches

This breakfast sandwich is inspired by the beloved Sausage McMuffin from McDonald's.

—muffins

2 large eggs

1 tablespoon melted unsalted butter (or avocado oil if dairy-free)

2 tablespoons unsweetened cashew milk (or hemp milk if nut-free)

½ cup pork dust (see page 363), or 2 tablespoons coconut flour

½ teaspoon baking powder

¼ teaspoon fine sea salt

—eggs

2 large eggs

¼ teaspoon fine sea salt

⅛ teaspoon ground black pepper

—sausage patties

4 ounces ground pork

¼ teaspoon fine sea salt

¼ teaspoon ground black pepper

¼ teaspoon dried ground sage

¼ teaspoon dried ground thyme

2 ounces cheddar cheese, thinly sliced (omit for dairy-free)

1. Preheat the oven to 400°F. Grease four 4-ounce ramekins.

2. Make the muffins: Crack the eggs into a medium-sized bowl. Add the melted butter, milk, pork dust, baking powder, and salt and stir until well combined. Divide the batter between 2 of the ramekins. Bake for 12 to 15 minutes, until a toothpick inserted in the center of a muffin comes out clean. Allow the muffins to cool completely before removing them from the ramekins.

3. Meanwhile, make the eggs: Crack the remaining 2 eggs into the other 2 ramekins. Season with the salt and pepper. Bake for 7 to 8 minutes for eggs with set whites but still-runny yolks; if you want set yolks, bake for another 2 to 3 minutes. Remove from the oven and set aside.

4. Make the sausage patties: Place the ground pork, salt, pepper, sage, and thyme in a small bowl and mix with your hands to combine. Form into 2 patties (about 2½ inches in diameter). Heat a lightly greased large cast-iron skillet over medium heat. Fry the patties in the skillet for 2 minutes, then flip and fry for 3 minutes more, or until the sausage is cooked through. Remove from the skillet and set aside; leave the drippings in the pan.

5. Return the skillet to medium heat. Slice the muffins in half, place in the greased skillet, cut side down, and fry for 2 minutes, or until golden brown. Remove from the skillet.

6. To assemble the sandwiches: Place a slice of cheese on the bottom half of one of the muffins, then top the cheese with a sausage patty. Remove one of the eggs from its ramekin and place on top of the sausage patty. Place the top half of the muffin on the egg. Repeat with the remaining muffin, cheese, sausage patty, and egg. Store in an airtight container in the refrigerator for up to 4 days. To reheat, place on a rimmed baking sheet in a preheated 400°F oven or toaster oven for about 5 minutes.

busy family tip: *I make a double batch of these sandwiches to store in the refrigerator or freezer for easy breakfasts on the go.*

NUTRITIONAL INFO (per serving)				
calories	fat	protein	carbs	fiber
440	36g	29g	2g	0.5g

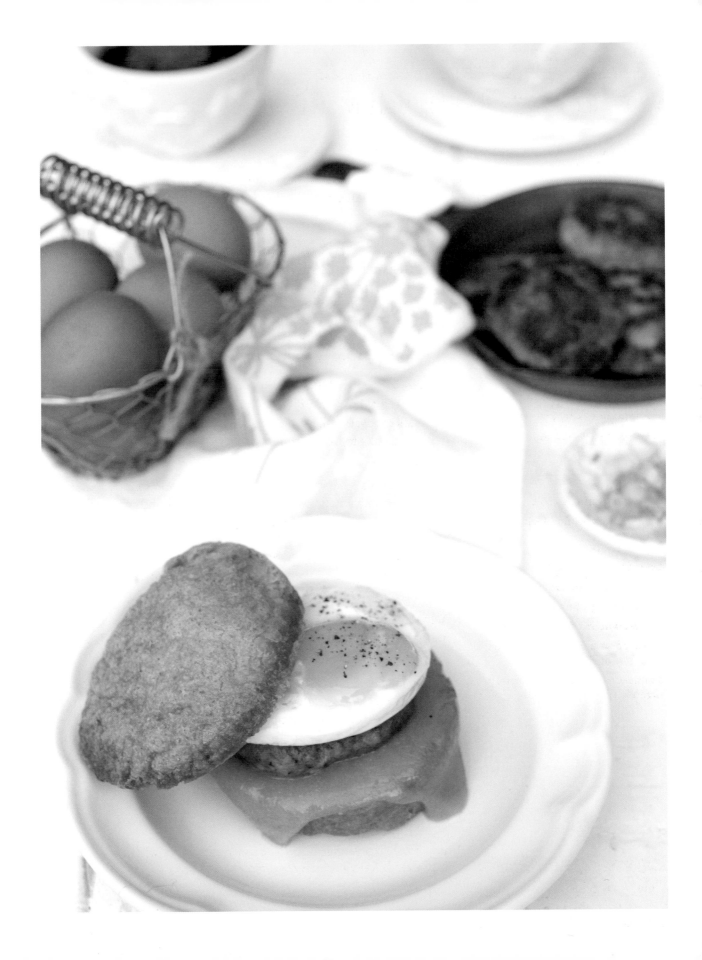

Mozzarella Sticks

$$\left(\begin{array}{c} \text{M} \\ \text{L} \curvearrowright \text{H} \\ \text{KETO} \end{array} \; \diagdown\hspace{-0.5em}\square \; \right)$$ **prep time:** 10 minutes, plus at least 2 hours to freeze (not including time to make marinara)
cook time: 2 minutes **yield:** 4 servings

1 large egg

½ cup powdered Parmesan cheese (see page 363)

¼ cup Italian seasoning

8 pieces string cheese

1 cup avocado oil or coconut oil, for frying

½ cup marinara, homemade (page 126) or store-bought, warmed

1. Crack the egg into a shallow baking dish and lightly beat with a fork. In a separate medium-sized shallow dish, combine the powdered Parmesan and Italian seasoning. Dip each cheese stick into the egg and roll to wet it. Then dip the cheese stick into the powdered Parmesan mixture and use your hands to coat it well. (Dip it again in both for a thicker coating.) Place the coated cheese sticks in an 8-inch square baking dish, cover, and freeze for a minimum of 2 hours, or until ready to fry. (*Note:* If the cheese sticks are not frozen, you will end up with a gooey mess instead of nicely formed cheese sticks.)

2. Heat the oil in a 4-inch deep (or deeper) cast-iron skillet or deep-fryer over medium heat to 350°F. The oil should be 2 inches deep; add more oil if needed.

3. Fry the cheese sticks in 2 batches, turning frequently, until the outsides are slightly crisp and golden brown, 1 to 2 minutes. Transfer to a platter; repeat with the remaining cheese sticks.

4. Serve with marinara. These are best served fresh, but extras can be stored in an airtight container in the refrigerator for up to 4 days. To reheat, place on a rimmed baking sheet in a preheated 350°F oven or toaster oven for about 3 minutes.

NUTRITIONAL INFO (per serving)				
calories	fat	protein	carbs	fiber
284	22g	20g	2g	1g

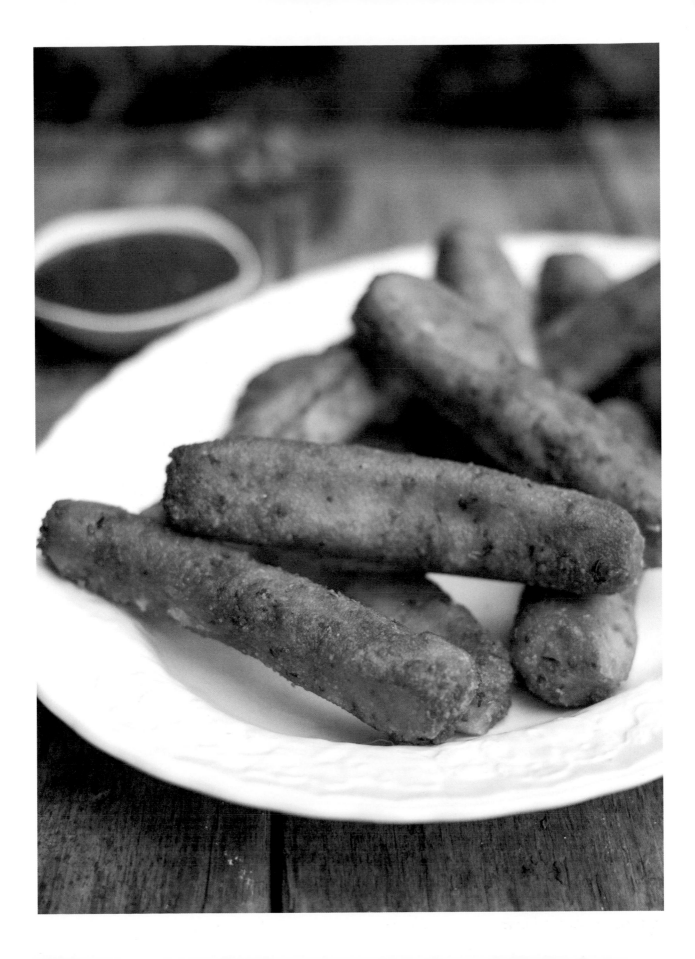

Taco Dip with Pepper Dippers

(L M H KETO / OPTION) **prep time:** 15 minutes **cook time:** 5 minutes **yield:** 4 servings

TGI Friday's has a creamy and delicious nine-layer dip that inspired this dish. I made this recipe quick and easy, but if you want to add another layer, prepare my Smoky Refried "Beans" (page 234) and spread them on the bottom of the serving dish, which would make the dip just like the TGI Friday's version, but without the carbs!

4 ounces ground beef

2 tablespoons tomato sauce

1½ teaspoons chili powder

1½ teaspoons ground cumin

½ teaspoon paprika

½ teaspoon fine sea salt

1 cup sour cream

1 cup cream cheese, at room temperature

1 cup guacamole, homemade (page 198) or store-bought

1 cup diced tomatoes (about 1 medium)

1 cup shredded lettuce

½ cup sliced black olives

Shredded cheddar cheese, for garnish (optional)

Chopped fresh cilantro, for garnish (optional)

2 large bell peppers or 6 mini bell peppers (any color), cut into 1-inch-wide strips, for serving

1. Place the ground beef, tomato sauce, chili powder, cumin, paprika, and salt in a small skillet over medium heat. Cook, stirring often to break up the beef with a spatula, until the beef is browned and cooked through, about 5 minutes. Remove from the pan and place in the refrigerator to cool.

2. In a medium-sized bowl, use a hand mixer to combine the sour cream and cream cheese until well blended. Spread the mixture in the bottom of a 9-inch pie pan.

3. Spread the guacamole over the sour cream and cream cheese layer. Top with the cooled beef mixture. Sprinkle the tomatoes, lettuce, and olives over the beef. Garnish with cheddar cheese and cilantro, if using. Serve with the sliced peppers. Store in an airtight container in the refrigerator for up to 4 days.

tip: *To make this recipe dairy-free, replace the sour cream and cream cheese with 2 cups of Kite Hill brand cream cheese style spread, at room temperature, thinned with a little cashew or hemp milk. Omit the cheddar cheese garnish.*

NUTRITIONAL INFO (per serving)				
calories	fat	protein	carbs	fiber
354	29g	9g	10g	3g

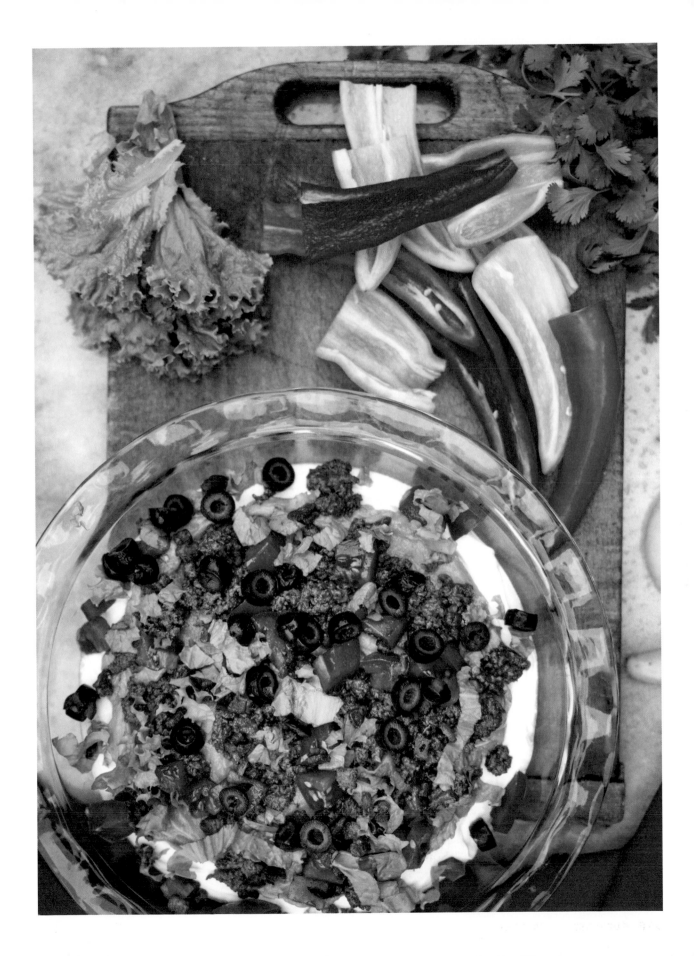

Parmesan Garlic Drummies

(L M H KETO   OPTION   OPTION)   **prep time:** 12 minutes   **cook time:** 30 minutes   **yield:** 12 servings

A popular fast-casual wing restaurant called Buffalo Wild Wings serves a delicious Parmesan garlic sauce with their wings. This keto-friendly version is sure to please your palate! Recipes like this one that involve deep-frying may call for a lot of coconut oil, but you can re-use the oil. I keep a large mason jar of oil reserved for frying in the refrigerator. When you're done frying the chicken, let the oil cool, strain it, and save it for future use.

2 cups coconut oil, for frying

—parmesan garlic sauce

½ cup mayonnaise, homemade (page 357) or store-bought

3 tablespoons chicken or beef bone broth, homemade (page 356) or store-bought

3 tablespoons coconut vinegar or apple cider vinegar

2 tablespoons grated Parmesan cheese

2 cloves garlic, smashed to a paste

¼ teaspoon fine sea salt

¼ teaspoon ground black pepper

2 pounds (about 24) chicken drumettes or wings

Fine sea salt and ground black pepper

1. Heat the oil in a 4-inch deep (or deeper) cast-iron skillet over medium heat to 350°F. The oil should be 2 inches deep; add more oil if needed.

2. While the oil is heating, make the sauce: Place the mayonnaise, broth, vinegar, Parmesan cheese, garlic, salt, and pepper in a small bowl. Stir well to combine. Taste and adjust the seasoning to your liking.

3. Fry about 6 drumettes or wings at a time until golden brown on all sides and cooked through, about 8 minutes. Remove from the skillet and season with a few pinches each of salt and pepper. Repeat with the remaining drumettes/wings.

4. Transfer the chicken to a platter and serve with the sauce. Store the drummies in an airtight container in the refrigerator for up to 4 days; the sauce can be stored in the fridge for up to a week. To reheat the drummies, place them on a rimmed baking sheet in a preheated 350°F oven for about 3 minutes.

note: *To make this recipe dairy-free, replace the Parmesan Garlic Sauce with 1 batch of Dairy-Free Ranch Dressing (page 358).*

busy family tip: *The sauce can be made up to 1 week ahead of time.*

NUTRITIONAL INFO (per serving)				
calories	fat	protein	carbs	fiber
383	45g	0.4g	0.2g	0g

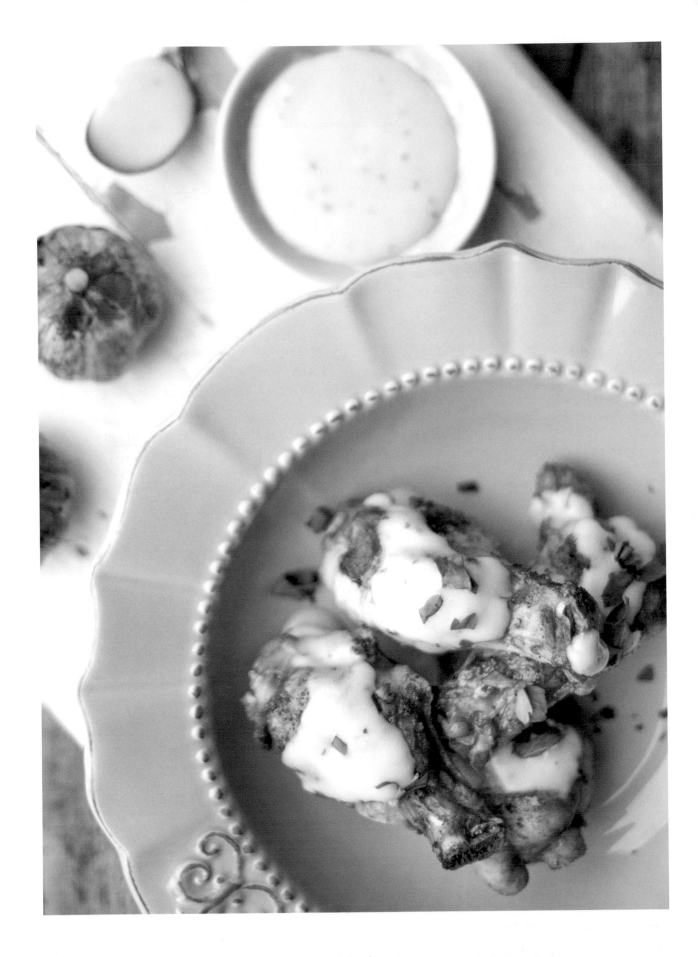

Baked "Potato" Soup

(L—M—H KETO OPTION 🍶) **prep time:** 6 minutes **cook time:** 15 minutes **yield:** 6 servings

Baked potato soup can be found at many fast-casual restaurants; this particular recipe is inspired by Panera's version. My soup is so decadent and creamy, you will never miss the potatoes!

3½ cups chopped cauliflower florets (about 2 pounds)

⅓ cup diced celery

⅓ cup finely chopped onions (about 1 small)

3¼ cups chicken bone broth, homemade (page 356) or store-bought

1 strip bacon, chopped, for garnish

½ teaspoon fine sea salt, or to taste

1 teaspoon ground black pepper

2½ ounces cream cheese (Kite Hill brand cream cheese style spread if dairy-free)

Sour cream, for garnish (omit for dairy-free)

Sliced fresh chives, for garnish

Melted ghee, for drizzling (omit for dairy-free)

1. Combine the cauliflower, celery, onions, and broth in a stockpot. Bring to a boil, then reduce the heat to medium and cook until the cauliflower is tender, 10 to 15 minutes. Meanwhile, fry the bacon in a small cast-iron skillet over medium heat until crisp, about 5 minutes; remove from the skillet and set aside for garnish.

2. Place half of the soup in a blender, add the cream cheese, and blend until very smooth. Return the pureed soup to the pot and season with the salt and pepper.

3. Divide the soup among 6 bowls and serve immediately, garnished with sour cream, bacon, chives, and a drizzle of melted ghee. Store in an airtight container in the refrigerator for up to 4 days. To reheat, place in a pot over medium heat for about 3 minutes.

NUTRITIONAL INFO (per serving)				
calories	fat	protein	carbs	fiber
113	8g	4g	5g	1g

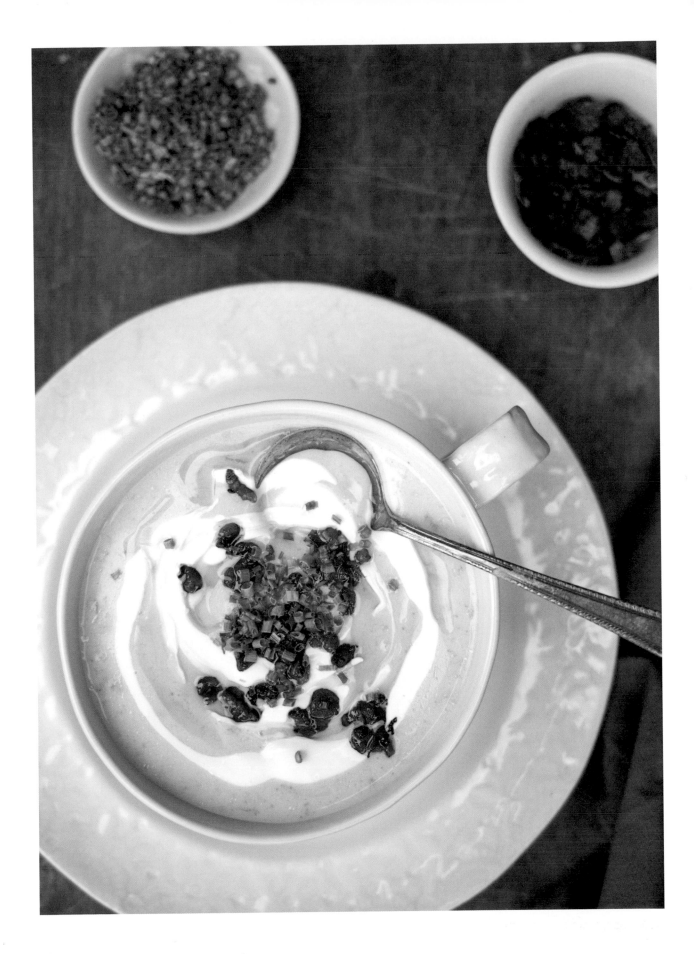

The Best Pub Salad

(L M H KETO OPTION) **prep time:** 15 minutes (not including time to make salads or dressing)
cook time: 5 minutes **yield:** 4 servings

You may be thinking, "Why a salad in a restaurant book?" But let me tell you, I ordered this salad years ago before I was strictly keto, and I still dream about it! About ten years ago, we were hiking along the north shore of Lake Superior over the Fourth of July and ventured into the closest town, the ever-so-charming Grand Marais, for the festivities. We decided to enjoy some lunch and music at the local pub. We sat in the rooftop dining area, where we had a glorious view of the lake, as well as the little parade going around and around the block. The group next to us had ordered an amazing-looking salad, and I told the waitress I wanted that. It just looked too decadent not to order. And you know what? It was so good, we went back to the pub for dinner and I ordered the same thing!

2 strips bacon, chopped

—blue cheese dressing (makes 1¼ cups)

8 ounces blue cheese, crumbled, plus extra if desired

¼ cup sour cream

¼ cup beef bone broth, homemade (page 356) or store-bought

¼ cup coconut vinegar or red wine vinegar

1½ tablespoons Swerve confectioners'-style sweetener or equivalent amount of liquid or powdered sweetener (see page 31) (optional)

1 tablespoon MCT oil or avocado oil

1 clove garlic

4 cups mixed greens, such as red leaf lettuce and spinach

1 tablespoon coconut vinegar

½ cup guacamole, homemade (page 198) or store-bought

½ cup curry chicken salad (page 304)

½ cup egg salad (page 304)

½ cup tuna salad (page 305)

4 ounces blue cheese, crumbled

Sunflower seeds, for garnish

Diced red onions, for garnish

1. In a medium-sized cast-iron skillet over medium heat, fry the bacon until crisp, about 5 minutes. Remove from the skillet and set aside.

2. Make the dressing: Place the blue cheese, sour cream, broth, vinegar, sweetener (if using), oil, and garlic in a food processor and blend until smooth. Stir in chunks of extra blue cheese if desired.

3. Place the mixed greens in a large bowl and toss with the vinegar. Divide among 4 serving plates. Scoop about 2 tablespoons each of the guacamole, curry chicken salad, egg salad, and tuna salad onto each plate. Sprinkle with the blue cheese and bacon and drizzle 2 tablespoons of the dressing over each plate. (You will have dressing left over.) Garnish with sunflower seeds and diced red onions.

4. Store the chicken, egg, and tuna salads in separate airtight containers in the refrigerator for up to 4 days. Store the dressing in an airtight container in the fridge for up to 12 days.

NUTRITIONAL INFO (per serving)				
calories	fat	protein	carbs	fiber
563	47g	28g	7g	3g

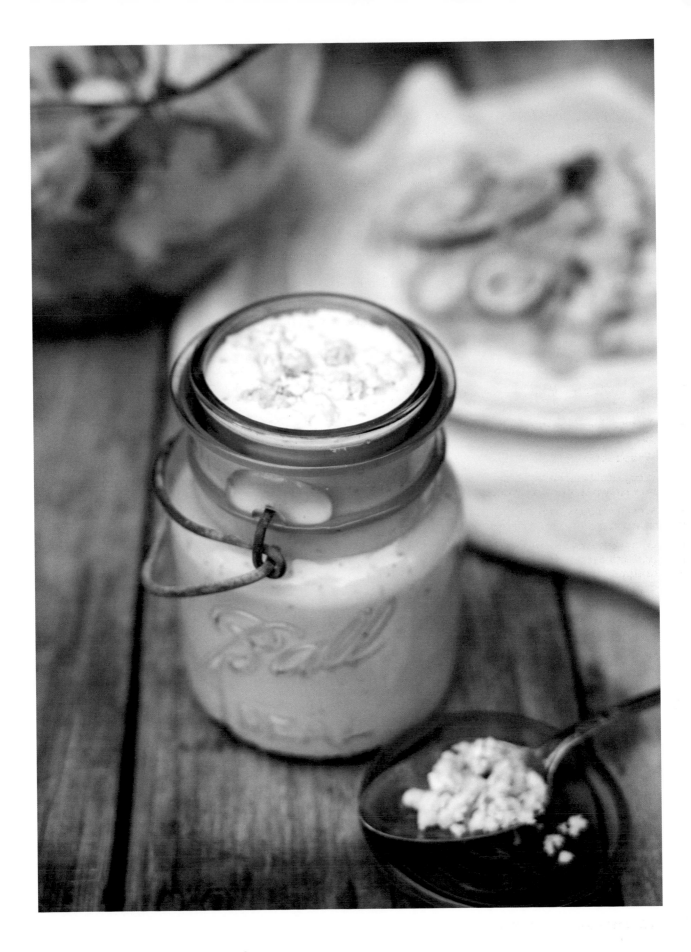

Curry Chicken Salad

(L M H KETO   OPTION   OPTION)   prep time: 10 minutes, plus time to chill   cook time: 12 minutes   yield: 4 servings

1 tablespoon ghee, lard, or bacon fat

1 pound boneless, skinless chicken thighs

1 teaspoon fine sea salt

½ teaspoon ground black pepper

¾ cup mayonnaise, homemade (page 357) or store-bought

2 tablespoons curry powder

¼ cup diced celery

¼ cup diced red onions

¼ cup chopped dill pickles

1. Heat the ghee in a deep sauté pan over medium-high heat. Season the chicken with the salt and pepper. Sauté the chicken in the pan for about 4 minutes per side, until golden brown and cooked through (there should be no pink remaining in the center).

2. Remove the chicken from the pan and let it cool slightly so that you can handle it. Dice the chicken into small pieces.

3. In a medium-sized bowl, whisk together the mayonnaise and curry powder. Add the celery, onions, pickles, and cooked chicken and stir to combine. Taste and adjust the seasoning to your liking, adding more salt or curry powder, if desired. Serve chilled. Store in an airtight container in the refrigerator for up to 4 days.

NUTRITIONAL INFO (per serving)				
calories	fat	protein	carbs	fiber
463	42g	20g	1g	0.3g

Egg Salad

(L M H KETO   OPTION)   prep time: 10 minutes, plus time to chill   cook time: 20 minutes   yield: 4 servings

8 large eggs

½ cup mayonnaise, homemade (page 357) or store-bought

2 tablespoons Dijon mustard

1 tablespoon chopped fresh dill, or 1 teaspoon dried dill weed

½ teaspoon fine sea salt

¼ teaspoon ground black pepper

1. Place the eggs in a medium-sized saucepan and cover with cold water. Bring to a boil, place the lid on the pan, and remove from the heat. Let the eggs stand in the hot water for 10 to 12 minutes. Transfer the eggs to a bowl of ice water, or rinse under cold running water, then peel and chop them.

2. In a large bowl, combine the eggs, mayonnaise, mustard, dill, salt, and pepper. Mash well with a fork or wooden spoon. Taste and adjust the seasoning to your liking, adding more salt or dill, if desired. Serve chilled. Store in an airtight container in the refrigerator for up to 4 days.

NUTRITIONAL INFO (per serving)				
calories	fat	protein	carbs	fiber
336	30g	13g	1g	0g

Tuna Salad

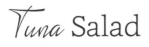

(L M>H KETO 🧂 🚫)   **prep time:** 7 minutes, plus time to chill   **yield:** 4 servings

2 (3¾-ounce) cans tuna packed in water, drained

¼ cup plus 2 tablespoons mayonnaise, homemade (page 357) or store-bought

½ teaspoon fine sea salt

⅛ teaspoon dried onion flakes, or 2 tablespoons chopped fresh chives

In a large bowl, combine the tuna, mayonnaise, salt, and onion flakes. Taste and adjust the seasoning to your liking, adding more salt or onion flakes, if desired. Serve chilled. Store in an airtight container in the refrigerator for up to 4 days.

variation: salmon salad. *I often use canned salmon in place of canned tuna because my dad often catches salmon and cans it for me. Canned salmon tastes just as good, but it has a better fat ratio for ketogenic eating, and it contains less mercury than canned tuna. To make salmon salad, simply replace the tuna with an equal amount of salmon.*

NUTRITIONAL INFO (per serving)				
calories	fat	protein	carbs	fiber
230	19g	14g	0.5g	0g

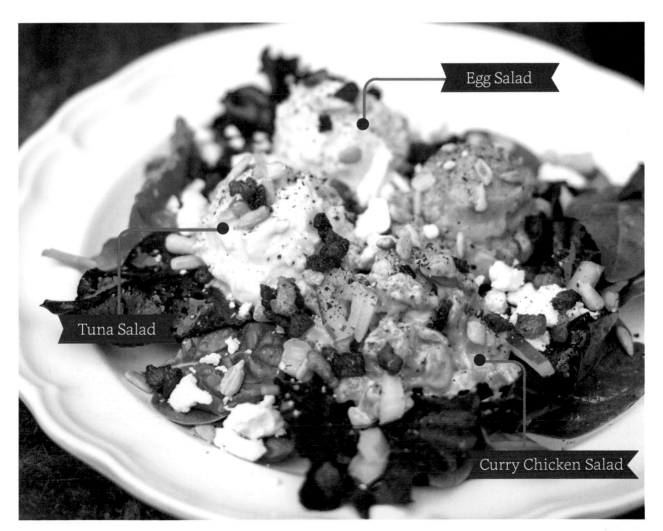

Egg Salad

Tuna Salad

Curry Chicken Salad

Chicken Lettuce Wraps with Satay Dipping Sauce

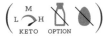 **prep time:** 8 minutes **cook time:** 11 minutes **yield:** 4 servings

This dish is a favorite at P. F. Chang's, a fast-casual Chinese restaurant. It is traditionally served with water chestnuts, but to my surprise, water chestnuts pack a lot of carbohydrates. I suggest skipping them.

1 tablespoon ghee or coconut oil

1 pound ground chicken or ground pork

¼ cup diced onions (about 1 small)

2 cloves garlic, minced

¼ teaspoon fine sea salt

—satay dipping sauce

¼ cup creamy almond butter, at room temperature

2 tablespoons wheat-free tamari, or ½ cup coconut aminos

2 tablespoons grated fresh ginger

2 tablespoons coconut vinegar or unseasoned rice vinegar

1 tablespoon hot sauce, or more to desired heat (optional)

1 teaspoon toasted (dark) sesame oil

½ teaspoon Chinese five-spice powder

2 scallions, thinly sliced on the diagonal, plus extra for garnish

2 small heads butter lettuce, leaves separated, for serving

1. Heat the ghee in a large cast-iron skillet over medium-high heat. Add the ground chicken, onions, garlic, and salt and cook, breaking up the chicken with a spatula, for 5 minutes, or until the chicken is browned and cooked through.

2. Make the sauce: In a medium-sized bowl, stir together the almond butter, tamari, ginger, vinegar, hot sauce, sesame oil, and five-spice powder until well combined. Add half of the sauce to the skillet with the chicken. Stir in the scallions and sauté for another minute, or until the scallions are softened.

3. To assemble the wraps, place a few tablespoons of the chicken mixture in each lettuce leaf and garnish with sliced scallions, if desired. Serve with extra sauce on the side. Store in an airtight container in the refrigerator for up to 4 days. To reheat the meat mixture, place in a lightly greased skillet and sauté over medium heat for about 3 minutes.

NUTRITIONAL INFO (per serving)				
calories	fat	protein	carbs	fiber
424	28g	36g	7g	2g

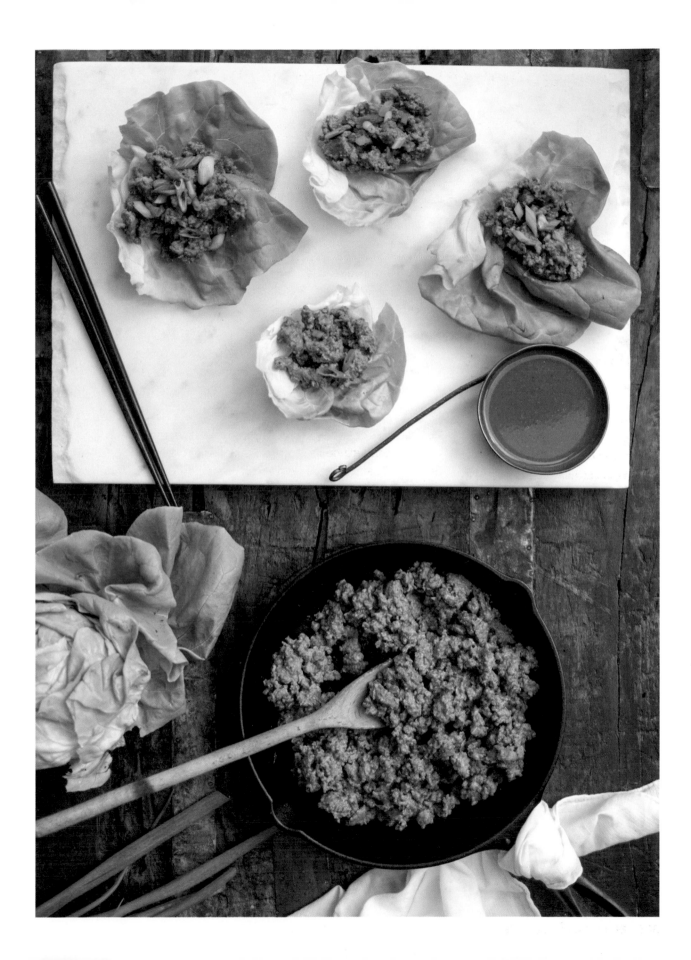

Chicken Nuggets

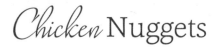

prep time: 8 minutes (not including time to make sauce)   **cook time:** 20 minutes
yield: 6 servings

2 large eggs

1 cup powdered Parmesan cheese (see page 363) (or pork dust if dairy-free; see page 363)

½ teaspoon dried oregano leaves (optional)

½ teaspoon dried parsley leaves (optional)

¼ teaspoon ground black pepper (optional)

1 pound boneless, skinless chicken thighs or breasts, cut into 1½-inch pieces

½ cup Keto Ketchup (page 290), Creamy "Honey" Mustard (page 291), or Aioli (page 328), for serving

1. Preheat the oven to 350°F. Line a rimmed baking sheet with parchment paper.

2. In a medium-sized bowl, lightly beat the eggs. In another medium-sized bowl, combine the powdered Parmesan with the oregano, parsley, and pepper, if using.

3. Dip the chicken pieces into the eggs, then into the Parmesan mixture. Use your hands to coat each nugget well. Place the coated nuggets on the prepared baking sheet. Bake for 20 minutes, or until golden brown.

4. Transfer the chicken nuggets to a platter and serve with the keto sauce(s) of your choice. Store in an airtight container in the refrigerator for up to 4 days. To reheat, place on a rimmed baking sheet in a preheated 350°F oven for about 3 minutes.

note: *You can also pan-fry the nuggets by heating ½ inch of coconut oil or ghee in a cast-iron skillet over medium heat to 375°F. When the oil is hot, fry the nuggets in batches until golden brown on all sides and cooked through, about 6 minutes.*

NUTRITIONAL INFO (per serving)				
calories	fat	protein	carbs	fiber
184	11g	20g	1g	0g

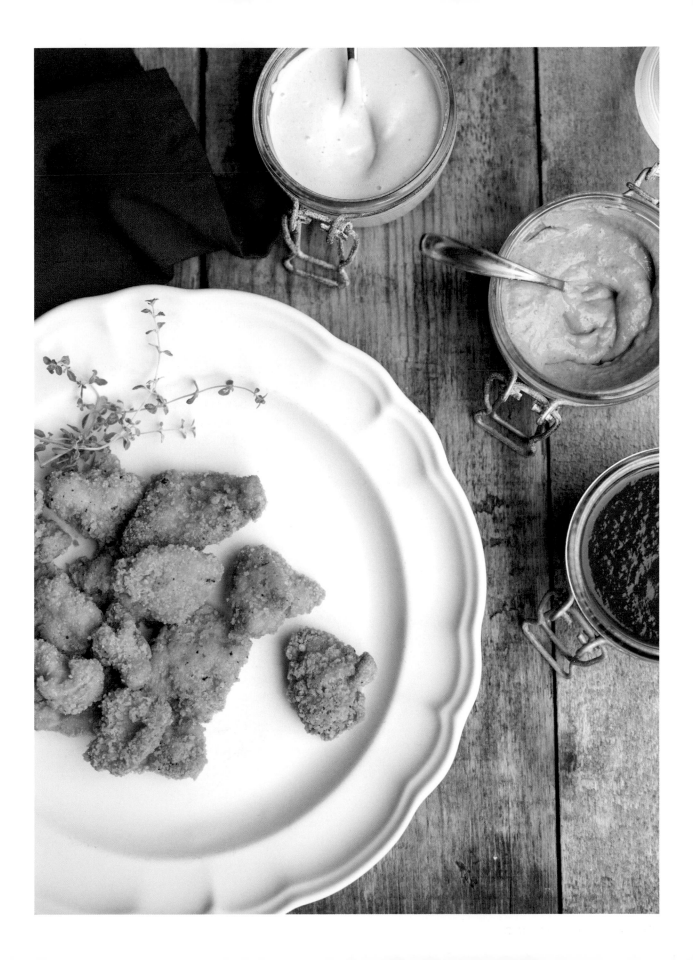

Bacon Cheeseburger

(L M H KETO OPTION OPTION OPTION) **prep time:** 4 minutes (not including time to make condiments)
cook time: 10 minutes   **yield:** 1 serving

2 strips bacon

1 (4-ounce) hamburger patty

Fine sea salt and ground black pepper

1 (1-ounce) slice sharp cheddar cheese (omit for dairy-free)

2 slices tomato

1 slice red onion

¼ avocado, sliced

2 large butter lettuce leaves

Condiments of your choice, such as Keto Ketchup (page 290), mustard, or mayonnaise, homemade (page 357) or store-bought

1. Fry the bacon in a medium-sized cast-iron skillet over medium heat until crisp, about 5 minutes. Remove the bacon but keep the drippings in the skillet.

2. Season the burger patty well with salt and pepper. Place the patty in the skillet and fry over medium-high heat for about 3 minutes per side for a medium-done burger, or longer if you prefer a more well-done burger.

3. Place the slice of cheese on the burger and cover the skillet to help the cheese melt. Remove the burger from the skillet and serve between the lettuce leaves, topped with the bacon, tomato, onion, avocado, and condiments of your choice.

NUTRITIONAL INFO (per serving)				
calories	fat	protein	carbs	fiber
619	51g	36g	7g	3g

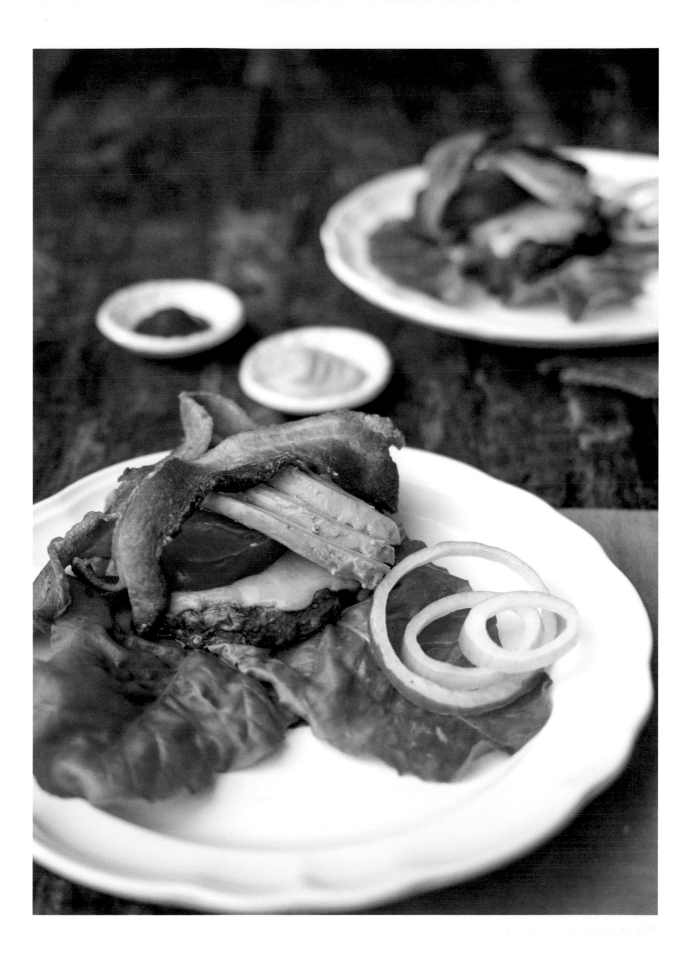

Juicy Lucy

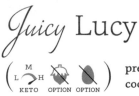

prep time: 8 minutes (not including time to make condiments)
cook time: 11 minutes   **yield:** 4 servings

If you've ever visited Minneapolis, you've probably heard about our classic Juicy Lucy, which is a mouthwatering burger with the cheese inside! It is served at the 5-8 Club and at Matt's. Both restaurants claim to be the creator of the Juicy Lucy, and they often have lighthearted battles over which restaurant makes a better version. The two restaurants even had a cook-off on the Food Network. For a decadent treat, serve these burgers with a Classic Diner Malt (page 342).

1 pound ground beef

4 slices American cheese

1 teaspoon fine sea salt

¼ teaspoon ground black pepper

4 Keto Buns (page 362)

2 tablespoons unsalted butter, at room temperature

—fixings (optional)

Lettuce leaves

Tomato slices

Red onion slices

Fried bacon strips

Dill pickle chips or spears

—condiments (optional)

Keto Ketchup (page 290)

Mustard

Mayonnaise, homemade (page 357) or store-bought

1. Divide the ground beef into 8 equal portions and form each portion into a ¼-inch-thick patty (about 3½ inches in diameter).

2. Fold the cheese slices in half and then in half again so that the cheese is about 1½ inches square. Place one stack of cheese in the center of a patty and top with another patty. Use your fingers to seal the patty around the cheese; be sure to seal the edges well or the cheese will melt out. Repeat with the remaining patties and cheese. Season the patties well on both sides with the salt and pepper.

3. Preheat a grill to medium-high heat, or heat up a large cast-iron skillet over medium-high heat. If using a grill, oil the grates with avocado oil; if using a skillet, pour 1 tablespoon of avocado oil into the hot skillet. Grill or fry the patties for 4 to 5 minutes per side for medium-done burgers, or longer if you prefer more well-done burgers. Let the burgers cool for a few minutes before consuming or the melted cheese will burn your mouth.

4. Slice the buns in half, spread the butter on the insides, and place the buns, cut side down, on the grill or in the skillet. Grill or fry for about 2 minutes, until golden brown.

5. Serve the burgers in the grilled or fried buns with the fixings and condiments of your choice. Store in an airtight container in the refrigerator for up to 4 days. To reheat, place in a lightly greased skillet over medium heat for about 3 minutes.

NUTRITIONAL INFO (per serving)				
calories	fat	protein	carbs	fiber
444	36g	27g	1g	0g

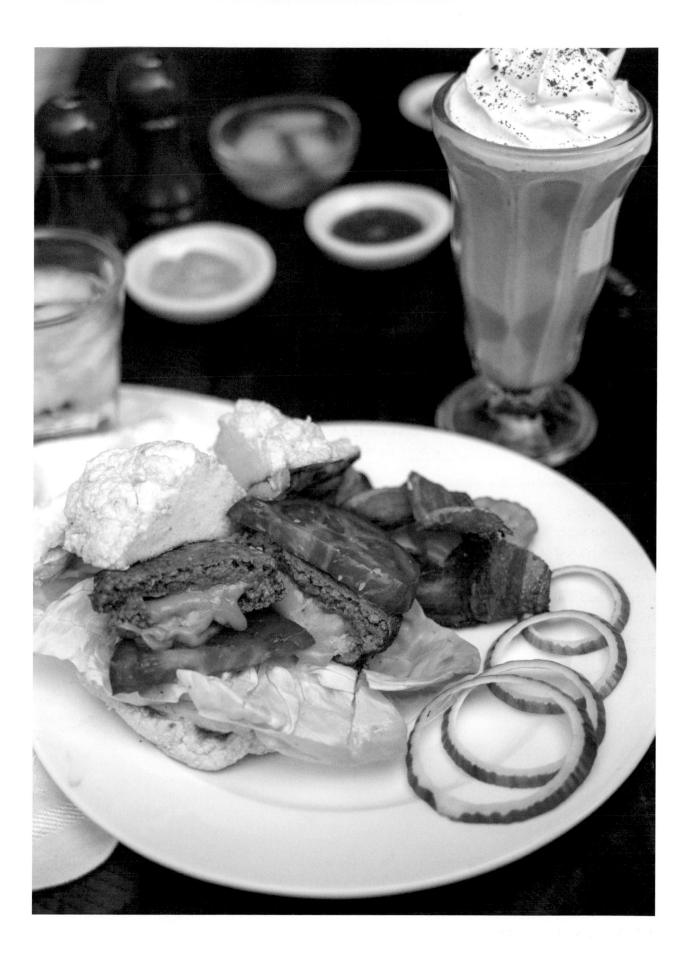

Fiesta Lime Chicken

(L M H | KETO OPTION) **prep time:** 8 minutes, plus 1 hour or overnight to marinate (not including time to make pico de gallo) **cook time:** 12 minutes **yield:** 4 servings

If you have ever been to Applebee's, you know that fiesta lime chicken is one of their classic menu items and is a huge hit with their patrons. When I asked my blog followers which restaurant recipes they wanted me to include in this book, many of them asked for a keto version of this dish. Here it is!

1 cup chicken bone broth, homemade (page 356) or store-bought

½ cup fresh lime juice (3 to 4 limes)

3 tablespoons Swerve confectioners'-style sweetener or equivalent amount of liquid or powdered sweetener (see page 31)

1 tablespoon plus 1 teaspoon wheat-free tamari, or ⅓ cup coconut aminos

3 cloves garlic, smashed to a paste or minced

1 teaspoon liquid smoke

½ teaspoon fine sea salt

¼ teaspoon grated fresh ginger

4 boneless, skinless chicken thighs

—dressing

¼ cup mayonnaise, homemade (page 357) or store-bought

¼ cup sour cream

2 tablespoons Pico de Gallo (page 197) or store-bought sugar-free chunky salsa

1 tablespoon chicken bone broth, homemade (page 356) or store-bought

1 teaspoon Cajun seasoning (see note)

¼ teaspoon dried parsley leaves

¼ teaspoon hot sauce

⅛ teaspoon ground cumin

1 cup shredded Colby Jack cheese (about 4 ounces)

Chopped fresh parsley or cilantro leaves, for garnish

1. Place the broth, lime juice, sweetener, tamari, garlic, liquid smoke, salt, and ginger in a large shallow dish and stir well to combine. Add the chicken, cover the dish, and place in the refrigerator to marinate for at least 1 hour or overnight.

2. Preheat the oven broiler to high. Remove the chicken from the marinade and place in a large cast-iron skillet or 9-inch square baking dish (discard the marinade). Broil for 5 minutes per side, or until the chicken is cooked through.

3. Meanwhile, make the dressing: Place the mayo, sour cream, pico de gallo, broth, Cajun seasoning, parsley, hot sauce, and cumin in a small bowl and stir well to combine. Pour the sauce over the chicken.

4. Sprinkle the chicken with the cheese and broil for 1 minute more, or until the cheese is bubbly and melted. Serve garnished with parsley. Store in an airtight container in the fridge for up to 3 days. To reheat, place on a rimmed baking sheet in a 350°F oven for about 5 minutes.

note: *When purchasing Cajun seasoning, check the ingredients label for harmful additives, such as a common filler called maltodextrin, and sugar. Or you can make your own keto Cajun seasoning; I have a tasty recipe in my book* The 30-Day Ketogenic Cleanse.

NUTRITIONAL INFO (per serving)				
calories	fat	protein	carbs	fiber
541	41g	37g	5g	0.4g

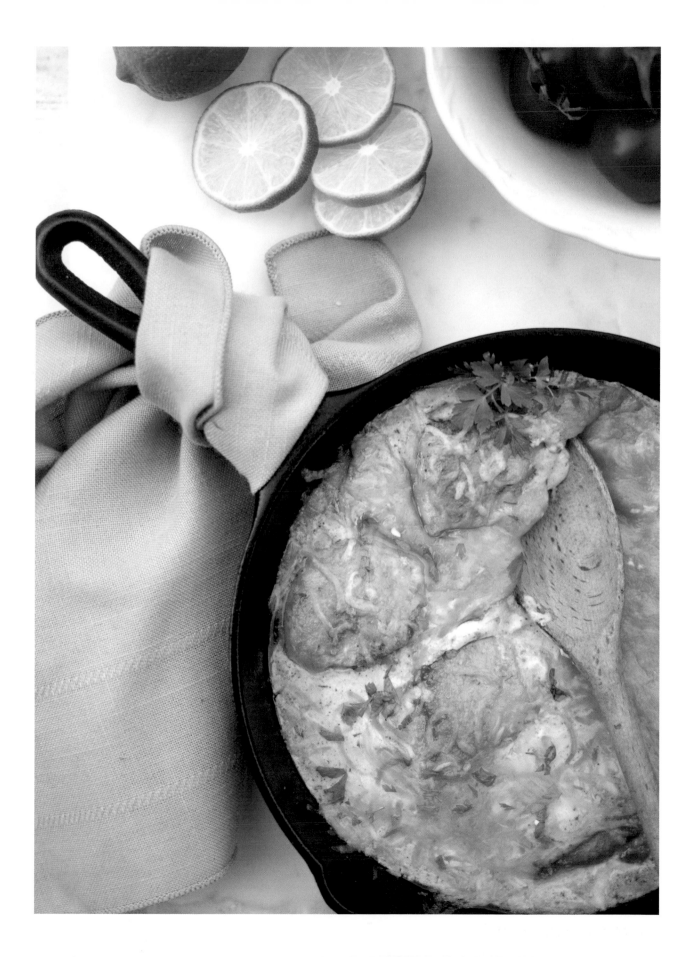

Easy Mini Corn Dogs

(L M H KETO OPTION OPTION) **prep time:** 5 minutes (not including time to make ketchup) **cook time:** 12 minutes
yield: 4 servings

4 large eggs

1 cup pork dust (see page 363), or 2 tablespoons coconut flour

2 tablespoons unsweetened cashew milk (or hemp milk if nut-free)

1 tablespoon unsalted butter, melted (or avocado oil if dairy-free)

½ teaspoon baking powder

⅛ teaspoon fine sea salt

4 uncured hot dogs, cut into 1½-inch slices (I prefer Applegate Farms organic hot dogs)

½ cup Keto Ketchup (page 290), for serving

1. Preheat the oven to 400°F. Grease a 24-well mini muffin pan.

2. Crack the eggs into a medium-sized bowl. Add the pork dust, milk, melted butter, baking powder, and salt and stir well to combine. Divide the batter among the muffin cups.

3. Place 1 hot dog slice in the center of each muffin cup and press down gently so that only the tip of the hot dog is sticking out. Bake for 12 to 15 minutes, until a toothpick inserted in the center of a muffin comes out clean. Allow to cool slightly before removing from the pan. Serve with ketchup.

4. Store in an airtight container in the refrigerator for up to 4 days. To reheat, place on a rimmed baking sheet in a preheated 350°F oven for about 3 minutes.

busy family tip: *I make a triple batch of these mini corn dogs and store them in the freezer for easy lunches for my boys.*

NUTRITIONAL INFO (per serving)				
calories	fat	protein	carbs	fiber
246	17g	17g	2g	1g

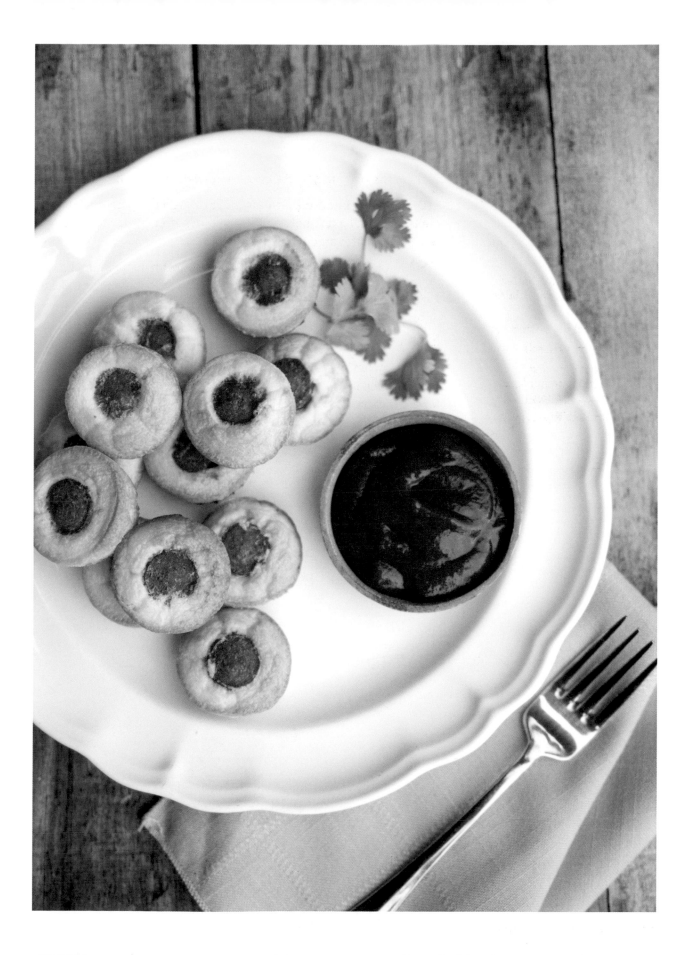

Deep-Fried Breaded Shrimp with Spicy Mayo

(L M H KETO · OPTION · OPTION)   prep time: 8 minutes   cook time: 6 minutes   yield: 4 servings

This Asian-inspired dish is the creation of the fast-casual chain Bonefish Grill. They call it Bang Bang Shrimp, and it's one of the most popular items on their menu. This is my keto take on it. I like to serve it on a bed of Cabbage Pasta (page 361).

—spicy mayo

½ cup mayonnaise, homemade (page 357) or store-bought

¼ cup beef or chicken bone broth, homemade (page 356) or store-bought

½ teaspoon hot sauce

½ teaspoon cayenne pepper

—dry coating

½ cup powdered Parmesan cheese (see page 363) (or pork dust if dairy-free; see page 363)

½ teaspoon garlic powder

½ teaspoon ginger powder

¼ teaspoon cayenne pepper

—wet coating

1 large egg

1 teaspoon hot sauce

1 cup coconut oil, for frying

1 pound large shrimp, peeled and deveined

8 lettuce leaves, for serving

Thinly sliced scallions, for garnish

1. Make the spicy mayo: Whisk together the mayonnaise, broth, hot sauce, and cayenne in a small bowl and set aside.

2. Make the dry coating: Place the powdered Parmesan, garlic powder, ginger powder, and cayenne in a shallow bowl and mix with a fork to combine.

3. Make the wet coating: In another small bowl, whisk together the egg and hot sauce.

4. Heat the oil in a 4-inch-deep (or deeper) cast-iron skillet over medium-high heat to 375°F. The oil should be about 2 inches deep; add more oil if needed. Line a plate with paper towels.

5. Meanwhile, bread the shrimp: Pat the shrimp dry. Place the shrimp in the wet coating, then dip them into the dry coating. Set the coated shrimp aside on a plate while the oil heats.

6. Fry the shrimp in batches in the hot oil until the breading is golden brown, about 3 minutes. Using a slotted spoon, remove the shrimp from the skillet and set on the paper towel–lined plate to drain. Repeat with the remaining shrimp.

7. To serve, place the lettuce leaves on a platter. Divide the shrimp among the lettuce leaves. Dollop the shrimp with the spicy mayo and garnish with scallions. Store in an airtight container in the refrigerator for up to 4 days. To reheat, place the shrimp on a rimmed baking sheet in a preheated 350°F oven or toaster oven for about 5 minutes.

note: *You can reserve the oil for future frying by straining it into a clean mason jar and storing it in the refrigerator for up to 1 month.*

NUTRITIONAL INFO (per serving)				
calories	fat	protein	carbs	fiber
398	28g	34g	1g	0.2g

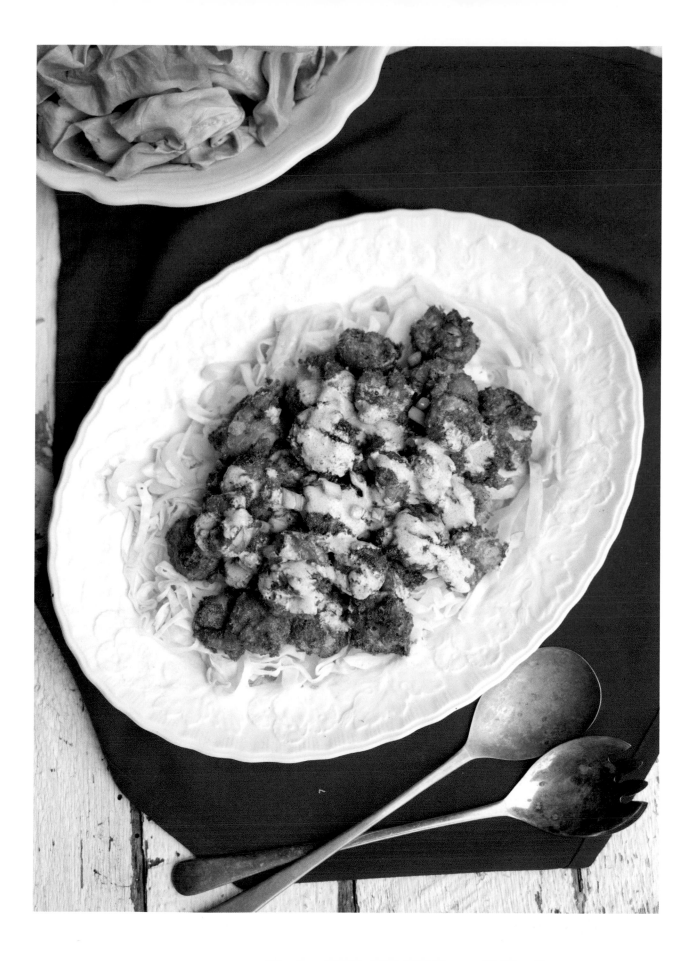

Tomato Basil Chicken Salad Wraps

(L M H T KETO ☐ ⊘ OPTION) **prep time:** 10 minutes (not including time to make marinara)
cook time: 5 minutes per tortilla, plus 5 minutes to fry bacon   **yield:** 10 wraps

When I was in high school, I worked at a cute coffee shop called Uncommon Ground. It was my favorite job (besides this job of writing cookbooks!). One of our specialties was tomato basil wraps. People would crowd into the tiny shop for them. If I ever opened a keto coffee shop, these wraps would be on my menu! If you prefer plain wraps, simply replace the pureed marinara with 1 cup of boiling hot water.

—tortillas

1¼ cups blanched almond flour, or ¾ cup coconut flour

3½ tablespoons psyllium husk powder (no substitutes)

1 teaspoon fine sea salt

2 large eggs (4 eggs if using coconut flour)

1 cup pureed Mama Maria's Marinara (page 126) or store-bought marinara, heated until boiling hot

—fillings

10 strips bacon

4 cups diced leftover cooked chicken (or organic rotisserie chicken)

¼ cup mayonnaise, homemade (page 357) or store-bought

2 cups torn or shredded leafy greens

½ cup shredded purple cabbage

1 small red onion, thinly sliced

1 avocado, sliced

busy family tip: *Make extras for easy lunches on the go!*

1. Make the tortillas: In a medium-sized bowl, combine the flour, psyllium husk powder, and salt. Add the eggs and mix until a thick dough forms. Add the marinara and mix until well combined. Let the dough sit for 1 to 2 minutes, until it firms up.

2. Lightly grease two 9-inch pieces of parchment paper. Separate the dough into 10 balls (about 2 inches in diameter). Place a ball of dough in the center of one of the greased pieces of parchment. Top with the other greased piece of parchment. Using a rolling pin, roll out each ball of dough into a circle that is an even ¹⁄₁₆ inch thick. This dough is very forgiving, so if you don't make a perfect circle with the rolling pin, you can use your hands to shape the tortilla. If you have a tortilla press, place the dough, sandwiched between the pieces of parchment, in the press and press down until the dough flattens to the edge of the press.

3. Grease a large skillet with ghee or coconut oil and set it over medium-high heat. Remove the tortilla from the parchment paper and place it in the skillet (if the dough sticks to the parchment, use your fingers to close up any holes). Cook until light brown, about 2 minutes, then flip and cook for another 2 minutes, until cooked through. While the tortilla cooks, roll out and press the second dough ball, regreasing the parchment paper as needed, then cook the tortilla as described above, adding more ghee or oil to the skillet if needed. Repeat until all the tortillas are pressed and cooked.

4. Prepare the fillings: In a large cast-iron skillet over medium heat, fry the bacon until crisp, about 5 minutes. Remove from the heat and set aside. Place the chicken in a large bowl. Add the mayonnaise and stir until the chicken is coated.

5. Place a tortilla on a flat work surface. Place a small handful of greens and a few teaspoons of cabbage in the center of the tortilla. Top with the chicken salad, 1 strip of bacon, some of the onion, and a slice of avocado. Roll up tightly and slice in half crosswise. Repeat with the remaining wraps and fillings. Store in an airtight container in the refrigerator for up to 4 days.

NUTRITIONAL INFO (per wrap)				
calories	fat	protein	carbs	fiber
470	31g	38g	10g	6g

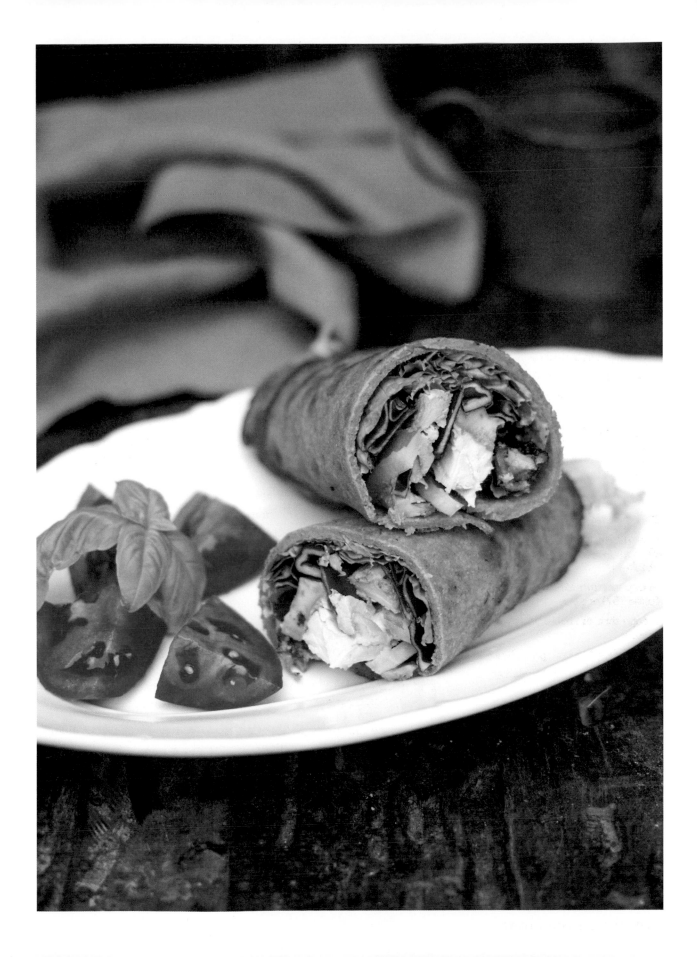

Fish Sticks with Homemade Tartar Sauce

(L → M → H KETO   OPTION   OPTION)   **prep time:** 10 minutes   **cook time:** 5 minutes   **yield:** 4 servings

—tartar sauce

¾ cup mayonnaise, homemade (page 357) or store-bought

2 tablespoons dill pickle juice

2 tablespoons finely diced dill pickles

¼ teaspoon fine sea salt

1 tablespoon Swerve confectioners'-style sweetener or equivalent amount of liquid or powdered sweetener (see page 31) (optional)

—fish sticks

1 large egg

1 cup powdered Parmesan cheese (see page 363) (or pork dust if dairy-free; see page 363)

¼ cup dried parsley leaves

1 pound cod fillets, cut into sticks about ½ inch wide by 2½ inches long

Avocado oil or coconut oil, for frying

1. Make the tartar sauce: Place the mayonnaise, pickle juice, pickles, salt, and sweetener, if using, in a small bowl and stir to combine. Cover the bowl and place in the refrigerator while you prepare the fish sticks.

2. Make the fish sticks: Crack the egg into a small shallow dish and beat lightly with a fork. Combine the powdered Parmesan and parsley in a separate medium-sized shallow dish. Dip the fish sticks in the egg just enough to wet them, then dip them in the Parmesan mixture and coat well; use your hands to press the mixture around each fish stick. (Dip again in both for a thicker coating.) Set the coated sticks aside on a large plate.

3. Heat the oil in a deep-fryer or a 4-inch-deep (or deeper) cast-iron skillet over medium-high heat to 350°F. The oil should be 3 inches deep; add more oil if needed.

4. Working in batches to avoid crowding, fry the coated fish sticks in the hot oil until golden brown, about 3 minutes, then turn them over and fry for another 2 minutes, or until the outsides are slightly crisp and the fish is cooked through.

5. Transfer to a platter and serve with the tartar sauce. Store the fish sticks in an airtight container in the refrigerator for up to 4 days or in the freezer for up to 1 month. Store the tartar sauce in an airtight container in the fridge for up to 2 weeks. To reheat the fish sticks, place on a rimmed baking sheet in a preheated 350°F oven for about 3 minutes.

busy family tip: *The tartar sauce can be made up to 2 weeks ahead. The fish sticks freeze well; I often make a double batch to store in the freezer for easy dinners for my boys.*

NUTRITIONAL INFO (per serving)				
calories	fat	protein	carbs	fiber
466	40g	23g	1g	0.3g

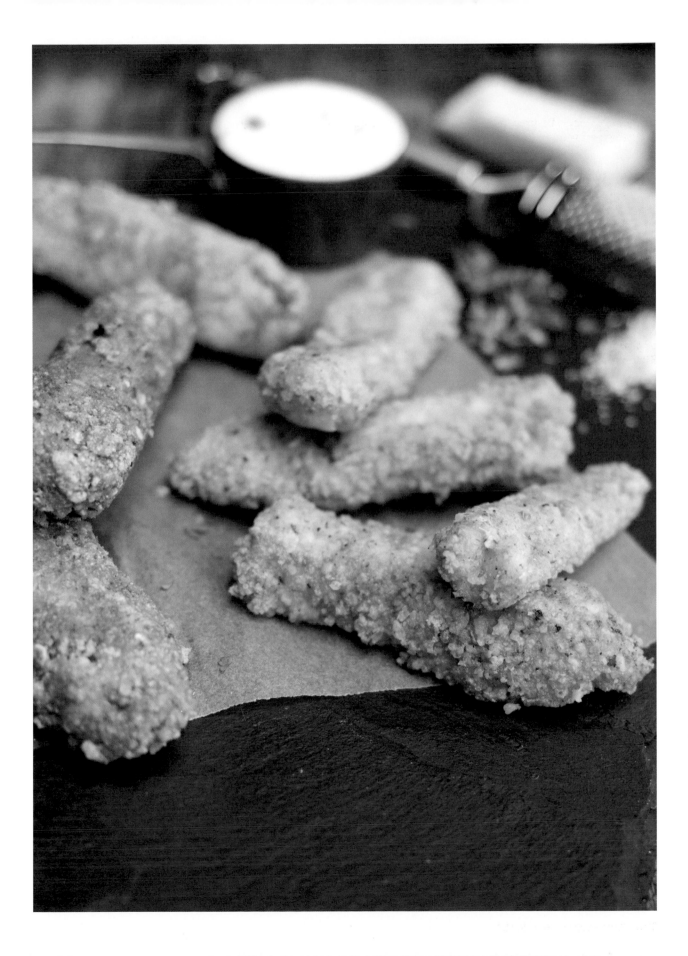

Cheeseburger Wraps with Special Sauce

 prep time: 10 minutes   cook time: 7 minutes   yield: 4 servings

My blogger and cookbook author friend Kyndra Holley posted a keto casserole based on the McDonald's Big Mac on her blog. I was inspired to make my own version for this book since the Big Mac is so popular around the world! These wraps are so amazing, you will never miss the bun.

—special sauce

½ cup baconnaise or mayonnaise, homemade (page 357) or store-bought

¼ cup chopped dill pickles

3 tablespoons tomato sauce

2 tablespoons Swerve confectioners'-style sweetener or equivalent amount of liquid or powdered sweetener (see page 31)

⅛ teaspoon fine sea salt

⅛ teaspoon fish sauce (optional, for umami taste)

—filling

2 teaspoons ghee or coconut oil

2 tablespoons minced onions

1 clove garlic, smashed to a paste or minced

1 pound ground beef

1 teaspoon fine sea salt

¼ teaspoon ground black pepper

1 cup shredded cheddar cheese

Toasted sesame seeds, for garnish

Boston leaf lettuce, for serving

Sliced dill pickles, for garnish

Cherry tomatoes, halved

1. Make the sauce: Combine the baconnaise, pickles, tomato sauce, sweetener, salt, and fish sauce, if using, in a pint-sized jar. Shake well.

2. Make the filling: Heat the ghee in a large cast-iron skillet over medium heat. Add the onions and sauté for 1 minute, or until slightly softened. Add the garlic and sauté for another minute, until fragrant. Add the ground beef, salt, and pepper and sauté, breaking up the ground beef with a spatula, for 4 minutes, or until browned and cooked through. Top the beef mixture with the cheese. Reduce the heat to low and cover the skillet until the cheese melts. Remove from the heat and garnish with toasted sesame seeds.

3. Serve with lettuce for wraps, along with pickles and cherry tomatoes. Drizzle the filling with the sauce. Store leftover filling and sauce in separate airtight containers in the refrigerator for up to 4 days. To reheat the filling, place in a lightly greased skillet over medium heat for about 3 minutes.

busy family tip: *The sauce can be made up to 2 weeks ahead and stored in the refrigerator.*

NUTRITIONAL INFO (per serving)				
calories	fat	protein	carbs	fiber
633	57g	27g	3g	0.3g

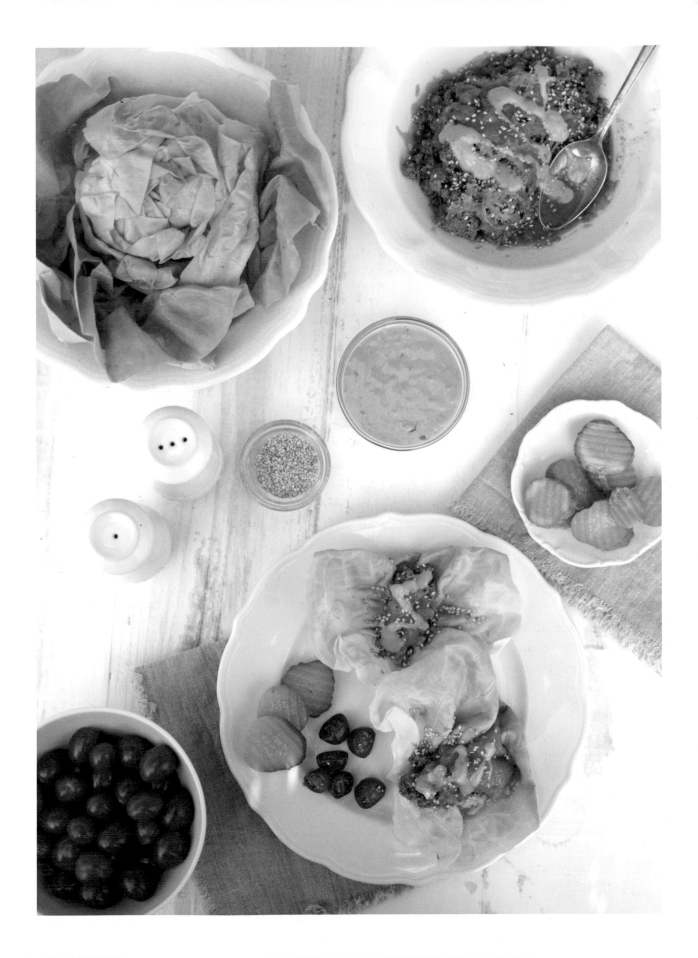

Bacon Cheeseburger Pizza

$\left(\begin{smallmatrix} & M & \\ L & \curvearrowright & H \\ & KETO & \end{smallmatrix}\right)$ **prep time:** 5 minutes (not including time to make dough)   **cook time:** 15 minutes
yield: 4 servings

2 strips bacon, diced

1 batch pizza dough from Craig's Special Pizza (page 182)

4 ounces ground beef

¼ teaspoon fine sea salt

¼ teaspoon ground black pepper

⅔ cup tomato sauce

2 tablespoons Swerve confectioners'-style sweetener or equivalent amount of liquid or powdered sweetener (see page 31)

2 tablespoons prepared yellow mustard

½ cup shredded mozzarella cheese (about 2 ounces)

½ cup shredded sharp cheddar cheese (about 2 ounces)

¼ cup chopped onions (about 1 small)

—for garnish

¼ cup sliced dill pickles (aka hamburger dill chips)

¼ cup shredded lettuce

1 small tomato or ½ cup cherry tomatoes, sliced

¼ red onion, sliced

Sesame seeds

1. Place a pizza stone in the oven and preheat the oven to 425°F. (You can use a baking sheet, but a pizza stone will bake the bottom better.) Grease a piece of parchment paper.

2. Place the bacon on a rimmed baking sheet and bake for 7 minutes (it may not be fully cooked at this point, but it will crisp up when you bake the pizza).

3. Place the pizza dough on the greased parchment. Use your hands to pat the dough into a large circle (about 10 inches in diameter). Slide the pizza on the parchment onto the hot pizza stone and set aside.

4. Heat a large cast-iron skillet over medium heat. Place the ground beef in the skillet, season with the salt and pepper, and cook, breaking up the meat with a spatula, until it is browned and cooked through, about 5 minutes. Set aside.

5. In a small bowl, combine the tomato sauce, sweetener, and mustard; spread the mixture over the pizza crust. Sprinkle the cheeses over the tomato sauce mixture and top with the ground beef, onions, and bacon.

6. Bake the pizza for about 10 minutes, until the cheeses are melted. Remove from the oven and garnish with the pickles, lettuce, tomato slices, onion slices, and sesame seeds. Store in an airtight container in the refrigerator for up to 4 days. To reheat, place on a rimmed baking sheet in a preheated 400°F oven or toaster oven for about 5 minutes.

NUTRITIONAL INFO (per serving)				
calories	fat	protein	carbs	fiber
457	36g	27g	10g	3g

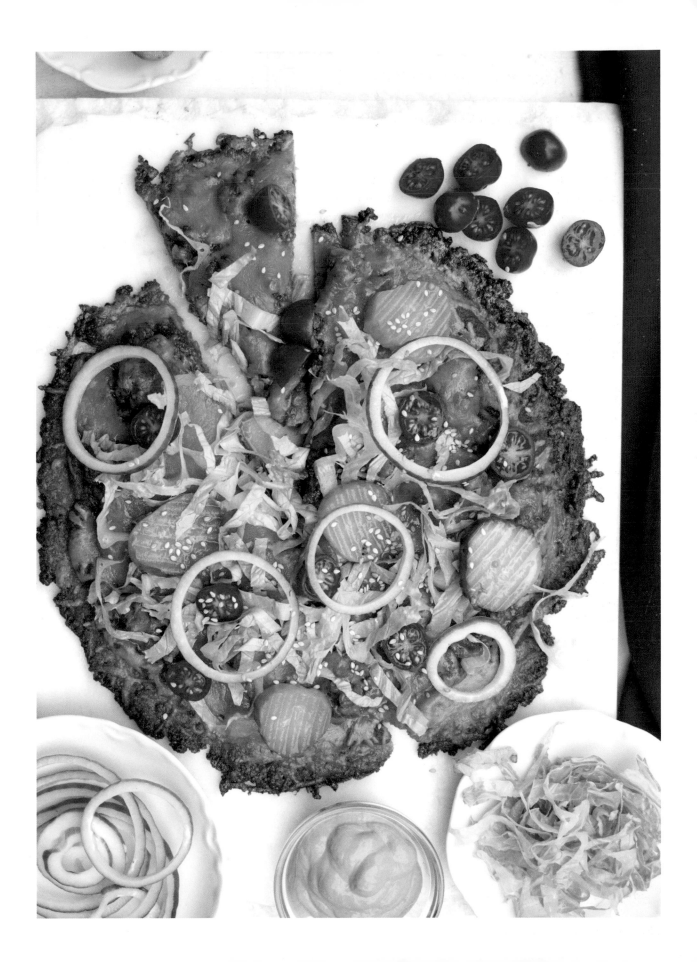

Keto Fries with Aioli

(LM→H KETO) (OPTION) **prep time:** 8 minutes **cook time:** 13 minutes **yield:** 8 servings

Outback Steakhouse serves fries with aioli; this is my delicious keto version!

3 large zucchini (about 2 pounds)

1 large egg

½ cup powdered Parmesan cheese (see page 363)

—aioli

1 cup mayonnaise, homemade (page 357) or store-bought

½ head roasted garlic (page 359), or 3 cloves raw garlic, smashed to a paste

2 teaspoons chopped fresh rosemary leaves

2 teaspoons chopped fresh thyme leaves

½ teaspoon fine sea salt

A few drops of hot sauce (optional)

Chopped fresh cilantro, thyme, or rosemary, for garnish

1. Preheat the oven to 450°F. Line 2 rimmed baking sheets with parchment paper. Grease the parchment with coconut oil spray and set aside.

2. Cut the zucchini into strips about ½ inch wide by 4 inches long.

3. Whisk the egg in a large bowl. Place the zucchini in the bowl and mix well with your hands, lightly coating all sides of the zucchini.

4. Place the powdered Parmesan in a large zip-top bag. Place half of the zucchini in the bag. Seal the bag with some air inside and shake well to coat the zucchini. Spread the zucchini fries on one of the baking sheets, not touching; repeat with the remaining zucchini. Bake the fries for 13 to 15 minutes, until golden brown.

5. Meanwhile, make the aioli: Place the mayonnaise, garlic, rosemary, thyme, salt, and hot sauce, if using, in a small bowl and whisk until smooth.

6. Remove the fries from the oven and garnish with cilantro. Serve with the aioli. The fries are best served fresh, but extras can be stored in an airtight container in the refrigerator for up to 4 days; the aioli can be stored in a separate airtight container in the fridge for up to 5 days. To reheat the fries, place on a rimmed baking sheet in a preheated 400°F oven or toaster oven for about 5 minutes.

busy family tip: *The aioli can be made up to 5 days ahead and stored in the refrigerator.*

NUTRITIONAL INFO (per serving)				
calories	fat	protein	carbs	fiber
228	22g	4g	3g	1g

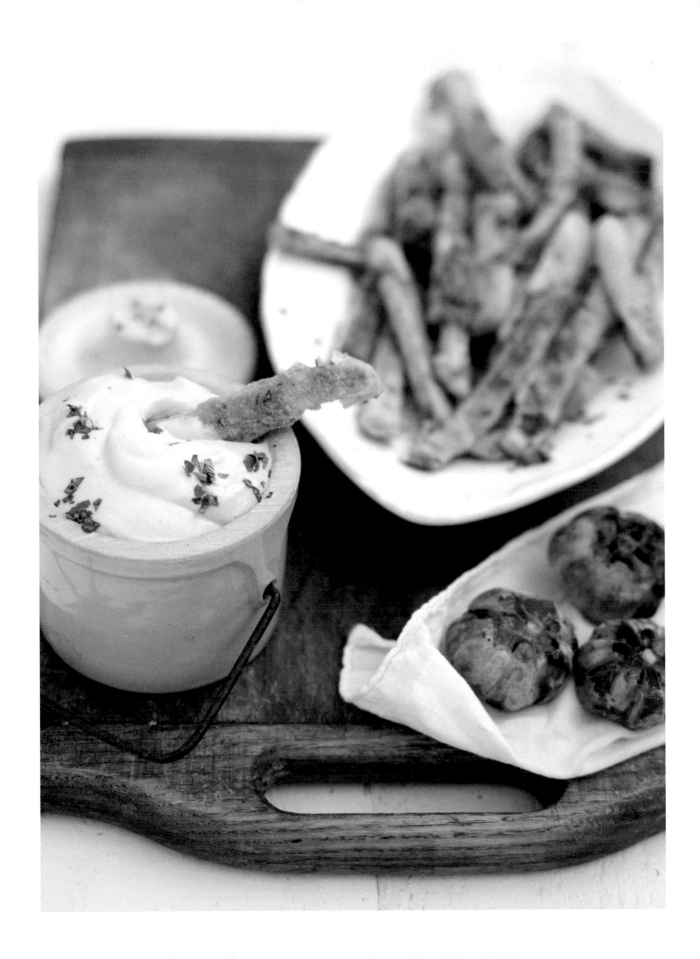

Waffle Fries with Cheese Sauce

(L M H KETO 🔪) **prep time:** 8 minutes **cook time:** 12 minutes **yield:** 4 servings

—waffle fries

3 cups shredded zucchini (about 2 medium)

1 teaspoon fine sea salt

1 cup powdered Parmesan cheese (see page 363)

2 tablespoons unsalted butter or coconut oil, melted but not hot

2 large eggs

—cheese sauce

¼ cup (½ stick) unsalted butter

1½ ounces cream cheese

¼ cup beef or chicken bone broth, homemade (page 356) or store-bought

1 cup shredded sharp cheddar cheese (about 4 ounces)

¼ cup grated Parmesan cheese (about 1 ounce)

Fine sea salt and ground black pepper

1. Heat a waffle iron to high heat.

2. Make the batter for the waffle fries: Place the shredded zucchini in a colander in the sink and sprinkle with the salt. Allow to drain for 4 minutes, then squeeze out any excess moisture. Place the zucchini in a medium-sized bowl. Add the powdered Parmesan, melted butter, and eggs. Mix well.

3. Cook the waffle fries: Grease the hot waffle iron with coconut oil spray. Place 3 tablespoons of the zucchini mixture in the center of the iron and close the top. Cook for 3 to 4 minutes, until the waffle is golden brown and crisp. Remove from the waffle iron, set in a warm oven to keep warm, and repeat with the remaining batter, making a total of 8 waffle fries.

4. Make the cheese sauce: Melt the butter in a medium-sized saucepan over medium heat. Stir in the cream cheese and broth. Cook, stirring, for 2 minutes, or until the sauce has thickened a bit. Reduce the heat to low and add the cheddar and Parmesan cheeses, stirring until the cheeses have melted. Season with salt and pepper to taste. Remove from the heat, pour over the waffle fries, and serve. These are best served fresh.

NUTRITIONAL INFO (per serving)				
calories	fat	protein	carbs	fiber
457	38g	22g	6g	1g

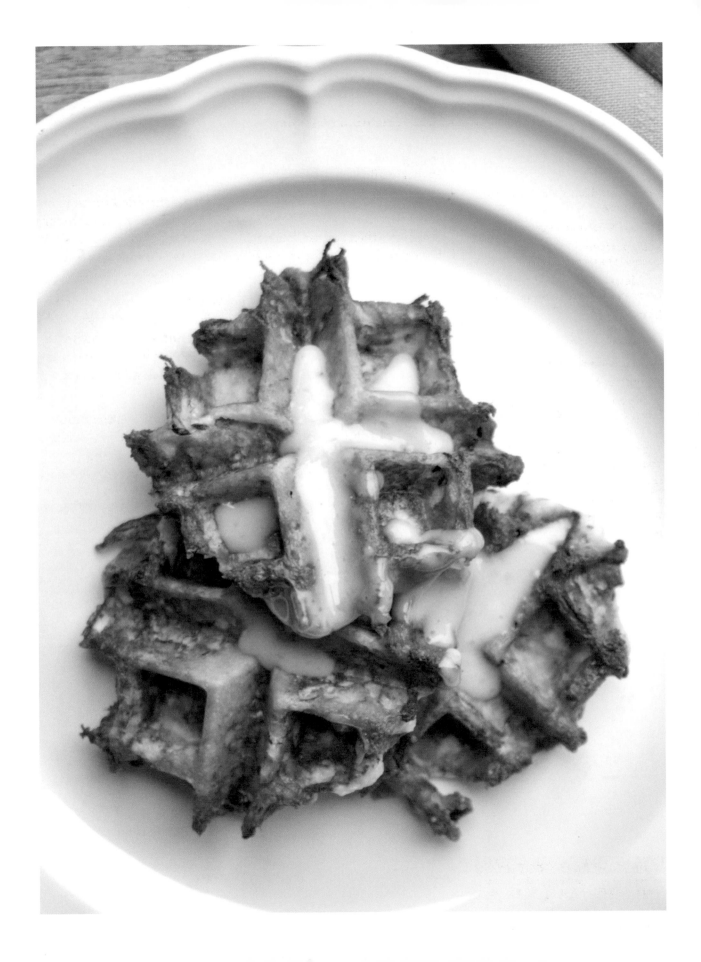

Poutine

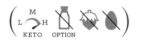

prep time: 10 minutes   cook time: 27 minutes   yield: 4 servings

Poutine is a diner classic in Canada. It usually consists of a basket of french fries topped with cheese curds and gravy. Here I've used cauliflower stems for the fries! You can use the other parts of the head of cauliflower as well if you like, but if you do, it won't look like french fries.

2 heads cauliflower

4 tablespoons (½ stick) melted butter, duck fat, leaf lard, or avocado oil, divided

Fine sea salt and ground black pepper

2 slices bacon, finely diced

½ cup thinly sliced onions

1 cup beef bone broth, homemade (page 356) or store-bought

1 cup cheese curds or cubed fontina or other melty cheese (omit for dairy-free)

Thinly sliced fresh chives, for garnish (optional)

Finely chopped fresh parsley, for garnish (optional)

1. To make the fries, preheat the oven to 425°F. Grease a rimmed baking sheet.

2. Cut the stems out of the cauliflower. Cut the stems into french fry shapes, about 2½ inches long by ¼ inch wide. Place on the greased baking sheet. Coat the "fries" with 1 tablespoon of the melted butter and sprinkle with salt and pepper. Bake for 25 minutes or until golden brown.

3. Meanwhile, make the gravy: Fry the bacon in a medium-sized cast-iron skillet over medium heat until crisp, about 5 minutes. Remove the bacon with a slotted spoon and set aside, leaving the fat in the skillet. Add the remaining 3 tablespoons of butter and the onions and sauté, stirring often, until the onions are just starting to cara-melize, 10 to 15 minutes. Add the broth and boil until the gravy is reduced by half.

4. Remove the fries from the oven and sprinkle the cheese over them. Place the fries back in the oven until the cheese is starting to melt, about 2 minutes. Transfer to a platter. Spoon the onion gravy over the fries and top with the bacon bits. Garnish with fresh chives and/or parsley, if desired.

5. Poutine is best served fresh, but extras can be stored in an airtight container in the refrigerator for up to 3 days. To reheat, place on a baking sheet in a preheated 350°F oven for about 3 minutes.

NUTRITIONAL INFO (per serving)				
calories	fat	protein	carbs	fiber
396	34g	19g	5g	2g

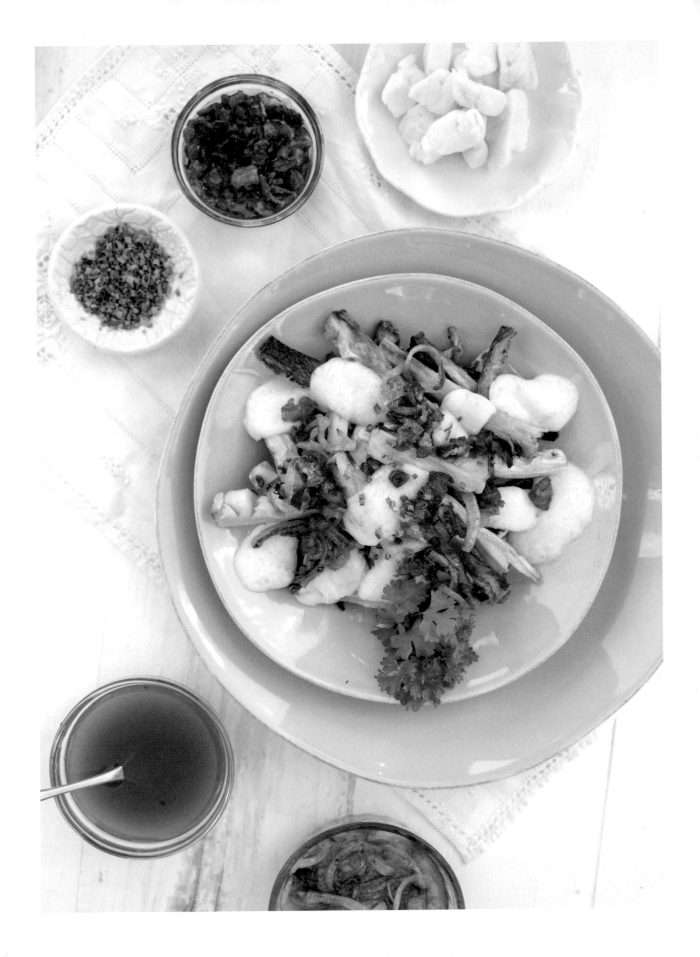

Frosted Lemonade

(L M H KETO 🚫 🚫) **prep time:** 5 minutes   **yield:** 4 servings

The chain restaurant Chick-fil-A has popularized this frosty treat, and you can find several knockoffs online. My keto version is refreshing and easy to make.

¾ cup heavy cream

½ cup lemon juice (2 to 3 lemons)

¼ cup Swerve confectioner's-style sweetener or equivalent amount of liquid or powdered sweetener (see page 31)

¼ teaspoon lemon-flavored liquid stevia (optional)

1 cup crushed ice

2 lemon slices, cut into half-moons, for garnish (optional)

Place all the ingredients in a blender and puree until smooth. Taste and adjust the sweetness to your liking. Pour into 4 glasses and hang a lemon slice on the rim of each glass, if desired. This is best served fresh; if you wait to serve it, the ice will melt and make it too watery.

NUTRITIONAL INFO (per serving)				
calories	fat	protein	carbs	fiber
158	18g	0.1g	3g	0.1g

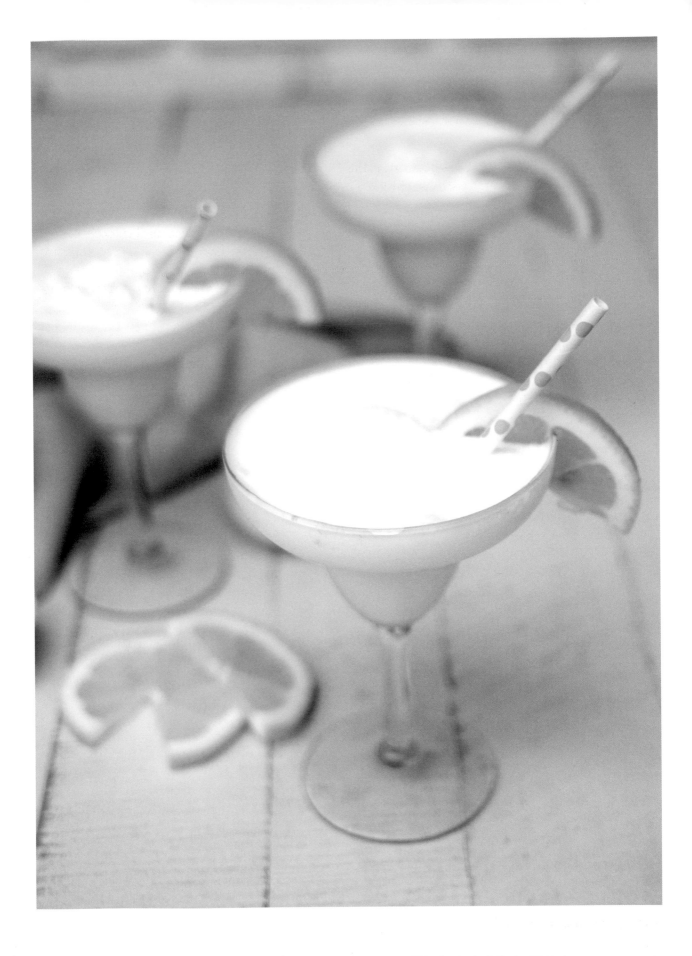

Frozen Hot Chocolate

(L —M→ H KETO   OPTION   OPTION)   **prep time:** 5 minutes   **cook time:** 2 minutes   **yield:** 4 servings

One of my favorite movies to watch during the holiday season is *Serendipity*, a cute romantic comedy about how life is serendipitous. I love watching the main characters, Jonathan and Sara, gallivant around New York City at Christmastime as they start to fall in love. At one point, they stop at the restaurant Serendipity for frozen hot chocolate. I often dream of owning a cute place like Serendipity where I would sell "healthified" desserts! Someday I hope to take my boys to New York during the holidays to see all the magic. But in the meantime, we can enjoy a little magic at home in the form of this tasty drink.

1 ounce unsweetened chocolate, finely chopped

2 tablespoons unsalted butter or coconut oil

¼ cup Swerve confectioners'-style sweetener or equivalent amount of liquid or powdered sweetener (see page 31)

2 teaspoons unsweetened cocoa powder

Seeds scraped from 1 vanilla bean (about 8 inches long), or 1 teaspoon vanilla extract

¼ teaspoon almond extract (omit for nut-free)

1½ cups unsweetened cashew milk, heavy cream, or full-fat coconut milk, divided

3 cups crushed ice

—for garnish

Sweetened whipped cream (see tip) (omit for dairy-free)

Shaved unsweetened baking chocolate or unsweetened cocoa powder

Avocado oil or extra-virgin olive oil, for drizzling

1. Melt the chocolate and butter in a small heavy-bottomed saucepan over medium heat, stirring constantly, or in a double boiler over simmering water, stirring occasionally. Add the sweetener and cocoa powder and heat, stirring constantly, until the cocoa powder is dissolved and blended into the chocolate.

2. Remove the pan from the heat. Add the vanilla bean seeds, almond extract (if using), and ½ cup of the milk and stir until smooth. Let cool to room temperature.

3. Place the remaining 1 cup of milk, the cooled chocolate mixture, and the ice in a blender and blend on high speed until the mixture is smooth and has a slushy consistency. Pour into 4 large goblets. Top with whipped cream (if using), a sprinkle of shaved chocolate or a dusting of cocoa powder, and a drizzle of oil. This is best served fresh; if you wait too long to serve it, the ice will melt and make it too watery.

tip: *I keep heavy cream in a whipped cream canister in my fridge at all times for easy additions to treats like this. I put 2 cups of cream and 2 tablespoons of powdered sweetener or ¼ teaspoon of liquid stevia in the canister and shake well to combine. Then it's presweetened and ready to go whenever I need it! If you don't have a whipped cream canister, a bowl and a hand mixer work just as well. For best results, use a chilled metal bowl and chilled beaters. Heavy cream roughly doubles in size when whipped, so for ½ cup of whipped cream, you'll need ¼ cup of heavy cream.*

NUTRITIONAL INFO (per serving)				
calories	fat	protein	carbs	fiber
115	10g	2g	3g	2g

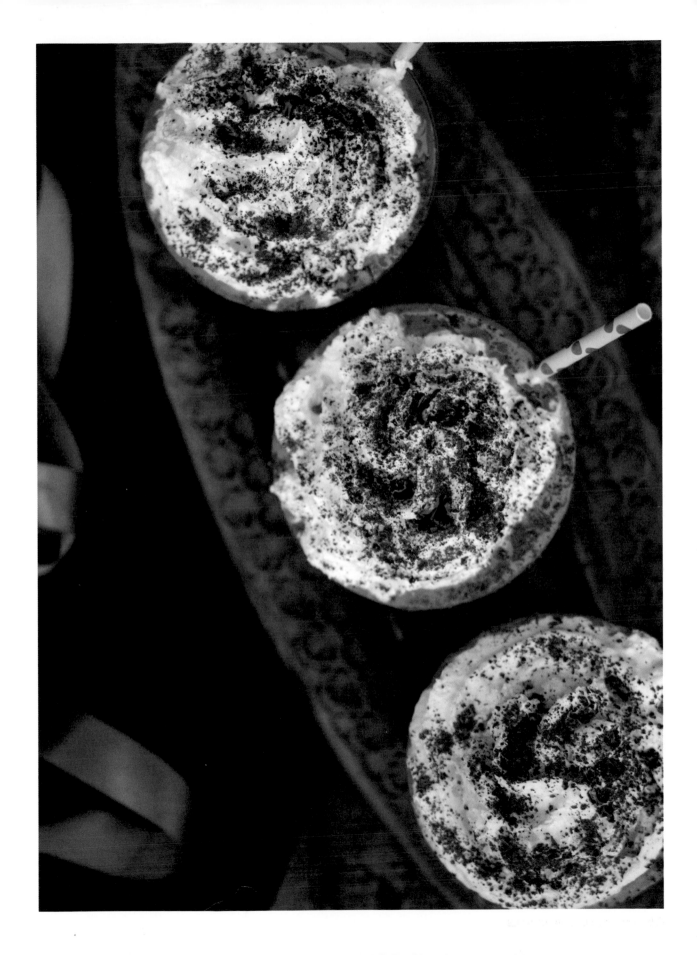

The Thickest Chocolate Shake Ever

(L M H KETO   OPTION   OPTION)   **prep time:** 8 minutes   **yield:** 4 servings

This recipe is inspired by Wendy's Frostys. You know the ones—they're so thick and creamy that you need a spoon to eat them. My keto version won't disappoint! Using a high-powered blender creates an ultra-smooth and thick texture.

1 cup heavy cream (or coconut cream if dairy-sensitive)

2 cups crushed ice

1 cup unsweetened cashew milk (or hemp milk if nut-free)

⅓ cup unsweetened cocoa powder

¼ cup plus 2 tablespoons Swerve confectioners'-style sweetener or equivalent amount of liquid or powdered sweetener (see page 31) or almond-flavored liquid stevia

1 teaspoon almond extract or vanilla extract

Pinch of fine sea salt

Place the cream in a blender and puree until it thickens and doubles in size. Add the ice, milk, cocoa powder, sweetener, extract, and salt and puree until smooth. Taste and adjust the sweetness to your liking. Pour into 4 glasses and serve. Store in an airtight container in the freezer for up to 1 month. Allow to thaw for a few minutes before enjoying.

variation: vanilla shake. *Use vanilla extract instead of almond extract and omit the cocoa powder.*

NUTRITIONAL INFO (per serving)				
calories	fat	protein	carbs	fiber
230	25g	2g	3g	1g

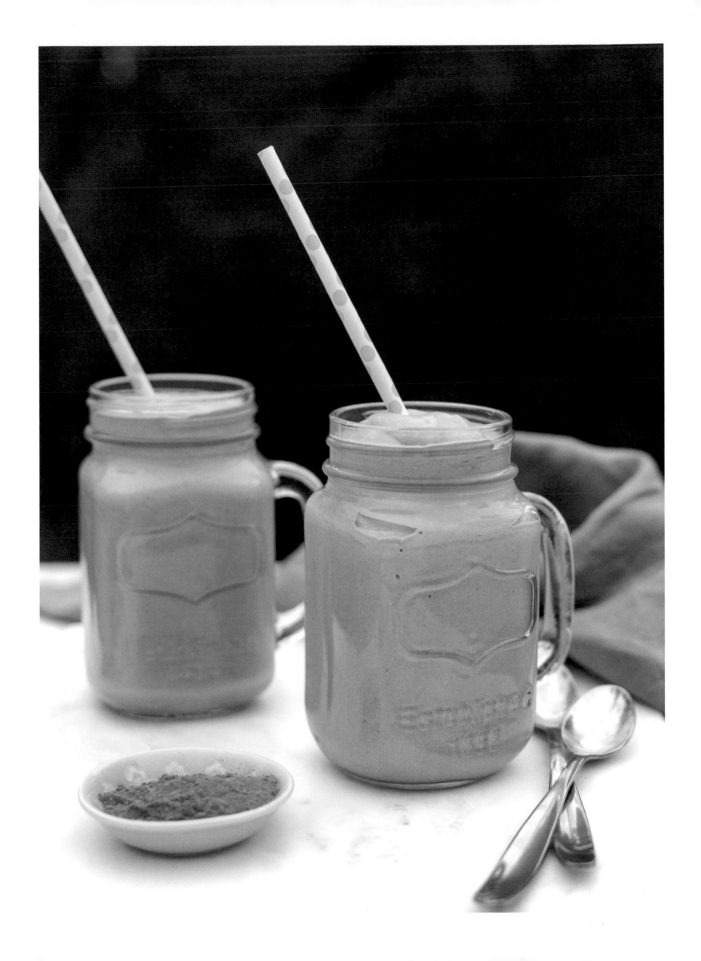

Leprechaun Shake

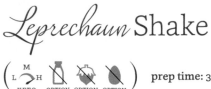

prep time: 3 minutes   **yield:** two 16-ounce servings

This recipe is inspired by the special shake that McDonald's rolls out around St. Patrick's Day: the famous Shamrock Shake. This keto version is protein-packed and good for you. The lovely green color comes from avocado rather than food dye.

When you think of sweets, salt is probably the last ingredient that comes to mind unless you once accidentally used salt in place of sugar! As contradictory as it may sound, salt truly changes a dessert, taking it from tasty to jaw-dropping. It adds complexity to the entire dish and can make your treats taste sweeter. Many famous pastry chefs say that you should double the salt in any classic dessert recipe and cut back on the sugar.

The takeaway here is that salt is a flavor enhancer. Even fast-food restaurants understand this concept: a small milkshake can have more sodium than a small order of fries!

1 cup crushed ice

¾ cup unsweetened almond milk or full-fat coconut milk

½ cup chopped avocado

¼ cup vanilla-flavored egg white or whey protein powder

¼ cup Swerve confectioners'-style sweetener or equivalent amount of liquid or powdered sweetener (see page 31)

2 tablespoons cream cheese (Kite Hill brand cream cheese style spread if dairy-sensitive), at room temperature

½ teaspoon fine sea salt

¼ teaspoon mint extract, or 1 tablespoon fresh mint leaves

¼ cup sweetened whipped cream, for topping (optional; see tip, page 336)

Place the ice, milk, avocado, protein powder, sweetener, cream cheese, ice, sweetener, salt, and mint extract in a blender and puree until smooth. Pour into 2 glasses. Top with sweetened whipped cream, if desired. Store in an airtight container in the freezer for up to 1 month. Allow to thaw for a few minutes before enjoying.

note: *You can use this same basic recipe to make any flavor of shake. Simply replace the mint extract with the flavored extract of your choice. My family loves mango!*

NUTRITIONAL INFO (per serving, made with coconut milk)				
calories	fat	protein	carbs	fiber
291	24g	14g	5g	2g

NUTRITIONAL INFO (per serving, made with almond milk)				
calories	fat	protein	carbs	fiber
167	11g	13g	4g	3g

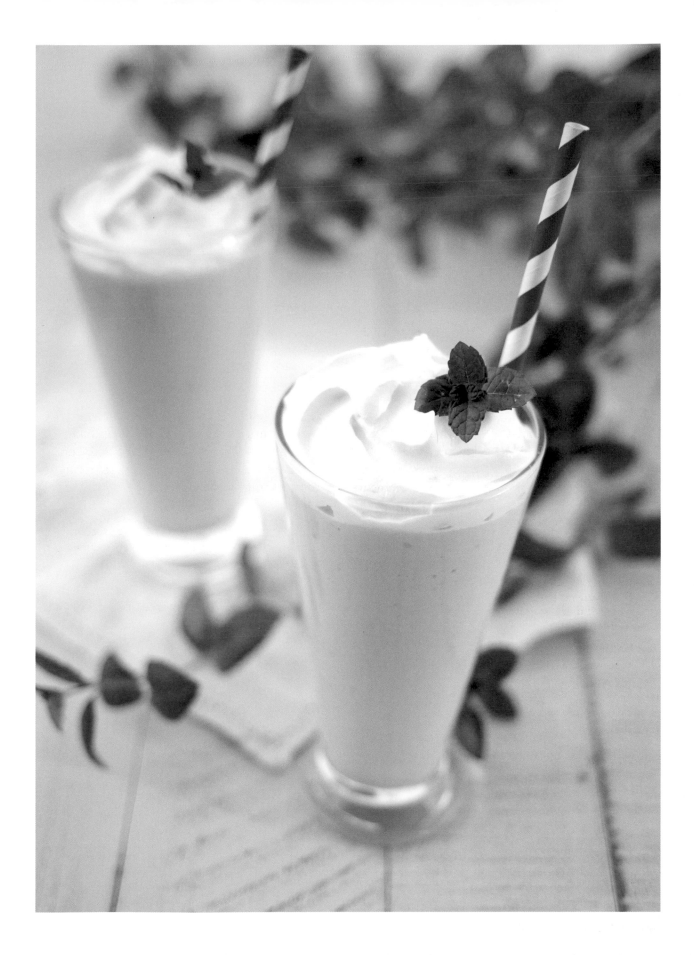

Classic Diner Malt

(L M H KETO) **prep time:** 5 minutes, plus time to churn ice cream   **yield:** 4 servings

When I was in high school, I worked at the front desk of a hotel across the parking lot from the Medford Café. I would get dinner from the café, and I always ordered the classic malt. I still love malts; I just make them keto now! The tricky part is getting that malt flavor without the barley. In this recipe, maca powder is the key to making it taste just like a classic diner malt! But skip the cherry on top. (*Note:* I always buy organic pastured eggs, so I am not fearful of consuming raw eggs. If you are concerned about making the ice cream with raw egg yolks, you can use the optional cooking method in Step 2.)

—keto vanilla ice cream

3 large egg yolks

¼ cup Swerve confectioners'-style sweetener or equivalent amount of liquid or powdered sweetener (see page 31)

½ cup heavy cream

½ cup unsweetened cashew milk or almond milk

Seeds scraped from 1 vanilla bean (about 8 inches long), or 1 teaspoon vanilla extract

⅛ teaspoon fine sea salt

—malts

1 cup unsweetened cashew milk or almond milk

¼ cup unsweetened cocoa powder (optional)

1 tablespoon maca powder, or more to taste

1 teaspoon vanilla extract

1 cup crushed ice

¼ cup Swerve confectioners'-style sweetener or equivalent amount of liquid or powdered sweetener

—for garnish (optional)

½ cup sweetened whipped cream (see tip, page 336)

Unsweetened cocoa powder

—special equipment

Ice cream maker

1. Make the ice cream: Place the egg yolks and sweetener in a large bowl. Using a hand mixer, whip the yolks until lightened in color and doubled in size. Stir in the heavy cream. If you're comfortable using raw eggs, stir in the milk, vanilla bean seeds, and salt, then skip ahead to Step 3. If you're not comfortable using raw eggs, follow Step 2 to cook the eggs.

2. To cook the custard, place the egg yolk mixture in a heavy-bottomed saucepan over medium-low heat. Cook, stirring constantly, until the custard is thickened and coats a wooden spoon. Remove from the heat and stir in the milk, vanilla bean seeds, and salt. Transfer the custard to a heatproof bowl and place the bowl in an ice bath. Let cool completely.

3. Pour the ice cream base into an ice cream maker and churn, according to the manufacturer's instructions.

4. To make the malts: Place the ice cream, milk, cocoa powder (if using), maca powder, vanilla powder, and ice in a blender and blend until smooth. Taste and add more maca powder if desired for a stronger malted milk flavor.

5. Pour into 4 malt glasses. Top each glass with a dollop of whipped cream and a dusting of cocoa powder, if desired. Serve immediately.

NUTRITIONAL INFO (per serving)				
calories	fat	protein	carbs	fiber
283	29g	4g	5g	2g

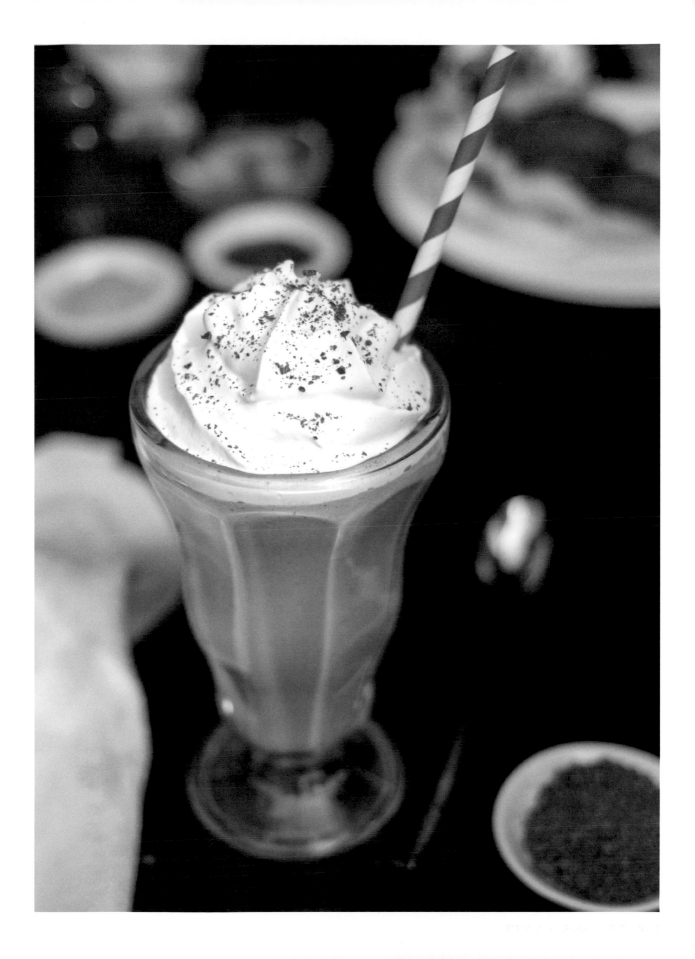

Lemon Loaf

$\left(\begin{smallmatrix} & \text{M} & \\ \text{L} & \curvearrowright & \text{H} \\ & \text{KETO} & \end{smallmatrix}\ \text{\bigg\rvert}\right)$ **prep time:** 15 minutes   **cook time:** 55 minutes   **yield:** one 9 by 5-inch loaf (16 servings)

This loaf cake is inspired by Starbucks' ever-popular iced lemon pound cake. Just like the popular coffee chain's, this loaf is a lovely afternoon indulgence with a cup of tea. But unlike theirs, my version is low-carb.

2 cups blanched almond flour

¼ cup coconut flour

1 teaspoon baking powder

1 teaspoon baking soda

1 teaspoon fine sea salt

6 large eggs

1¼ cups coconut oil, softened

1 cup Swerve confectioners'-style sweetener or equivalent amount of powdered sweetener (see page 31)

²/₃ cup lemon juice (3 to 4 lemons)

1 tablespoon lemon extract

2 teaspoons vanilla extract, or seeds scraped from 2 vanilla beans (about 8 inches long)

—lemon icing

½ cup coconut oil, melted

½ cup Swerve confectioners'-style sweetener or equivalent amount of powdered stevia or erythritol

2 tablespoons unsweetened almond milk

1 teaspoon lemon extract

1. Preheat the oven to 325°F and thoroughly grease a 9 by 5-inch loaf pan.

2. In a large bowl, whisk together the almond flour, coconut flour, baking powder, baking soda, and salt.

3. In a medium-sized bowl, beat the eggs and coconut oil until light and fluffy. Add the sweetener, lemon juice, lemon extract, and vanilla extract and combine well with a hand mixer.

4. Pour the wet ingredients into the dry ingredients and use the hand mixer to blend until smooth. Pour the batter into the greased loaf pan and cover with foil to prevent the top from burning.

5. Bake for 55 minutes or until a toothpick inserted in the center of the loaf comes out clean. Let cool completely in the pan.

6. While the loaf is cooling, make the lemon icing: Place all the icing ingredients in a blender and blend until smooth.

7. When the loaf is totally cool, remove it from the pan and top it with the icing. Place in the refrigerator for at least 1 hour for the icing to set before slicing and serving.

note: *The secret to success when baking with erythritol (either pure erythritol or erythritol-based sweeteners, such as Swerve or Organic Zero) is to cream the fat first (or the fat and eggs), then add the sweetener. In traditional baking recipes, sugar and butter are normally beaten together, and a chemical reaction between the two creates a lot of air. But because erythritol has a different chemical structure than regular sugar, in keto baking the butter (or other fat) should be beaten first until light and fluffy. Only after that point should the erythritol be added.*

NUTRITIONAL INFO (per serving)				
calories	fat	protein	carbs	fiber
319	33g	6g	4g	2g

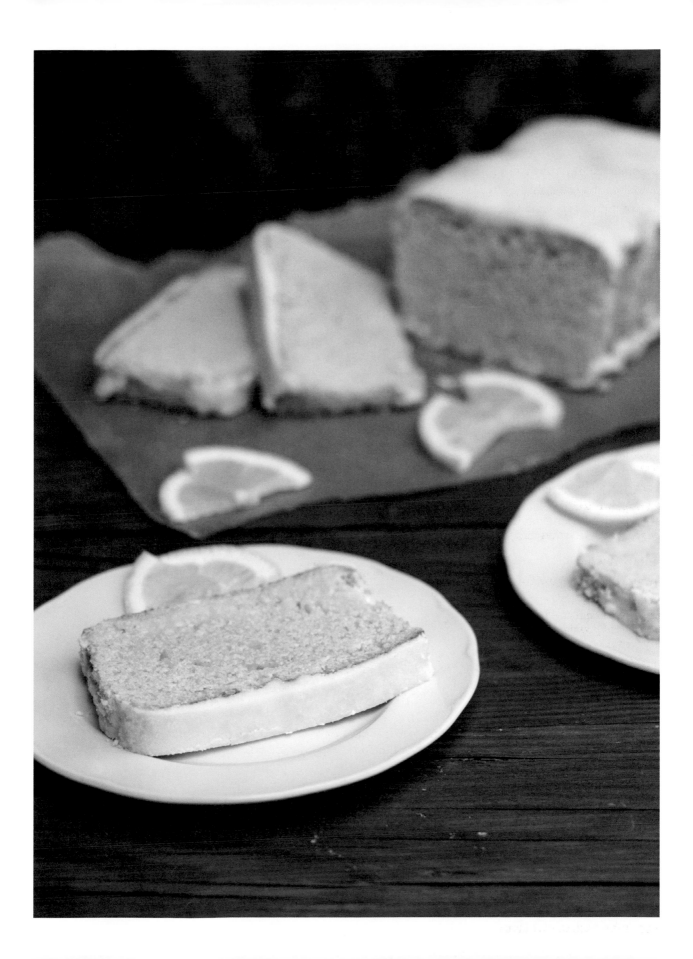

Tiramisu Cheesecake

(L $\overset{\text{M}}{\underset{\text{KETO}}{\curvearrowright}}$ H OPTION) **prep time:** 10 minutes, plus 4 hours to chill **cook time:** 1 hour 15 minutes
yield: one 8-inch cake (12 servings)

Tiramisu cheesecake is a classic at the Cheesecake Factory. This slice of heaven is sure to please! My boys are true Ethiopians; they love anything coffee-flavored. This was my son Kai's birthday cake of choice for his sixth birthday!

—ladyfinger crust

5 large egg whites

½ teaspoon cream of tartar

½ cup blanched almond flour

½ cup Swerve confectioners'-style sweetener or equivalent amount of liquid or powdered sweetener (see page 31)

¼ teaspoon fine sea salt

—espresso flavoring

1 cup brewed decaf espresso

¼ cup Swerve confectioners'-style sweetener or equivalent amount of liquid or powdered sweetener

2 teaspoons rum extract

—cream cheese filling

2 (8-ounce) packages mascarpone cheese (or Kite Hill brand cream cheese style spread if dairy-free), softened

2 (8-ounce) packages cream cheese (Kite Hill brand cream cheese style spread if dairy-free), softened

1¼ cups Swerve confectioners'-style sweetener or equivalent amount of liquid or powdered sweetener

Extra espresso flavoring (from above)

5 large egg yolks

—ganache

¾ cup heavy cream (or full-fat coconut milk if dairy-free)

⅓ cup Swerve confectioners'-style sweetener or equivalent amount of liquid or powdered sweetener

3 ounces unsweetened chocolate, finely chopped

1 teaspoon vanilla extract, or seeds scraped from 1 vanilla bean (about 8 inches long)

⅛ teaspoon fine sea salt

Unsweetened cocoa powder, for dusting

1. Preheat the oven to 325°F. Place a piece of parchment paper in an 8-inch springform pan, creasing the paper at the bottom so that it forms snugly into the pan. Grease the parchment well.

2. Make the ladyfinger crust: Place the egg whites and cream of tartar in the bowl of a stand mixer and whip until stiff peaks form. Add the almond flour, sweetener, and salt and fold into the egg whites. Spoon the dough into the prepared pan. Bake for 20 minutes or until light golden brown and cooked through.

3. Meanwhile, make the espresso flavoring: In a small bowl, stir together the espresso, sweetener, and rum extract. When the crust is done, remove it from the oven. Pour 1¼ cups of the espresso flavoring over the crust and set it aside to absorb the liquid.

4. Make the cream cheese filling: Place the mascarpone, cream cheese, and sweetener in a large bowl and, using a hand mixer, blend until smooth. Add the rest of the espresso flavoring and blend until combined. Add the egg yolks and mix until smooth. Pour the batter over the crust.

NUTRITIONAL INFO (per serving)				
calories	fat	protein	carbs	fiber
449	42g	10g	5g	2g

5. Bake the cheesecake for 55 minutes, or until the center is almost set (a water bath helps it cook evenly). If you are not using a water bath, I suggest placing a lined baking sheet under the cheesecake to catch any leaks or overflow. If you don't use a water bath, when done baking, turn off the oven and let the cheesecake cool in the oven for 5 to 6 hours; this prevents cracking. Let cool completely. Dust the top with unsweetened cocoa powder. Refrigerate for 4 hours or overnight. Gently remove the cake from the pan. Place on a platter and remove the parchment paper from the sides and bottom of the cake.

6. Make the ganache: Bring the heavy cream and sweetener to a simmer in a saucepan over medium heat. Remove from the heat and stir in the chocolate, vanilla bean seeds, and salt. Allow to sit for 3 minutes, then stir again until completely smooth. Let cool for a few minutes, then drizzle over the chilled cheesecake.

7. Store in an airtight container in the refrigerator for up to 3 days.

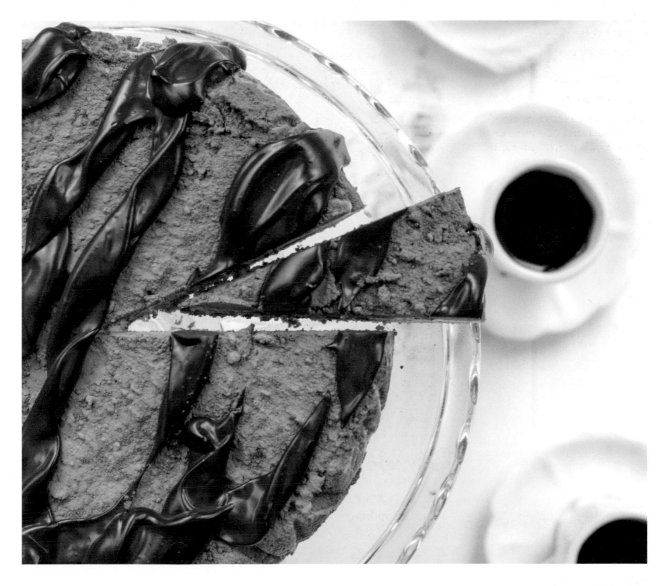

Zero-Carb Pie Crust

(L M H KETO) 🍶 🚫 **prep time:** 10 minutes, plus 1 hour to rest in the oven   **cook time:** 1 hour
yield: one 9-inch crust (12 servings)

This crust is made with meringue. It may sound odd, but it makes an excellent crust for custards and other creamy pie fillings. Please note that meringues and humidity do not mix. If your kitchen is very humid, you will not end up with a crispy crust.

3 large egg whites

¼ teaspoon cream of tartar

¾ cup Swerve confectioners'-style sweetener or equivalent amount of powdered sweetener (see page 31)

1 teaspoon vanilla extract, or a few drops of lemon oil

1. Preheat the oven to 275°F. Thoroughly grease a 9-inch pie pan with butter or coconut oil.

2. In a small bowl, use a hand mixer to beat the egg whites and cream of tartar until soft peaks form. With the mixer on low, slowly sprinkle in the sweetener until completely incorporated. Add the vanilla and continue to beat until stiff peaks form.

3. Spoon the mixture into the greased pie pan, then smooth the mixture across the bottom, up the sides, and onto the rim to form a shell. Bake for 1 hour, then turn off the oven and let the crust sit in the oven for another hour. Store in an airtight container in the refrigerator for up to 3 days before filling.

NUTRITIONAL INFO (per serving)				
calories	fat	protein	carbs	fiber
4	0g	1g	0g	0g

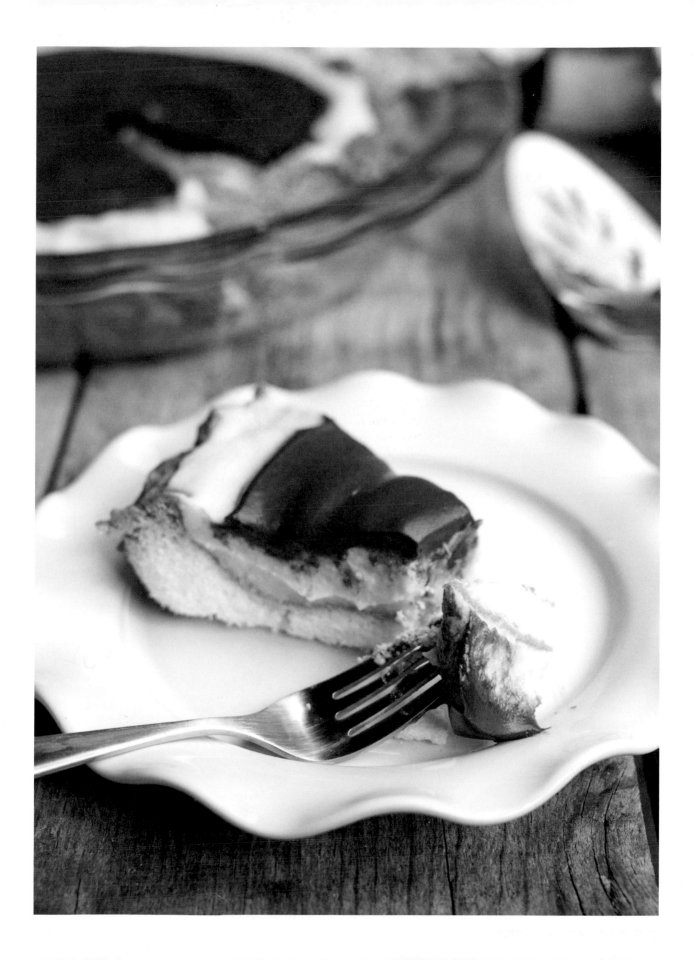

Boston Cream Pie

(L M→H KETO / OPTION / OPTION) prep time: 15 minutes, plus 15 minutes to chill (not including time to make crust)
cook time: 5 minutes   yield: one 9-inch pie (12 servings)

When I think of diner food, I always think of the amazing pies. Boston cream pie is one of my all-time favorites. The creamy custard with a chocolate topping is so decadent and lovely. This custard filling is so good, it can be eaten on its own, warm or chilled!

—custard filling

6 large egg yolks

½ cup unsweetened cashew milk (or hemp milk for nut-free)

¼ cup Swerve confectioners'-style sweetener or equivalent amount of liquid or powdered sweetener (see page 31)

¼ cup melted unsalted butter or coconut oil

Seeds scraped from 1 vanilla bean (about 8 inches long), split lengthwise, or 1 teaspoon vanilla extract

1 prebaked Zero-Carb Pie Crust (page 348)

—ganache topping

¾ cup heavy cream or full-fat coconut milk

⅓ cup Swerve confectioners'-style sweetener or equivalent amount of liquid or powdered sweetener

2 ounces unsweetened chocolate, finely chopped

Seeds scraped from 1 vanilla bean (about 8 inches long), or 1 teaspoon vanilla extract

1. Make the custard filling: Place the egg yolks, milk, and sweetener in a medium-sized heatproof bowl and whisk to blend. Whisking constantly, drizzle in the melted butter slowly so that the eggs don't cook. Set the bowl over a saucepan of simmering water and stir the custard vigorously and constantly until it coats the back of a spoon and an instant-read thermometer inserted into the mixture registers 140°F, about 3 minutes. Remove the custard from the heat and stir in the vanilla bean seeds.

2. Serve the custard warm or chilled. To cool the custard, set the bowl in a larger bowl of ice water. Pour the cooled custard into the prepared crust and place the pie in the refrigerator to chill for 15 minutes to allow the custard to set.

3. Meanwhile, make the ganache topping: Place the cream, sweetener, and chocolate in a double boiler or in a heatproof bowl set over a pan of simmering water. Heat on low, stirring, just until the chocolate melts, then remove from the heat. Add the vanilla bean seeds and stir to combine. Use immediately or let cool, then cover and refrigerate until ready to serve.

4. Remove the pie from the refrigerator and cover with the ganache. Serve immediately or set in the fridge for 10 minutes to allow the ganache to set. Store in an airtight container in the fridge for up to 3 days.

busy family tip: *All the components for this pie can be made ahead and stored in the refrigerator until the day of assembly and serving: the ganache can be made up to 4 days ahead (or 2 months ahead if frozen!), and both the custard filling and the pie crust can be made up to 3 days ahead.*

NUTRITIONAL INFO (per serving)				
calories	fat	protein	carbs	fiber
222	22g	4g	3g	2g

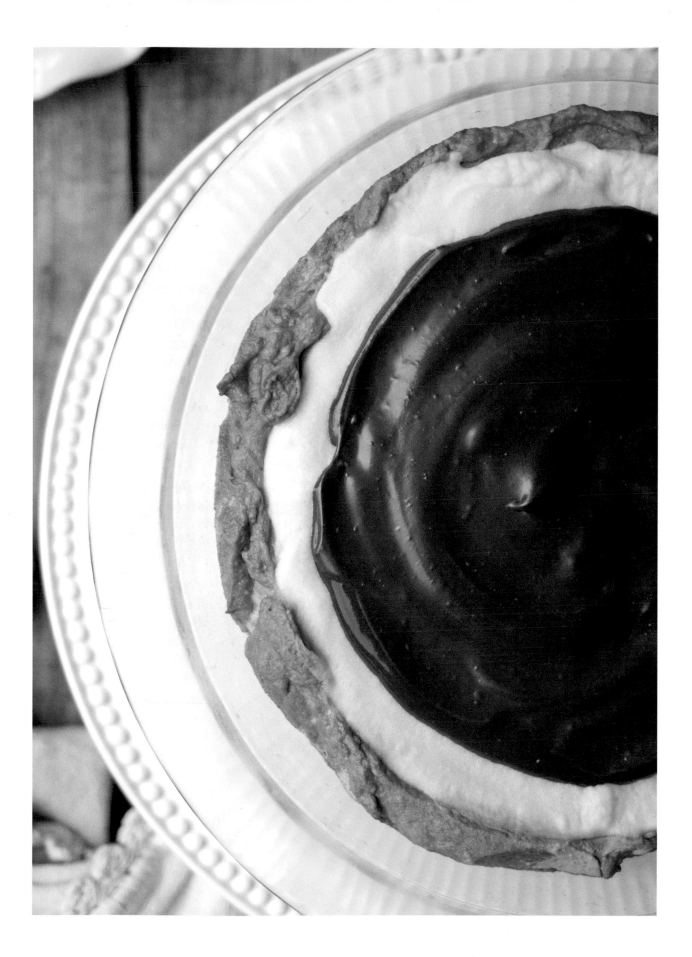

Upside-Down Lemon Meringue Pie

(L $\overset{M}{\underset{H}{\curvearrowright}}$ 🧂 🚫)   **prep time:** 10 minutes, plus 15 minutes to chill curd filling (not including time to make
KETO OPTION   crust)   **cook time:** 12 minutes   **yield:** one 9-inch pie (12 servings)

My favorite book is *A Walk in the Woods* by Bill Bryson, which probably doesn't surprise most of my readers. It is about a man who hikes the Appalachian Trail with an old college roommate who is anything but an avid hiker. Hilarity ensues, as does hunger. I can understand how camp food could get quite boring after hiking in the wilderness for weeks. In the book, Bill and his companion hitchhike to town, where they devour a delicious meal at a local diner. Their dessert is a lemon pie that Bill describes as so sweet and so bright yellow that "your eyes roll to the back of your head." Sounds like a winner to me! My version is eye-rolling good, too. But to make it keto, I've inverted it. Instead of topping the pie with meringue, as it's usually done, here the meringue goes under the pie filling, serving as a zero-carb pie crust.

—lemon curd

1 cup Swerve confectioners'-style sweetener or equivalent amount of liquid or powdered sweetener (see page 31)

4 large eggs

1 tablespoon grated lemon zest

½ cup lemon juice (about 3 lemons)

½ cup (1 stick) unsalted butter (or coconut oil if dairy-sensitive)

1 prebaked Zero-Carb Pie Crust (page 348)

Sweetened whipped cream (see tip, page 336), for garnish (omit for dairy-free)

1. Make the lemon curd: Combine the sweetener, eggs, lemon zest, and lemon juice in a medium-sized heavy saucepan and whisk to blend. Add the butter and set the pan over medium heat. Cook, whisking constantly, until the curd thickens and coats the back of a spoon (do not allow it to boil), about 12 minutes.

2. Pour the curd through a fine-mesh strainer into the prepared pie crust. Place in the refrigerator to chill completely before serving, about 15 minutes. Garnish with whipped cream, if desired, then cut into slices and serve. Store in an airtight container in the refrigerator for up to 3 days.

busy family tip: *The lemon curd and crust can be made up to 3 days ahead and stored separately in the refrigerator.*

NUTRITIONAL INFO (per serving)				
calories	fat	protein	carbs	fiber
104	10.8g	3.1g	0.4g	0g

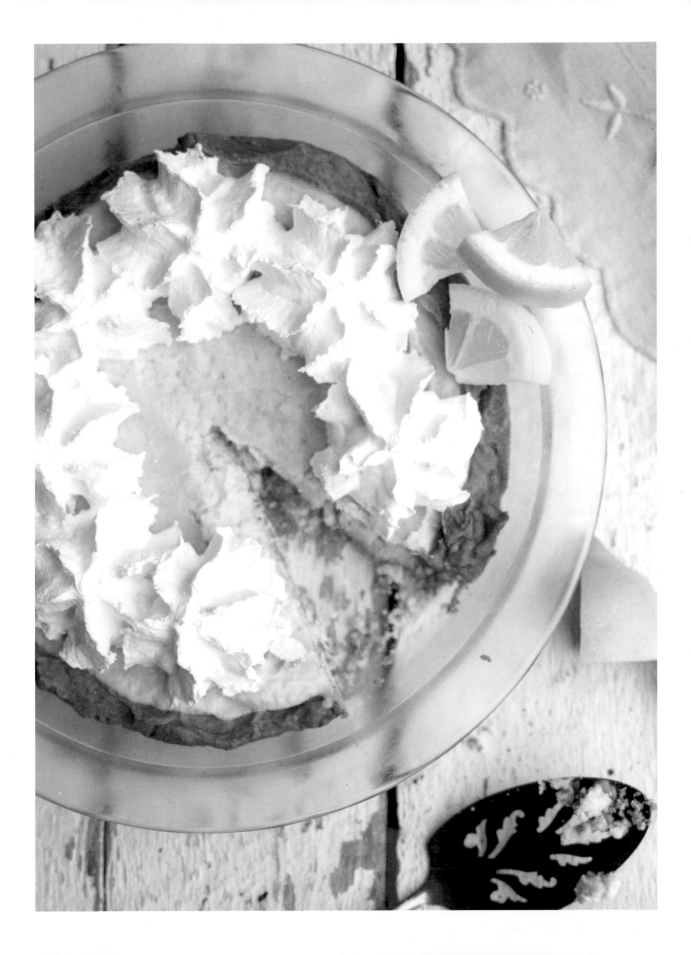

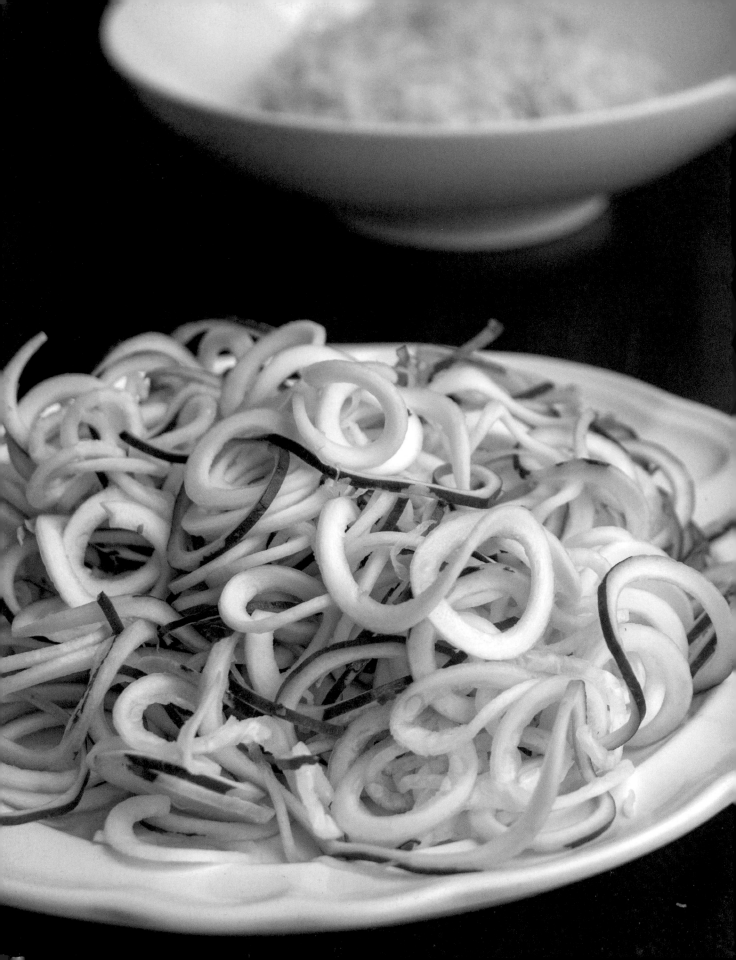

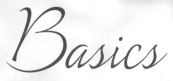

Basics

Bone Broth: Beef or Chicken

(L—M—H KETO 🥛 🥜 🌾)   prep time: 10 minutes   cook time: 1 to 3 days   yield: 4 quarts (1 cup per serving)

Nothing could be more fundamental to keto cooking or easier to make than this broth. With slight adjustments to the flavorings, it will serve you for all your cooking needs, whether you're making a bowl of ramen (page 50) or posole soup (page 212) or a plate of Chicken Piccata (page 160). You can use this broth to make soups and sauces or drink it as a nourishing beverage. Once you get all the ingredients into the slow cooker, it does all the work for you. The longer you cook the broth, the thicker and more nutritious it will become. If you roast the beef bones before making the broth, you will get a darker, more flavorful broth (see note below).

4 quarts cold water (filtered or reverse-osmosis water is best)

4 large beef bones (about 4 pounds), or leftover bones and skin from 1 pastured chicken (ideally with the feet)

1 medium onion, chopped

2 stalks celery, sliced ¼ inch thick

2 tablespoons coconut vinegar or apple cider vinegar

2 tablespoons fresh rosemary

2 teaspoons finely chopped garlic

2 teaspoons fine sea salt

1 teaspoon fresh thyme leaves, or ¾ teaspoon dried thyme leaves

1. Place the ingredients in a 6-quart slow cooker. Cover the slow cooker and set it to high, then, after 1 hour, turn it to low. Simmer the broth for a minimum of 1 day and up to 3 days. The longer it cooks, the more nutrients and minerals will be extracted from the bones.

2. Pour the broth through a strainer and discard the solids, but do not skim the fat off the top after it cools. The fat makes this broth even more ketogenic.

3. Store the broth in the refrigerator for up to 5 days or in the freezer for up to several months.

note: *For a richer, more deeply flavored beef broth, before adding the bones to the slow cooker, roast large beef bones on a rimmed baking sheet at 375°F for 50 to 60 minutes and smaller bones for 30 to 40 minutes.*

variation: bone broth for use in asian recipes. *Follow the instructions above, but replace the onion with 6 scallions, cut into thirds; add 2 teaspoons finely chopped fresh ginger; and omit the rosemary and thyme.*

busy family tip: *Make a double batch in two slow cookers and freeze the broth in freezer-safe jars to have on hand as needed.*

NUTRITIONAL INFO (per serving)				
calories	fat	protein	carbs	fiber
10	2g	0.7g	0.8g	0g

Mayonnaise

(L M H KETO / OPTION)   prep time: 5 minutes   yield: 1½ cups (about 1 tablespoon per serving)

Homemade mayonnaise is so much tastier and healthier than store-bought mayo! You can personalize this basic mayo to your taste by adding garlic paste, roasted garlic (page 359), or your favorite herb.

2 large egg yolks

2 teaspoons lemon juice

1 cup MCT oil or other neutral-flavored oil, such as macadamia nut oil or avocado oil

1 tablespoon Dijon mustard

½ teaspoon fine sea salt

—special equipment

Immersion blender

1. Put the ingredients in the order listed in a wide-mouth pint-sized jar. Place an immersion blender at the bottom of the jar. Turn the blender on and very slowly move it to the top of the jar. Be patient! It should take you about a minute to reach the top. Moving the blender slowly is the key to getting the mayonnaise to emulsify.

2. Store the mayo in a jar in the refrigerator for up to 5 days.

note: *To make this mayo nut-free, don't use a nut-based oil.*

variation: baconnaise. *Replace the MCT oil with melted, but not hot, bacon fat. Taste and add salt if needed (it may be salty enough from the bacon fat).*

NUTRITIONAL INFO (per serving)				
calories	fat	protein	carbs	fiber
92	10g	0.3g	0.1g	0g

Dairy-Free Ranch Dressing

prep time: 3 minutes, plus 2 hours to chill

yield: 1¾ cups (2½ scant tablespoons per serving)

Ranch is the new ketchup at fast-casual restaurants. Yes, you can use this to dress a salad, but you can also dunk fries into it, dip chicken nuggets or wings into it, or smother a hamburger with it!

1 cup mayonnaise, homemade (page 357) or store-bought

¾ cup chicken or beef bone broth, store-bought or homemade (page 356) (or vegetable broth for vegetarian)

½ teaspoon dried chives

½ teaspoon dried dill weed

½ teaspoon dried parsley

¼ teaspoon garlic powder

¼ teaspoon onion powder

⅛ teaspoon fine sea salt

⅛ teaspoon ground black pepper

Place the ingredients a 16-ounce (or larger) jar and shake vigorously until well combined. Cover and refrigerate for 2 hours before serving (it will thicken up as it rests). Store in the refrigerator for up to 5 days.

NUTRITIONAL INFO (per serving)				
calories	fat	protein	carbs	fiber
145	16g	0.3g	0.5g	0.2g

Roasted Garlic

$\left(\begin{smallmatrix} & M & \\ L & \curvearrowright & H \\ & KETO & \end{smallmatrix}\right.$ 🥛 🥜 🥑 $\left.\right)$ **prep time:** 5 minutes   **cook time:** about 35 minutes   **yield:** 12 heads

Roasted garlic can be used in any recipe that calls for raw garlic; it adds a rich but mellow garlic flavor. As garlic roasts, it caramelizes and develops a sweet flavor and silky-smooth texture. To use it, simply squeeze the roasted garlic out of the cloves—no need to chop or mince it. To substitute roasted garlic for raw, use about half a head of roasted garlic for every two cloves of raw garlic. I love to use it in Guacamole (page 198), in Parmesan Garlic Sauce (page 298), and whenever I want to add garlic flavor to a dish without the pungent bite of raw garlic.

12 heads garlic

¼ cup avocado oil

½ teaspoon fine sea salt

1. Preheat the oven to 350°F.

2. Slice ⅛ inch off the top of the heads of garlic to expose the cloves and place the heads in a baking dish. Pour the oil over the tops of the heads, letting it sink down into the cloves, then sprinkle the tops with the salt. Cover the baking dish with parchment paper, then a layer of foil, and tightly crimp the edges all around to seal.

3. Roast the garlic for 25 to 35 minutes. It is done when a center clove is completely soft when pierced with a paring knife. Even after it's soft, you can continue roasting the garlic until it is deeply golden for a more caramelized flavor—check it every 10 minutes. The exact roasting time will depend on the size of your heads of garlic, the variety, and their age.

4. Allow the garlic to cool, then squeeze the cloves from the skins as needed. Store unused roasted garlic in the skins in an airtight container in the refrigerator for up to 3 days or in the freezer for up to 3 months.

busy family tip: *I keep roasted garlic in my freezer at all times for easy use in recipes.*

NUTRITIONAL INFO (per clove)				
calories	fat	protein	carbs	fiber
263	5g	9g	45g	3g

Zoodles—Two Ways

(L $\overset{M}{\underset{KETO}{\frown}}$ H ⬜ 🚫 ◗)   prep time: 5 minutes (plus 5 minutes to drain if making salted, raw noodles)
cook time: 20 minutes (if making baked noodles)   yield: 4 servings (1 cup per serving)

Noodles can be part of a ketogenic lifestyle if they are made from zucchini or other low-carb vegetables. Zucchini noodles, in particular, are neutral enough to be used with just about any type of cuisine. That is why you'll find them throughout this book: they're an equally good choice for Pad Thai as they are for a creamy Alfredo sauce.

One of the tricks to making zoodles is to use zucchini that are no larger than 12 inches long and 2 inches wide. The seeds in a larger zucchini can make a mess of your spiral slicer. The other trick is to remove some of the water from the zoodles so that your sauce doesn't become a watery mess when tossed with the zoodles. The two easiest ways to remove the excess water are to salt and drain the raw zoodles (salt draws out water) or to bake them in a low-temperature oven (essentially dehydrating them). If you are a visual learner like me and would like to see how zoodles are made, check out the video on my site, MariaMindBodyHealth.com (type the word *video* in the search field).

To increase the ketogenic level to high, toss the zoodles with melted butter or a keto sauce.

2 large zucchini, not more than 12 inches long

1 tablespoon fine sea salt (if making salted and drained zoodles)

—special equipment

Spiral slicer

busy family tip: *To enjoy zoodles throughout the week, prepare a double or triple batch of raw zoodles by completing Steps 2 and 3 above. Store the raw zoodles in an airtight container in the refrigerator for up to 5 days. Following Step 4 above, bake or salt and drain the amount of zoodles you need just before serving them.*

1. If making baked zoodles, preheat the oven to 250°F. Place a paper towel on a rimmed baking sheet.

2. To prepare the zucchini for either method: Cut the ends off the zucchini to create nice, even edges. If you desire white zoodles, peel the zucchini.

3. Using a spiral slicer, swirl the zucchini into long, thin noodle-like shapes by gently pressing down on the handle while turning it clockwise.

4. To make baked zoodles: Spread out the zucchini noodles on the paper towel–lined baking sheet and bake for 20 minutes. Serve immediately.

5. To make salted and drained zoodles: Place the raw zucchini noodles in a colander over the sink and sprinkle with the salt. Allow to sit for 5 minutes, then press to squeeze out the excess water. Serve immediately.

6. Store leftover zoodles, unsauced, in an airtight container in the refrigerator for up to 5 days. Wait to sauce salted and drained or baked zoodles until ready to serve. (Once sauced, the noodles get a little soggy when stored.) Freezing is not recommended; frozen zoodles tend to get soggy.

NUTRITIONAL INFO (per serving)				
calories	fat	protein	carbs	fiber
16	0.2g	1g	3g	1g

Cabbage Pasta

(L M H KETO   OPTION)   **prep time:** 10 minutes   **cook time:** 15 minutes
yield: 4 servings (¾ cup per serving)

I prefer cabbage pasta over zoodles. One of the reasons is that cabbage pasta does not get soggy when sauced. It also can be stored with the sauce; not only will it hold up well, but it also grabs onto flavors and tastes even better as leftovers!

4 tablespoons (½ stick) unsalted butter or coconut oil

4 cups very thinly sliced green cabbage (about 1 small head)

Melt the butter in a large sauté pan over medium heat. Add the cabbage and sauté until the cabbage is very tender, about 15 minutes, stirring often so it doesn't burn. Store leftover pasta, unsauced, in an airtight container in the refrigerator for up to 5 days.

NUTRITIONAL INFO (per serving)				
calories	fat	protein	carbs	fiber
117	11g	1g	4g	2g

Keto Bread

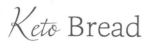

prep time: 10 minutes   cook time: 45 minutes
yield: one 9 by 5-inch loaf (14 slices, 2 slices per serving)

Keto Bread is handy for so many things. In this book, it is used in my recipes for Fried Ice Cream (page 237) and Juicy Lucy (page 312); you also can use it for Garlic Bread (page 134) if you prefer to stick to a lower-carb bread.

6 large eggs

1 teaspoon cream of tartar

¼ cup unflavored egg white protein powder (or ½ cup unflavored whey protein powder if not dairy-sensitive)

1. Preheat the oven to 325°F. Grease a 9 by 5-inch loaf pan.

2. Separate the eggs, placing the whites in a medium-sized bowl and the yolks in a small bowl. Whip the egg whites with the cream of tartar until very stiff peaks form, about 4 minutes. Slowly fold in the protein powder until just combined. In a small bowl, lightly beat the egg yolks. Then gently fold the yolks into the whipped whites (making sure the whites don't deflate).

3. Fill the prepared pan with the "dough." Bake for 40 to 45 minutes, until golden brown. Let cool completely in the pan before cutting or the bread will fall. Cut into 14 slices. Store in an airtight container in the refrigerator for up to 5 days or in the freezer for up to 2 months.

variation: keto buns. *To make buns instead of a loaf, line two baking sheets with parchment paper and grease the paper. To form hamburger buns, use a spatula to gently scoop up about ⅓ cup of the dough and place it on one of the prepared baking sheets. Using a spatula, form it into a round bun, about 3½ inches in diameter. Repeat with the rest of the dough, placing 7 buns on each baking sheet. Bake the buns for 15 to 20 minutes, until golden brown. Let cool completely on the baking sheets before removing or cutting. Store in an airtight container in the refrigerator for up to 5 days or in the freezer for up to 2 months. Makes about 14 buns.*

NUTRITIONAL INFO (per serving)				
calories	fat	protein	carbs	fiber
77	4g	8g	1g	0g

How to Rice Cauliflower

Cauliflower rice is a godsend to the low-carb lifestyle. Unlike conventional rice, it requires an additional preliminary step: before you can make cauliflower rice, you have to "rice" the cauliflower. Luckily, this task does not take long to do—all of about 5 minutes. Food manufacturers have caught on to cauliflower rice's rising popularity and have begun to offer pre-"riced" cauliflower in the frozen food and fresh produce sections of grocery stores. This is another option, which will save you a few minutes of prep time.

To rice cauliflower, place small florets, about 1 inch in size, in a food processor. Pulse until you have small pieces of "rice." To make 2 cups of riced cauliflower, you will need about 3 cups of small (1-inch) florets, or 1 small head of cauliflower. Store riced cauliflower in the refrigerator for up to 3 days.

How to Make Powdered Parmesan Cheese

Powdered Parmesan is simply Parmesan cheese that has been grated to the point of being light, fluffy, and powdery. One of my favorite ways to use it is for making chips for nachos.

Fresh pregrated Parmesan cheese available at supermarket cheese counters usually has a powdery texture and can be a convenient option in recipes that call for powdered Parmesan. To make powdered Parmesan at home, place grated Parmesan in a food processor or spice grinder and pulse until it is fluffy and powdery.

How to Make Pork Dust

Pork dust is a great zero-carb substitute for breadcrumbs or flour. Pork dust is made from pork rinds that are ground to the texture of fine breadcrumbs. You can purchase pork dust from a company called Bacon's Heir, or you can make your own pork dust by grinding pork rinds in a food processor. Just be sure to buy pork rinds without harmful additives; I prefer Epic or Bacon's Heir. To make ½ cup of pork dust, you will need about 2 cups of pork rinds. Store the dust in an airtight container at room temperature for up to 1 month.

Quick Reference

• omits this ingredient   O option

RECIPES	PAGE	KETO	DAIRY FREE	NUT FREE	EGG FREE
Stir-Fry Sauce	42	M	•	•	•
Ginger Sauce	42	H	•	•	•
Asian Dipping Sauce	43	L	•	•	•
Sweet-and-Sour Sauce	43	L	•	•	•
Zero-Carb Fried "Rice"	44	H	•	•	
Cauliflower Fried Rice	46	H	O	•	
Scallion Pancakes	48	H	O	•	
Break-Your-Fast Ramen	50	M	•	•	O
Cucumber Kimchi	52	M	•	•	•
Gyoza Meatballs	53	H	•	•	
Pot Stickers	54	L	•	O	
Crab Rangoon Puffs	56	H	O	•	
Gyoza (Japanese Dumplings)	58	H	•	•	•
Cream Cheese Wontons	60	H	O	•	
Crab Rangoon Fritters	62	H	O	O	
General Tso's Chicken Drummies	64	H	•	•	•
Chinese Sticky Rib Bites	66	H	•	•	•
Po Ho Thng	68	H	•	•	•
Hot-and-Sour Soup	70	M	•	•	
Simple Egg Drop Soup	72	H	•	•	
Gyoza Meatball Soup	74	M	•	•	
Pot Sticker Soup	76	L	•	O	
Udon Soup with Bok Choy and Poached Eggs	78	H	•	•	
Asian Slow Cooker Short Ribs	80	H	•	•	•
Moo Shu Pork and Pancakes	82	H	O	•	
Crispy Almond Chicken (Soo Guy)	84	H			
Chicken Chow Mein	86	M	•	•	•
Chicken and Mushrooms	88	M	•	•	•
Beef and Broccoli Stir-Fry	90	H	•	•	•
Teriyaki Salmon	92	M	•	•	•
Bulgogi Wraps	94	H	•	•	•
Sweet-and-Sour Chicken	96	H		•	
Chop Suey	98	M	•	•	O
Singapore Noodles	100	M	•	•	
Szechuan Beef	102	L	•	•	
Bourbon Chicken	104	H	•	•	O
Char Siu	106	H	•	•	
Moo Go Gai Pan	108	H	•	•	
Kung Pow Shrimp	110	H	•	O	
Chinese Lemon Chicken	112	H		•	
Sushi Rolls	114	L	O	•	O
Deconstructed Pot Sticker Bowl	118	H	•	•	
Green Tea Ice Cream	120	H	O	O	
Italian Dressing	124	H		O	
Alfredo Sauce	125	H		•	•
Mama Maria's Marinara	126	L	O	•	•
Mama Maria's Pizza Sauce	128	L	O	•	•
Italian Wedding Soup	129	H	O	•	
Zuppa Toscana	130	H	O	•	•
Italian Restaurant Salad	132	M		O	
Garlic Bread	134	L	O		
Mama Maria's Stuffed Mushrooms	136	M	O	•	•
Mama Maria's Meatballs	138	M	O	•	
Cheesy Zucchini Agnolotti	140	L	O	•	•
Five-Cheese "Ziti"	142	M	O	•	
Chicken Scaloppine	144	H	O	•	•
Gnocchi—Three Ways	146	H		•	

RECIPES	PAGE	KETO (L–M–H)	DAIRY FREE	NUT FREE	EGG FREE
Spaghetti and Meatballs	148	L	O	•	
Chicken Parmigiana	150	M		•	
Shrimp Caprese Pasta	152	H		•	•
Sausage and Pepper Rustica	154	M	O	•	•
Stuffed Manicotti	156	H		•	
Steak Gorgonzola Alfredo	158	H		•	•
Chicken Piccata	160	H	O	•	•
Sugo Bianco	162	H		•	•
Protein Noodle Lasagna	164	H		•	
Chicken Milanese	166	H			
Chicken Cacciatore	168	L	•	•	•
Shrimp Portofino	170	H	O	•	•
Toscana Paglia e Fieno	172	H		•	
Salmon Sorrento	174	H	O	•	•
Prosciutto-Stuffed Chicken	176	H			•
Chicken Scarpariello	178	M	O	•	•
Pasta Carbonara	180	L		•	
Craig's Special Pizza	182	H			
Calzones	184	H			
Deconstructed Chicken Parm Pizza	186	H		•	
Keto Cannoli	188	H			•
Dessert Pizza	190	H			
Traditional Tiramisu	192	H			
Easy Blender Enchilada Sauce	196	L	•	•	•
Pico de Gallo	197	L	•	•	•
"Tortilla" Chips with Guacamole	198	L		•	•
Soft Tortillas	200	M	O	O	
Keto Tortillas	201	H	O	•	
Breakfast Burritos	202	H	O	•	
Empanadas	204	H		•	•
Chicken Quesadilla	206	H		O	
Tortilla Soup	208	L	O	O	O
Carne en su Jugo	210	M	O	O	
Slow Cooker Posole Soup	212	H	O	O	
Chicken Enchilada Soup	214	L	O	O	
Easy Burrito Bowls	216	H	O	O	•
Burritos	218	M	O	O	
Enchiladas	220	M		O	O
Steak Fajitas	222	L	O	O	
Cheesy Chile Rellenos	224	H		•	
Enchiladas Verdes Lasagna	226	H	O	O	O
Chicken Thigh Chili Verdes	228	H	O	•	•
Simple Pollo Asado	229	H	•	•	•
Mouthwatering Carnitas	230	H	O	•	•
Carne Asada Tacos	232	M	O	O	O
Smoky Refried "Beans"	234	L	O	•	•
Piña Colada	236	H	•	•	•
Fried Ice Cream	237	H			
Flan	238	H	O	•	
Churros	240	H			
Tres Leches Cake	242	H			
Sinangag	246	M	O	•	•
Thai Basil Fried "Rice"	247	M	O	•	
Vietnamese Imperial Rolls	248	H	•	•	•
Tom Ka Gai (Coconut Chicken Soup)	250	M	•	•	•
Tom Yum Gai (Hot-and-Sour Chicken Soup)	252	H	•	•	•
Pho	254	M	•	•	•
Pho Gà (Vietnamese Chicken Noodle Soup)	256	H	•	•	•
Vietnamese Salad	257	M	•	O	•
Thai Curry Stew	258	M	•	•	•
Crab Curry "Rice"	260	H	O	•	
Pad Thai	262	M	•	O	

RECIPES	PAGE	KETO	DAIRY FREE	NUT FREE	EGG FREE
Larb	264	M	•	•	•
Yellow Chicken Thighs Adobo	266	H	•	•	•
Chicken Korma	268	M		○	•
Green Curry Chicken	270	L	○	•	•
Red Curry Shrimp	272	H	○	•	•
Coconut Curry Chicken and Pancakes	274	H	○	•	
Kofta with Cilantro Sauce	276	H	○	•	•
Malai Curry Shrimp	278	L	○	•	•
Fish Palak	280	L	○	•	•
Thai Red Beef Curry	282	M	•	•	•
Oven-Baked Curried Turkey Legs	284	H	○	•	•
Coconut and Thai Basil Ice Cream	286	H	○	○	
Keto Ketchup	290	M	•	•	•
Creamy "Honey" Mustard	291	H	•	○	
Sausage Breakfast Sandwiches with Zero-Carb English Muffins	292	H	○	○	
Mozzarella Sticks	294	H		•	
Taco Dip with Pepper Dippers	296	L	○	•	•
Parmesan Garlic Drummies	298	H	○	○	
Baked "Potato" Soup	300	M	○	•	•
The Best Pub Salad	302	H		○	
Curry Chicken Salad	304	H	○	○	
Egg Salad	304	H	•	○	
Tuna Salad	305	H	•	•	
Chicken Lettuce Wraps with Satay Dipping Sauce	306	H	○		•
Chicken Nuggets	308	H	○	○	
Bacon Cheeseburger	310	H	○	○	○
Juicy Lucy	312	H		○	○
Fiesta Lime Chicken	314	H		○	
Easy Mini Corn Dogs	316	H	○	○	
Deep-Fried Breaded Shrimp with Spicy Mayo	318	M	○	○	
Tomato Basil Chicken Salad Wraps	320	M	•	○	
Fish Sticks with Homemade Tartar Sauce	322	H	○	○	
Cheeseburger Wraps with Special Sauce	324	H		○	
Bacon Cheeseburger Pizza	326	H			
Keto Fries with Aioli	328	H		○	
Waffle Fries with Cheese Sauce	330	H		•	
Poutine	332	H	○	•	•
Frosted Lemonade	334	H		•	•
Frozen Hot Chocolate	336	H	○	○	•
The Thickest Chocolate Shake Ever	338	H	○	○	•
Leprechaun Shake	340	H	○	○	○
Classic Diner Malt	342	H			
Lemon Loaf	344	H	•		
Tiramisu Cheesecake	346	H	○		
Zero-Carb Pie Crust	348	H	•	•	
Boston Cream Pie	350	H	○	○	
Upside-Down Lemon Meringue Pie	352	H	○	•	
Bone Broth: Beef or Chicken	356	M	•	•	•
Mayonnaise	357	H	•	○	
Dairy-Free Ranch Dressing	358	H	•	○	
Roasted Garlic	359	L	•	•	•
Zoodles—Two Ways	360	L	•	•	•
Cabbage Pasta	361	M	○	•	•
Keto Bread	362	M	○	•	

Recipe Index

Chinese, Japanese, and Korean Delights

44
Zero-Carb Fried "Rice"

46
Cauliflower Fried Rice

48
Scallion Pancakes

50
Break-Your-Fast Ramen

52
Cucumber Kimchi

53
Gyoza Meatballs

54
Pot Stickers

56
Crab Rangoon Puffs

58
Gyoza (Japanese Dumplings)

60
Cream Cheese Wontons

62
Crab Rangoon Fritters

64
General Tso's Chicken Drummies

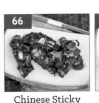
66
Chinese Sticky Rib Bites

68
Po Ho Thng

70
Hot-and-Sour Soup

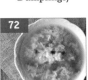
72
Simple Egg Drop Soup

74
Gyoza Meatball Soup

76
Pot Sticker Soup

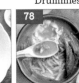
78
Udon Soup with Bok Choy and Poached Eggs

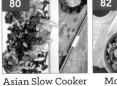
80
Asian Slow Cooker Short Ribs

82
Moo Shu Pork and Pancakes

84
Crispy Almond Chicken (Soo Guy)

86
Chicken Chow Mein

88
Chicken and Mushrooms

90
Beef and Broccoli Stir-Fry

92
Teriyaki Salmon

94
Bulgogi Wraps

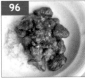
96
Sweet-and-Sour Chicken

98
Chop Suey

100
Singapore Noodles

102
Szechuan Beef

104
Bourbon Chicken

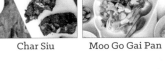
106
Char Siu

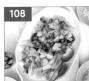
108
Moo Go Gai Pan

110
Kung Pow Shrimp

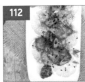
112
Chinese Lemon Chicken

114
Sushi Rolls

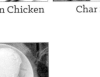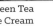
118
Deconstructed Pot Sticker Bowl

120
Green Tea Ice Cream

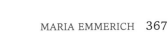

Italian Classics

124 Italian Dressing

125 Alfredo Sauce

126 Mama Maria's Marinara

128 Mama Maria's Pizza Sauce

129 Italian Wedding Soup

130 Zuppa Toscana

132 Italian Restaurant Salad

134 Garlic Bread

136 Mama Maria's Stuffed Mushrooms

138 Mama Maria's Meatballs

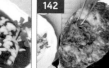
140 Cheesy Zucchini Agnolotti

142 Five-Cheese "Ziti"

144 Chicken Scaloppine

146 Gnocchi—Three Ways

148 Spaghetti and Meatballs

150 Chicken Parmigiana

152 Shrimp Caprese Pasta

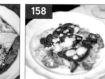
154 Sausage and Pepper Rustica

156 Stuffed Manicotti

158 Steak Gorgonzola Alfredo

160 Chicken Piccata

162 Sugo Bianco

164 Protein Noodle Lasagna

166 Chicken Milanese

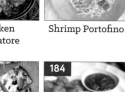
168 Chicken Cacciatore

170 Shrimp Portofino

172 Toscana Paglia e Fieno

174 Salmon Sorrento

176 Prosciutto-Stuffed Chicken

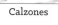
178 Chicken Scarpariello

180 Pasta Carbonara

182 Craig's Special Pizza

184 Calzones

186 Deconstructed Chicken Parm Pizza

188 Keto Cannoli

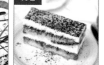
190 Dessert Pizza

192 Traditional Tiramisu

Mexican and Latin American Fare

196
Easy Blender
Enchilada Sauce

197
Pico de Gallo

198
"Tortilla" Chips
with Guacamole

200
Tortillas

202
Breakfast Burritos

204
Empanadas

206
Chicken
Quesadilla

208
Tortilla Soup

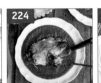
210
Carne en su Jugo

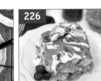
212
Slow Cooker
Posole Soup

214
Chicken
Enchilada Soup

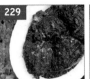
216
Easy Burrito Bowls

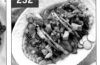
218
Burritos

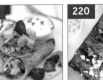
220
Enchiladas

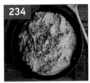
222
Steak Fajitas

224
Cheesy Chile
Rellenos

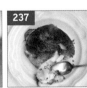
226
Enchiladas Verdes
Lasagna

228
Chicken Thigh
Chili Verdes

229
Simple
Pollo Asado

230
Mouthwatering
Carnitas

232
Carne Asada Tacos

234
Smoky Refried
"Beans"

236
Piña Colada

237
Fried Ice Cream

238
Flan

240
Churros

242
Tres Leches Cake

Indian, Thai, and Other Southeast Asian Cuisine

246
Sinangag

247
Thai Basil Fried "Rice"

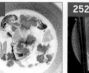
248
Vietnamese Imperial Rolls

250
Tom Ka Gai (Coconut Chicken Soup)

252
Tom Yum Gai (Hot-and-Sour Chicken Soup)

254
Pho

256
Pho Gà (Vietnamese Chicken Noodle Soup)

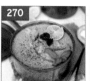
257
Vietnamese Salad

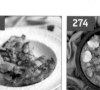
258
Thai Curry Stew

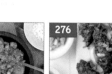
260
Crab Curry "Rice"

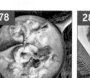
262
Pad Thai

264
Larb

266
Yellow Chicken Thighs Adobo

268
Chicken Korma

270
Green Curry Chicken

272
Red Curry Shrimp

274
Coconut Curry Chicken and Pancakes

276
Kofta with Cilantro Sauce

278
Malai Curry Shrimp

280
Fish Palak

282
Thai Red Beef Curry

284
Oven-Baked Curried Turkey Legs

286
Coconut and Thai Basil Ice Cream

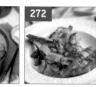
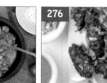
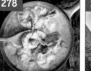

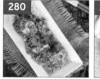
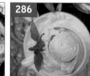

Fast-Casual Favorites

290
Keto Ketchup

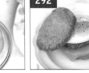
291
Creamy "Honey" Mustard

292
Sausage Breakfast Sandwiches

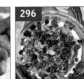
294
Mozzarella Sticks

296
Taco Dip with Pepper Dippers

298
Parmesan Garlic Drummies

300
Baked "Potato" Soup

302
The Best Pub Salad

304
Curry Chicken, Egg, & Tuna Salad

306
Chicken Lettuce Wraps with Satay Dipping Sauce

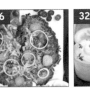
308
Chicken Nuggets

310
Bacon Cheeseburger

312
Juicy Lucy

314
Fiesta Lime Chicken

316
Easy Mini Corn Dogs

318
Deep-Fried Breaded Shrimp with Spicy Mayo

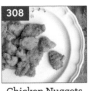
320
Tomato Basil Chicken Salad Wraps

322
Fish Sticks with Homemade Tartar Sauce

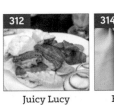
324
Cheeseburger Wraps with Special Sauce

326
Bacon Cheeseburger Pizza

328
Keto Fries with Aioli

330
Waffle Fries with Cheese Sauce

332
Poutine

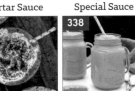
334
Frosted Lemonade

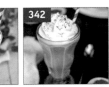
336
Frozen Hot Chocolate

338
The Thickest Chocolate Shake Ever

340
Leprechaun Shake

342
Classic Diner Malt

344
Lemon Loaf

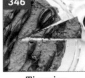
346
Tiramisu Cheesecake

348
Zero-Carb Pie Crust

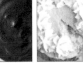
350
Boston Cream Pie

352
Upside-Down Lemon Meringue Pie

General Index

Gratitude

I, like many of you, have had some difficult times. Life is like waves of the ocean; we all have highs as well as lows. I have learned to accept the lows and have gratitude for the highs. The hardships have taught me amazing life lessons; after all, it was during those low points that I had to stop spending money at restaurants and start cooking at home, which helped shape me into the healthy ketogenic cook I am today! I struggled out of the cocoon, and it made me a butterfly with strong wings.

First, I am grateful to my love and best friend, Craig, who never complains even though I often mess up the kitchen as soon as he cleans it. He has also been a huge part of this book, picking up all the groceries, testing recipes, as well as adding the detailed nutritional information for all the recipes.

I am grateful for my boys, Micah and Kai, who love to help me in the kitchen. Even though it takes twice as long to get dinner on the table when they help me, it is totally worth it. When we had to put our adoption on hold, I was devastated, but I remember my mom telling me that my children just weren't born yet. I cry as I write this because she was totally right. These two boys were meant for me!

I am grateful for Jimmy Moore. Jimmy called me to write *The Ketogenic Cookbook* with him, and I am forever grateful for his support!

I also need to express my gratitude to the whole Victory Belt team, who offer me such amazing support and kindness.

Holly and Pam, you all are truly a huge part of making this book a piece of art. You all have such amazing ideas and attention to detail. I am forever grateful for both of you! You both worked very long days and weekends to get the edits done on time, and I can't think you enough for your amazing work!

Susan, I am grateful for your passion and how magnificently you promote my books! I get a smile on my face whenever I receive an email from you. Your happiness shines through!

Erich, your praise and fun outlook made this journey extraordinary and totally worth the hard work and long days of writing, editing, cooking, and photographing! I appreciate your caring phone calls just to check in on me and make sure everything is going smoothly.

Wendy and Kristie, I am grateful for you, and I know my readers are, too! You spent many hours testing my recipes and making sure that they were worthy of being included in this book. Your hard work helped create a tasty cookbook.

Bill and Haley, I am honored to have your photo for the cover for this book. I've always been a big fan of your photos and cookbooks. My first Victory Belt cookbook was your *Gather* book. I was in love with your artistry from the beginning. Thank you for taking the time to make my recipes and shoot the cover.

Finally, I want to express my gratitude to you, my readers. I can't thank you enough for all your love and support through my journey!